Stress in Health and Disease

Editors

DANIEL L. KIRSCH
MICHEL A. WOODBURY-FARIÑA

PSYCHIATRIC CLINICS
OF NORTH AMERICA

www.psych.theclinics.com

December 2014 • Volume 37 • Number 4

ELSEVIER

1600 John F. Kennedy Boulevard • Suite 1800 • Philadelphia, Pennsylvania, 19103-2899

http://www.theclinics.com

PSYCHIATRIC CLINICS OF NORTH AMERICA Volume 37, Number 4
December 2014 ISSN 0193-953X, ISBN-13: 978-0-323-32676-6

Editor: Joanne Husovski
Developmental Editor: Stephanie Carter

Psychiatric Clinics of North America (ISSN 0193-953X) is published quarterly by Elsevier Inc., 360 Park Avenue South, New York, NY 10010-1710. Months of issue are March, June, September, and December. Business and Editorial Offices: 1600 John F. Kennedy Blvd., Suite 1800, Philadelphia, PA 19103-2899. Periodicals postage paid at New York, NY and additional mailing offices. Subscription prices are $300.00 per year (US individuals), $546.00 per year (US institutions), $150.00 per year (US students/residents), $365.00 per year (Canadian individuals), $687.00 per year (Canadian Institutions), $455.00 per year (foreign individuals), $687.00 per year (foreign institutions), and $220.00 per year (international & Canadian students/residents). Foreign air speed delivery is included in all *Clinics*' subscription prices. All prices are subject to change without notice. **POSTMASTER:** Send address changes to *Psychiatric Clinics of North America*, Elsevier Health Sciences Division, Subscription Customer Service, 3251 Riverport Lane, Maryland Heights, MO 63043. Customer Service: 1-800-654-2452 (US). From outside the United States, call 1-314-447-8871. Fax: 1-314-447-8029. E-mail: journalscustomerservice-usa@elsevier.com (for print support) and journalsonlinesupport-usa@elsevier.com (for online support).

Reprints. For copies of 100 or more, of articles in this publication, please contact the Commercial Reprints Department, Elsevier Inc., 360 Park Avenue South, New York, New York 10010-1710. Tel.: 212-633-3874, Fax: 212-633-3820, E-mail: reprints@elsevier.com.

Psychiatric Clinics of North America is covered in *MEDLINE/PubMed (Index Medicus), Current Contents/Social and Behavioral Sciences, Social Science Citation Index, Embase/Excerpta Medica,* and PsycINFO.

Printed in the United States of America.

Contributors

EDITORS

DANIEL L. KIRSCH, PhD, DAAPM, FAIS
President, The American Institute of Stress, Fort Worth, Texas

MICHEL A. WOODBURY-FARIÑA, MD, DFAPA, FAIS
Clinical and Research Psychiatrist; Associate Professor, Department of Psychiatry, University of Puerto Rico School of Medicine, San Juan, Puerto Rico

AUTHORS

JOALEX L. ANTONGIORGI, MD
Psychiatry Resident, Department of Psychiatry, University of Puerto Rico School of Medicine, San Juan, Puerto Rico

YVES BUREAU, PhD
Statistics Consultant, Statistics Adjunct Faculty; Lawson Scientist, Lawson Health Research Institute, University of Western Ontario, London, Ontario, Canada

ALEXANDER BYSTRITSKY, MD, PhD
Director, UCLA Anxiety and Related Disorders Program; Professor, Department of Psychiatry and Biobehavioral Sciences, Semel Institute for Neuroscience and Human Behavior, David Geffen School of Medicine, University of California, Los Angeles, Los Angeles, California

ROBBIE CAMPBELL, MD, FRCP
Associate Professor, Lawson Health Research Institute, University of Western Ontario, London, Ontario, Canada

ZACK CERNOVSKY, PhD, CPQ, ASPB
Professor of Emeritus Psychiatry, University of Western Ontario, London, Ontario, Canada

SIMON CHIU, MD, PhD, FRCP, ABPN
Associate Professor, Department of Psychiatry; Research Scientist, Lawson Health Research Institute, University of Western Ontario, London, Ontario, Canada

JOHN COPEN, MD, MSc, FRCP
Director Bioinformatics, Vancouver Island Health Authority; Assistant Professor, Department of Psychiatry, University of British Columbia, British Columbia, Canada

MISTY EATON, PhD
Professor, Department of Biochemistry, Universidad Central Del Caribe, Bayamón, Puerto Rico

FRANCES FIGUEROA-FANKHANEL, PsyD
Clinical Psychologist, Primary Care Mental Health Integration Program, Caribbean Healthcare System, San Juan, Puerto Rico

MICHAEL J. GONZALEZ, DSc, NMD, PhD, FANMA, FACN
Professor, Nutrition Program, Department of Human Development, School of Public Health, University of Puerto Rico, Medical Sciences Campus, San Juan, Puerto Rico

POLARIS GONZALEZ, BA
Ponce School of Medicine, Ponce, Puerto Rico

ANA HATEGAN, MD, FRCP
Geriatric Psychiatry Division, Department of Psychiatry, McMaster University Health Sciences, Hamilton, Ontario, Canada

J. JURUI HOU, PhD
Lawson Scientist, Lawson Health Research Institute, London, Ontario, Canada

MARIWAN HUSNI, MD, MRC (Psy), FRCP
Associate Professor, Northern Ontario Medical School, Thunderbay, Ontario, Canada; Faculty of Medicine, Senior Lecturer, Imperial College London, London, United Kingdom

MIKE KAUSHAL, MD
Lawson Research Assistant, Lawson Health Research Institute, London, Ontario, Canada

DAVID KRONEMYER, MA
Researcher, UCLA Anxiety and Related Disorders Program, Department of Psychiatry and Biobehavioral Sciences, Semel Institute for Neuroscience and Human Behavior, David Geffen School of Medicine, University of California, Los Angeles, Los Angeles, California

R. GREGORY LANDE, DO
Colonel (Retired), Medical Corps, US Army; Director, Psychiatry Continuity Service, Walter Reed National Military Medical Center, Bethesda, Maryland

KAREN G. MARTINEZ, MD, MSc
Assistant Professor; Director, Center for the Study and Treatment of Fear and Anxiety, Department of Psychiatry, University of Puerto Rico, Medical Sciences Campus, San Juan, Puerto Rico

JORGE R. MIRANDA-MASSARI, BS, BSPharm, RPh, PharmD
Professor, Department of Pharmacy Practice, School of Pharmacy, University of Puerto Rico, Medical Sciences Campus, San Juan, Puerto Rico

HANA RAHEB, BA Honors
Lawson Research Graduate Student, Lawson Health Research Institute, London, Ontario, Canada

EDGARDO RODRIGUEZ-VALLECILLO, MD, FAAD
Dermatologist, Private Practice, San Juan; Consultant, Dermatology, HIMA, San Pablo Hospital, Bayamon, Puerto Rico

VERONICA SANCHEZ, MSc
Department of Psychiatry, Lawson Health Research Institute, University of Western Ontario, London, Ontario, Canada

MUJEEB U. SHAD, MD, MSCS
Supervising Psychiatrist, Oregon State Hospital; Associate Professor of Psychiatry, Oregon Health & Science University, Portland, Oregon

SERGUEI N. SKATCHKOV, PhD
Distinguished Research Professor, Department of Biochemistry, Universidad Central Del Caribe; Department of Physiology, Universidad Central Del Caribe, Bayamón, Puerto Rico

KRISTEN TERPSTRA, BA Honors, MSc (Neurosciences)
McMaster University, Hamilton, Ontario, Canada; Nursing Program, University of Toronto, Toronto, Ontario, Canada

RICARDO M. VELA, MD
Director of Child Psychiatry; Psychiatrist-in-Chief, Child and Family Services, North Suffolk Mental Health Association; Assistant in Psychiatry, Massachusetts General Hospital, Chelsea, Massachusetts

MICHEL A. WOODBURY-FARIÑA, MD, DFAPA, FAIS
Clinical and Research Psychiatrist; Associate Professor, Department of Psychiatry, University of Puerto Rico School of Medicine, San Juan, Puerto Rico

Contents

factors such as genes and early traumatic experiences. In PTSD, enhanced fear learning and poor extinction are common. Fear is manifested through autonomic responses and persistent memories of the traumatic event. These manifestations are related to stress responses modulated by the hypothalamic-pituitary-adrenal axis. This article evaluates the role of fear and stress in the course of PTSD. Findings on fear learning and extinction are presented in order to guide future treatments of patients with PTSD.

Military service differs from civilian jobs in the stressors that service members experience, including frequent deployments (eg, to an area of combat operations), obedience, regimentation, subordination of self to the group, integrity, and flexibility. The military culture emphasizes teamwork and peer support. In some cases, service members cannot adapt to military life, become overwhelmed by stress, or cannot overcome a traumatic experience. Clinicians should conduct a thorough evaluation guided by an understanding of the military culture. Every effort should be made to identify the stress and the maladaptive response and provide early clinical interventions to prevent progression.

Humor has not been taken as seriously and should be considered another of the legitimate therapeutic tool used in therapy. Humor has many positive effects in the daily lives of patients and clinicians need to take advantage of these. Many indices of stress are attenuated and this serves to improve the therapeutic alliance. Freudian, rational emotive therapy, and Kleinian views are presented, as well as examples of how to use playful therapy. In addition, advice on how to develop humor is given.

Stress refers to a reaction given a particular stimulus. Stress is a common problem in most modern societies. Stress creates greater physiologic demands. Unhealthy eating patterns will only result in an increased level of stress, followed by further health problems if in the future if the issues are not resolved. Prolonged stress increases the metabolic needs of the body and causes many other changes. The increased metabolism can also cause an increase in the use and excretion of many nutrients. Although stress alters nutrient needs, if marginally deficient in a nutrient, stress can make that deficiency even worse.

Converging evidence identifies stress-related disorders as putative risk factors for Alzheimer Disease (AD). This article reviews evidence on the complex interplay of stress, aging, and genes-epigenetics interactions.

The recent classification of AD into preclinical, mild cognitive impairment, and AD offers a window for intervention to prevent, delay, or modify the course of AD. Evidence in support of the cognitive effects of epigenetics-based diet, and nutraceuticals is reviewed. A proactive epigenetics diet and nutraceuticals program holds promise as potential buffer against the negative impact of aging and stress responses on cognition, and can optimize vascular, metabolic, and brain health in the community.

This article explores the way stress affects the skin, both at the molecular level, where the skin has an intricate connection to the neurocutaneous and immune systems, and at the clinical level. The concept of psychodermatology is reviewed with regard to the way skin reacts to stress, how stress is a trigger for several common skin diseases, and how neuropsychiatric disorders may have skin manifestations. The article is directed at making the dermatologist, the psychiatrist, the psychologist, and the primary physician familiar with the brain-skin mechanisms involved in stress and the resultant clinical expressions on the skin.

This review focuses on the roles of glia and polyamines (PAs) in brain function and dysfunction, highlighting how PAs are one of the principal differences between glia and neurons. The novel role of PAs, such as putrescine, spermidine, and spermine and their precursors and derivatives, is discussed. However, PAs have not yet been a focus of much glial research. They affect many neuronal and glial receptors, channels, and transporters. They are therefore key elements in the development of many diseases and syndromes, thus forming the rationale for PA-focused and glia-focused therapy for these conditions.

Glia are starting to be accepted as the equal of neurons. Glia's role in stress and disease as well as the latest glial modulators are reviewed. Environmental enrichment and exercise can increase intelligence, a buffer against stress, most likely via glial involvement. Cerebral dominance is also related to how glia respond to stress resulting in psychiatric illness. Glial effects on depression and schizophrenia are reviewed. Astrocytes, microglia, NG2 cells, and oligodendrocytes all contribute. Suicidal ideation can increase the permeability of the BBB resulting in the increase in serum levels of a glial protein S100B that has become a marker for the intensity of suicidal risk. Microglia form one of the bases of the inflammatory theory of psychiatric disorders. Minocycline, adenosine and cAMP inhibitors, such as PDE-4 inhibitors, have been used to modulate the microglia, with positive results in psychiatric illness. Controlling the microglia can even be protective against drug abuse. Recently a "glymphatic" system has been discovered in mice that if applicable to humans means that we clean out our brains in sleep.

PSYCHIATRIC CLINICS OF NORTH AMERICA

FORTHCOMING ISSUES

Mental Health in the Medical Setting: Delivery, Workforce Needs, and Emerging Best Practices
Peter F. Buckley, *Editor*

Young-onset Dementia
Chiadi Onyike, *Editor*

Clinical Advances in Psychiatry
David Baron and
Lawrence Gross, *Editors*

Bipolar Depression
John Beyer, *Editor*

RECENT ISSUES

September 2014
Obsessive Compulsive and Related Disorders
Wayne K. Goodman, *Editor*

June 2014
Sexual Deviation: Assessment and Treatment
John M.W. Bradford and
A.G. Ahmed, *Editors*

March 2014
Neuropsychiatry of Traumatic Brain Injury
Ricardo E. Jorge and
David B. Arciniegas, *Editors*

December 2013
Late Life Depression
W. Vaughn McCall, *Editor*

RELATED INTEREST

Veterinary Clinics of North America
March 2009 (Vol. 39, No.2), Pages 293–326
The Human—Companion Animal Bond: How Humans Benefit
Erika Friedmann and Heesook Son, *Editors*

Preface

If Life Were Easy They Would Have Asked For Volunteers

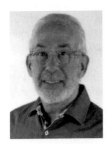 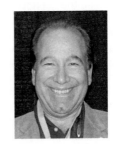

Daniel L. Kirsch, PhD, DAAPM, FAIS   Michel A. Woodbury-Fariña, MD, DFAPA, FAIS
Editors

Stress is ubiquitous and follows us everywhere. Since there is simply no avoiding it, the task for psychiatrists has become to further our understanding to improve management in our patients and in ourselves. We see the goal in this is to have a more preventive health care system and consequently a happier and healthier population. We hope to contribute to that end, having made the detailed description of this common occurrence and its impact on the body and mind the focus of this issue.

Dr Daniel L. Kirsch is a neuroscientist who has been in the forefront of pain and stress management for 40 years. He was asked to edit this issue in his role as the President of the American Institute of Stress (AIS), a nonprofit organization founded at the request of the father of the stress concept, Dr Hans Selye, in 1978. Dr Kirsch replaced the legendary stress specialist, Dr Paul J. Rosch, as president of AIS, although Dr Rosch remains with the AIS as Chairman of the Board and continues to write the member-only newsletter, *Health and Stress*. AIS offers many free resources to practitioners and patients alike at its Web site: www.stress.org. Those resources include the free emagazines *Contentment* and *Combat Stress*. *Contentment* is for everyone, while *Combat Stress* is devoted to the special needs of military service members and veterans. Since 2005, Dr Kirsch has been actively working with the US military in teaching pain and stress management to uniformed practitioners and working with health care professionals on their own compassion fatigue. He also works with the Army Substance Abuse Program and is a member of the Board of Scientific and Professional Advisors of the Institute for Traumatic Stress.

Coeditor Dr Michel A. Woodbury-Fariña is a Lifetime Distinguished Fellow of the American Psychiatric Association and board-certified Child and Adult Psychiatrist who has been in private practice, academia, and pharmaceutical research for over 30 years. He is also the Chairman of the AIS Daily Life Stress Board. Dr Woodbury-Fariña teaches his residents to use a technique he developed to provide a simple explanation to their patients on how the mind works when under stress. He tells

Psychiatr Clin N Am 37 (2014) xi–xvi
http://dx.doi.org/10.1016/j.psc.2014.09.002
0193-953X/14/$ – see front matter © 2014 Elsevier Inc. All rights reserved.

them to hold one fist up and the other hand open next to the fist. The fist represents the primitive (or the unconscious, limbic/brainstem, or immature) brain. The open hand is the adult (or conscious, prefrontal, or mature) brain. He then instructs them to cover the fist with the open hand and say that this is the state of the mind at peace, where the adult brain covers or controls the primitive brain. In this way, we can calmly go about our daily business. The primitive brain will be more active when there is stress, represented by opening the fist and hiding the other hand. The newly opened hand is there to fight or take flight as it takes over. The problem is that the fight/flight response means the primitive brain is under the impression that there is real danger lurking, even the possibility of being killed. The primitive brain sends waves of intense emotions to the adult brain because it does not communicate with words. The adult brain does not know what to do with these intense emotions, so it tries to make sense of them by attributing a real cause to them. Thus, all the distortions described by cognitive psychology come into play, such as, "I failed the exam and my life is over!"

We need to use psychotherapy, relaxation techniques, biofeedback and Alpha-Stim cranial electrotherapy stimulation, supplements or medications, and exercise, among other options, to give enough strength to the adult brain to maintain control of the primitive brain. You can then have the hand representing the primitive brain close to a fist again and have the open hand/adult brain move back over to cover the primitive brain/fist. This simple exercise has helped psychiatric residents communicate the reasons for the interventions used in their therapy sessions. The goal of this issue is to give more explicit details on this subject.

The first article is an overview of how to measure stress. The author of this article has extensive experience with these kinds of measurements as she is a collocated collaborative health behavior provider who has been working in the Primary Care Mental Health Program at the VA Caribbean Healthcare System since 2012. Before this, she completed her APA-accredited internship at the VA Hospital in San Juan Puerto Rico and shortly after began working at the Brief Individual and Family Psychotherapy Clinic. Within the context of her work, Dr Figueroa-Fankhanel has focused on brief interventions that aim toward early detection, disease prevention, and health promotion. At present, her clinical setting affords her the opportunity to work collaboratively with primary care staff in providing consultation for the treatment of stress-related and anxiety-related disorders within the medical settings of the veteran population. In addition, she helps providers effectively engage with their patients and implement motivational interviewing techniques, supportive interventions, and crisis management with veterans who possibly display heightened stress and anxiety states during medical appointments. Aside from her interdisciplinary work, she is a clinical supervisor in the Primary Care Mental Health Fellowship Program and co-leads a health behavior training seminar for psychology trainees focusing on health-related issues such as stress. In addition to staff engagement and education, she provides evidence-based therapies for patients with stress-related and anxiety-related disorders. Cognitive behavioral, acceptance, and commitment therapies, as well as a mindfulness-based stress reduction group are among the treatment modalities she implements. In sum, she has a special interest in measuring how stress affects a person's quality of life, including the documentation of health behaviors, treatment adherence, and treatment outcomes. In her article, she identifies the psycho-immunologic, psychological, and environmental models of stress as being the most influential theories in stress research and proceeds to describe how they are measured. She also includes the advantages and disadvantages of each evaluation modality.

Dr Alexander Bystritsky has been the Director of the Anxiety Related Disorders Program in the Department of Psychiatry and Biobehavioral Sciences, Semel Institute for

Neuroscience and Human Behavior, David Geffen School of Medicine, University of California at Los Angeles for the last 30 years. He has very broad experience in researching, teaching, and treating stress, anxiety, and related disorders, including treatments using psychopharmacology, behavior therapy, and various types of brain stimulation. Dr Bystritsky developed the ABC dynamical theory of anxiety, which he is using in research, patient education, and practice. For the past 4 years, Dr David Kronemyer has been a researcher at the Anxiety Related Disorders Program. There he specializes in nonlinear dynamical processes associated with belief revision, translational cognitive neuroscience, and phenomenological psychology. In their article, they present the concept that stress and anxiety are so interrelated that the two should be considered on a continuum. This increases the understanding of the brain's response and helps to delineate intervention strategies as well as provide directions for future research.

The article on the developing brain and the effects of severe stress is written by Dr Ricardo Vela, who has had many years of experience studying this relationship. For 36 years, as a child and adolescent psychiatrist, he has worked with inner-city populations and treated hundreds of children with extensive trauma histories. In fact, during his 9-year tenure at Boston Medical Center/Boston University School of Medicine, he spent more than 4 years at the neuroanatomy lab of Dr Thomas Kemper, a neuroanatomist, neuropathologist, and pediatric neurologist, going at least once a week to study brain anatomy. From this experience and independent study, he organized an advanced neuroscience course for psychiatry residents as well as developed the course/seminar, "Neuroanatomy of Emotions," at the American Psychiatric Association's Annual Meeting, which he has taught for the past 9 years. At present, he teaches child psychiatry residents the neuroanatomy of emotions, child abuse/development, autism, schizophrenia, and attentional problems at Massachusetts General Hospital. In his article, he tells us how the neuronal development of the limbic system, which is used to develop emotions and attachment, is extremely vulnerable to abuse and neglect in the first year of life. If such abuse continues, by 3 years of age there will be more negative than positive emotions expressed. The author proposes that we try to understand these effects so that we can present what he has called a *psychoanatomical formulation* on how the impact of severe stress has impacted the brains of our patients.

For the last 3 years, Dr Karen G. Martinez has been the Director of the Center for the Study and Treatment of Fear and Anxiety of the Department of Psychiatry, School of Medicine of the University of Puerto Rico Medical Sciences Campus, where she is also an assistant professor. Polaris Gonzalez is the Chief Psychology Student of the Ponce School of Medicine and is rotating through CETMA. Afterwards, she plans to continue her training in neuropsychology. For the past couple of years, Dr Martinez's lab has been coordinating research efforts with the lab of Dr Gregory Quirk, famous for his work on extinction learning. The efforts of her lab are an attempt to do translational research in stress and anxiety, going from the study of fear in the murine population to humans, and using these insights to understand pathologic anxiety states such as posttraumatic stress disorder (PTSD). This article, in fact, focuses on how fear and stress can build up to PTSD, giving us the knowledge that will be necessary to set up research projects that will increase the probably of being able to find how to successfully treat this condition.

Dr R. Gregory Lande is the Director of the Psychiatry Continuity Service (PCS) at Walter Reed National Military Medical Center (WRNMMC) in Bethesda, Maryland. As the nation's premier military medical center, WRNMMC is both a national and an international referral resource, providing care for some of the more complex medical and psychiatric cases. The PCS provides both adult partial and intensive outpatient psychiatric care for beneficiaries requiring this level of care, with specialty practice areas for the treatment of combat-related PTSD, treatment refractory depression, and a wide range of complementary medical practices. The PCS also conducts research in a broad range of clinical areas. Before assuming his current role, Dr Lande was the chief medical officer of a large public hospital. Dr Lande's knowledge of the military life and its unique stresses can in part be attributed to his 20-year career as a medical officer in the US Army. Dr Lande is the author of numerous articles, chapters, and books. His interest in history is reflected in the recent publication of "The Abraham Man," which traces the historical origins of medical expert witness testimony in America.

Humor is a particular interest of ours as we use it daily with patients, when indicated, of course. Dr Woodbury-Fariña has said that Freud's interest in wit, which is based on punning, probably helped him to use this kind of association to analyze dreams and the unconscious. We see wit as having two meanings of the words used. This is what forms the basis of his interpretations: what one person says has another meaning. While it is done without humor, the response of cathartic insight is due to the same rules of humor: incongruity. Joalex Antongiorgi Torres, MD is a third-year psychiatric resident of the Department of Psychiatry, School of Medicine of the University of Puerto Rico Medical Sciences Campus and actively participates in many extracurricular activities and associations regarding mental health and training of future residents. He has trained under Dr Woodbury-Fariña, where he has effectively learned and incorporated humor into his interview style. Dr Antongiorgi intends to specialize in the field of Child and Adolescent Psychiatry, in which he expects to maintain his style of using humor to aid the general population. The article is a review of different types of humor and how they help modulate stress. There are also examples on how to use humor under the rubric of play therapy. Everyone is encouraged to recommend Laughter Yoga to their patients and to start such a group in their area if none exist. It is very interesting that humor helps to decrease stress and anxiety by changing the locus of control from external to internal. Therapists are encouraged to see humor as a bona fide therapy technique and to develop this skill with their patients.

Dr Michael J. Gonzalez is Professor at the Nutrition Program, School of Public Health in the Medical Sciences Campus, University of Puerto Rico and adjunct faculty at the University of Western States. He earned a Masters in Cellular Biology and Biophysics (Nova University) and another Masters in Nutrition and Public Health (University of Puerto Rico Medical Sciences Campus). He has a Doctorate in Nutritional Medicine (John F. Kennedy University), a Doctorate in Health Sciences (Lafayette University), and a Doctorate in Nutritional Biochemistry and Cancer Biology (Michigan State University). He completed a Post-Doctoral Fellowship in Geriatrics at the University of Puerto Rico School of Medicine. Dr Gonzalez is a Fellow of the American College of Nutrition and has authored over 150 scientific publications. He has obtained several research awards for his work on nutrition and cancer. He is currently Co-Director of RECNAC II project, and Research Director of the InBioMed Project Initiative. Dr Gonzalez also serves as a nutrition consultant to the Puerto Rican Basketball National Team and is part of the Medical Commission of the Puerto Rican Basketball Federation. He is in a part-time clinical practice with Dr Miguel J. Berdiel in Ponce, Puerto Rico. Dr González and Dr Jorge Miranda-Massari, founders of InBioMed, are leaders in the development of nontoxic chemotherapy treatments for cancer. The findings of their work with intravenous vitamin C as an anticancer agent, published in 2002, were confirmed by the National Institutes of Health in 2005. They have brought many new concepts into the scientific field, such as the bioenergetic theory of carcinogenesis, the systemic saturation phenomenon of intravenous vitamin C, and the metabolic correction concept for disease treatment and prevention. Currently, they are finishing a book on vitamin C and cancer for Springer-Larger. In their article in this issue, they were chosen to bring us up-to-date on the relationship between diet and stress.

Dr Simon Chiu is a psychiatrist who, for the past 8 to 10 years, has successfully developed and cemented a very cohesive research team committed to the CNS Target-Driven Drug and Nutraceuticals Discovery Platform Program. He has headed, conducted, and completed translational and clinical trials of bioactive agents exhibiting neuroprotective activities through the epigenetics system. His team has studied such compounds as ginsenosides, which are active at the Transcription Regulator (PPAR) complexes, curcumin, which is a pan-HDAC inhibitor, and *Sceletium tortuosum* (an indigenous South African plant), which is a PDE-4 modulator. The article on epigenetics points out how diets can effect changes at the molecular and DNA level, with one goal being to try to use these insights to prevent Alzheimer disease.

Anything that affects the skin will cause stress and often the reverse is equally true. Dr Rodriguez Vallecillo is a dermatologist who has been in private practice for 31 years. In the article reviewing how stress affects the skin, he reviews conditions that can cause skin pathology as well as psychiatric syndromes that can express themselves by mutilating skin. The term psychodermatology is introduced to help understand the skin's relationship with the brain and stress. Dr Michel A. Woodbury Fariña contributed the psychiatric treatment approaches to this article and has been using hypnosis in his psychiatric practice for over 25 years. While the article ends by underlining the need to have an interdisciplinary approach, with psychiatrists, dermatologists, and primary care physicians working together to improve the skin care of patients, the main thrust of the conclusion is that all dermatologic problems have a stress component that can be summarized as pointing out that since the skin has the same stress system as the mind, any attempt to improve the skin has to include calming the mind.

This issue includes two articles on glia. Glia are a hot topic in basic science research but are only now starting to develop interest in clinical circles. The first article is an original research article on how polyamines (PA) might be the answer to how stress makes glia communicate. PAs include putrescine, spermidine, and spermine and their precursors and derivatives, which are reviewed. PAs are not synthesized by glia but are stored in them. Glia use PAs to regulate neuronal activity. Dr Skatchkov feels that understanding PA function might form the basis of understanding disease states and their treatment. While PAs have not been studied much, they are a focus of research at the lab of Dr Serguei N. Skatchkov at the Universidad Central del Caribe in Bayamon, Puerto Rico. He received his PhD in Biology and Biophysics from the Saint Petersburg State University, Saint Petersburg, Russia and is a Distinguished Research Professor of the Departments of Biochemistry and of Physiology of the Universidad Central del Caribe (UCC) Medical School in Bayamon, Puerto Rico. He is funded by NINDS and is studying the neurobiology of neuronal glial networks, with a particular interest in how glia participate in the regulation of neuronal signaling and neuronal communication by such means as PA and ATP release. He is also working on Kir channels and light signaling. In fact, he was the 2007 recipient of the Cozzarelli Prize for having discovered that glial cells act as light cables, a previously unknown function of glia. Misty Eaton received her PhD in Physiology from the University of Texas Southwestern Medical School and is a full Professor at the UCC Medical School. She is very interested in understanding the relationship between potassium channels and glia and has run research projects funded by NINDS and NIGMS that have demonstrated the role of Kir4.1 and TREK-2 channels in establishing potassium and glutamate homeostasis in astrocytes. She has gone on to elucidate the role of glial potassium channels in epilepsy, ischemia, and stress. Drs Skatchkov and Eaton have hosted national and international symposia as well as an IBRO workshop on glia on their university campus. Drs Skatchkov (Director) and Eaton (Associate Director) of the Integrative Center for Glial Research in Puerto Rico have brought together an impressive group of researchers from departments of other institutions to collaborate as a team so as to maximize the study of glia on the island.

The second article is an update on the clinical aspects of glia. Dr Woodbury-Fariña has been studying the effects of glia in psychiatric illness for a few years. He is experimenting with potassium and taurine, important solutes in glia, to see if it can be manipulated by the external administration of these substances. There is no doubt that glia have historically taken a back seat to neurons as previous theories suggested that all of the brain's functions are due to neurons. It is ironic that the neuronal mechanisms used to explain the learning process, such as long-term potentiation, were done using only neurons in very simple animals that did not have many glia. We now know glia is intimately involved in intelligence in humans, which in fact increases with environmental enrichment and exercise. We hope that by seeing how this helps to modulate stress, and by reviewing glia's role in psychiatric disorders, psychiatrists will have a better understanding of glia. To understand the role of inflammation in stress states, the role of microglia is included as well as the medications and supplements that control them so as to promote clinical research into these areas. Dr Woodbury Fariña has even included a glia biomarker that predicts suicidal behavior, the S100B, to encourage the inclusion of this biomarker in a suicide workup.

Through the understanding of the stress phenomenon, medical professionals and all people everywhere will be in a better position to marshal the positive aspects of this phenomenon. Our collective hope for humankind is that this will improve health care as well as life itself. It is a fact that we program ourselves for disappointment as many expectations remain unfulfilled throughout the day. Such is life, yet we need not be so reactive, as this is not healthy. We must make every effort to recognize fear, eat better, laugh it off when things don't go as we hoped, and, as professionals, measure and bring to the attention of our patients what all this means. After all, rarely are we chased by saber-toothed tigers in the urban jungles of the twenty-first century. This is the age of information overload. It is simply not in our best interests to keep acting so prehistorically. It is time to understand how to increase the modulation of our primitive brains so we can become better, more tolerant neighbors on this planet that we all call home.

Daniel L. Kirsch, PhD, DAAPM, FAIS
The American Institute of Stress
6387B Camp Bowie Boulevard, #334 Fort Worth
TX, USA, 76116

Michel A. Woodbury-Fariña, MD, DFAPA, FAIS
University of Puerto Rico School of Medicine
307 Eleanor Roosevelt Street
San Juan, PR, USA 00918-2720

E-mail addresses:
dkirsch@stress.org (D.L. Kirsch)
michel.woodbury@upr.edu (M.A. Woodbury-Fariña)

Measurement of Stress

Frances Figueroa-Fankhanel, PsyD

KEYWORDS

- Stress • Stressor • Measurement of stress • Assessment • Physiologic tradition
- Psychological tradition • Environmental tradition • Mind-body

KEY POINTS

- The popular definition of stress is very different from the scientific definition, and even in the scientific community different fields and specialties define stress in different ways.
- Stress affects how a person performs (behaviors), how a person feels (emotions), and what bodily responses (neurophysiological) are endorsed. All 3 components should be evaluated using a heuristic/holistic approach to understanding health and disease.
- Life changes affect physical and emotional health. Those who experience more life stress are at increased risk for health problems. Specifically, increased life stressors can lead to weakened immune systems and increased vulnerability for chronic diseases.
- There several ways to measure stress. However, the exact way depends on several factors including the questions being raised, the chief complaints of the person affected, the potential impact on a stated person, the socioeconomic experience of the person, the different kind of life events to which the person is exposed, coping resources, resilience, and opportunity for growth.
- Physiological changes in response to stress can be easily evaluated through blood, urine, saliva, and proxy autonomic measures. The psychological impact of stress, on the other hand, can be obtained through observation, checklists, self-report methods, and interviews.

Disclosure Statement: The author certifies that the VA Caribbean Healthcare System has no relevant financial interest in this article and that the content of this article in no way represents the views on opinions of stated organization. The author alone is responsible for the content and writing of this article.
Primary Care Mental Health Integration Program, Caribbean Healthcare System, 10 Casia Street, San Juan, PR 00921, USA
E-mail address: Frances.Figueroa-Fankhanel@va.gov

Abbreviations	
ACTH	Adrenocorticotropic hormone (corticotropin)
BF	Biofeedback
DHS	Daily Hassles Scale
DUS	Daily Uplifts Scale
ECG	Electrocardiogram
FPG	Finger plethysmography
GAS	General adaptation syndrome
HPA	Hypothalamic-pituitary-adrenal
HRV	Heart rate variability
IBA	Investigator-based assessment
IBR	Interview-based rating
LDL	Low-density lipoprotein
LEDS	Life Events and Difficulties Schedule
PCP	Primary care physician
RR	Respiratory rate
SAM	Sympathetic-adrenal-medullary
SRE	Schedule of Recent Experiences

THE STRESS PERSPECTIVES

CLINICAL VIGNETTE: RITA

Rita is a 32-year-old woman who recently had a baby boy. She is breastfeeding at this time. Rita has always been a healthy woman. Before getting pregnant, Rita would be cautious about what she ate and would work out 5 times a week. She was also very careful about her health during pregnancy and would participate in yoga classes 3 times a week. On a personal level, Rita has been married for 7 years. Her baby boy is the couple's first child. Her husband is the CEO of at a large corporation, which requires him to work around 60 hours a week. Rita herself has been a very driven woman when it comes to her career. For the past 10 years, she has worked as a lawyer at a high-powered firm that specializes in corporate fraud and other white-collar crimes. For years, she worked 12-hour days and had proved herself to be a top-notch competitor for the next opening as partner in the firm (which is scheduled to take place within the next 10 months of the evaluation). For Rita, having taken time off from work because of maternity leave was a strange sensation. In reality, she had never been away from work for more than 1 consecutive week. After the 3-month leave, Rita was finally back in the office. She had been hoping for this day for a couple of weeks and had expected it to be a joyous occasion. It was not. In fact, today she arrived to see her primary care provider (PCP) reporting several changes in her body and overall health. "Something is terribly wrong," she exclaimed. She noticed that these changes began 2 weeks after returning to work 2 months ago. She is concerned about what these changes might mean. Specifically, she is worried that she might have a terrible illness and that she may not be able to take care of her family nor have success in her professional life. She seeks medical advice, wanting to understand the etiology of such complaints and eager to discuss possible treatment alternatives.

Stress

Stress is a popular topic nowadays and has long been a subject of study.[1–4] Despite its popularity the concept of stress is not properly understood by all, and has therefore been conceptualized in different ways. Commonly stress is a term that comes from physics, and is thus conceptualized as a pressure, force, or demand placed on the body of an organism. It is a force that triggers a type of reaction that might indicate that a person is feeling some sort of strain.[5] This pressure allows a person to respond either by adapting or adjusting to these life demands. In scientific terms, stress has been operationalized as more than just an outside force. For instance, it involves anything that activates the biological stress system; this could be a perceived threat, a distressing event, or life hassles. In other words, here stress is seen as a reaction in response to a stressor.[6]

Stress researcher Hans Selye coined the term general adaptation syndrome (GAS) (later called the stress response)[7] to describe a common biological response pattern seen in prolonged or excessive stress. In 1929, Walter Cannon[8] renamed this response pattern the fight-or-flight response. What both models suggest is that the human body acts like an alarm system that helps in responding to threatening situations. The GAS model consists of 3 processes important for survival: the alarm reaction, the resistance stage, and the exhaustion phase. The alarm reaction mobilizes the body to prepare for a challenge. In this stage, the body reacts by recruiting the help of both the central nervous and endocrine systems.[9] Specific hormones called cortisol, adrenaline, and noradrenaline are released to provide instant energy so that the body can confront a stressor. If a stressor persists, the resistance state comes into being and the body tries to adapt. The endocrine and sympathetic system respond to this need by releasing additional hormones and renewing spent energy. Eventually a person reaches exhaustion, whereby the body's resources are spent and the parasympathetic system dominates.

Stress responses arise to help an individual cope with certain demands. It is a normal physical response that takes place in the body to help thrive, meet challenges, and succeed. This condition is called eustress. However, if it is prolonged it alters the body's harmony, balance, and overall homeostatic and allostatic processes. In time, it can also limit an organism's problem-solving abilities and affect its well-being. Continued activation harms the body and also leads to overload, burnout, adrenal fatigue, maladaptation, or dysfunction.[10] When this occurs, stress is no longer adaptive. Rather, it contributes to distress, a state of physical or mental pain and suffering.

Based on the aforementioned definitions, stress is a highly individualistic experience that depends on a particular event and on specific psychological determinants that trigger a particular response.[11] The activator of the stress process is called a stressor, which is a source of stress that has a specific set of responses within the body of a living organism.[12] A stressor is any physical or psychological challenge that is perceived to have the potential to threaten the stability of the internal milieu of the organism.[13] In short, stressors are things we respond to. It involves psychosocial resources and learned patterns of coping. Stressors include anything from psychological challenges (eg, IQ or personality traits) to life changes and daily hassles (eg, divorce). Physical and environmental demands (eg, subtle changes in temperature or noise levels or complex social situations) are also sources of stress. On average, the amount of stress a person feels is determined by 4 important ingredients: the numerical degree or intensity of the stressor, the length of time exposed to the stressor, the evaluation of the stressor as a threat, and a person's coping abilities (**Table 1**).[14,15]

Conceptualizing Models of Stress

There are several scientific definitions within the literature that comprise the foundations for the understanding of stress. The most salient of these definitions are based on 3 important models: response-based, transactional, and stimulus-based. These theories focus on the specific relationship between bodily process, psychological components, and external demands.[16]

Table 1
Common life stressors

Stressors	Examples
Daily hassles	Traffic; transportation problems; exams; training sessions; caregiving; difficult work shifts; job burnout; conflicts with coworkers
Life changes	Death; divorce; separation from family; job loss; unexpected/unwanted transfer; marriage; childbirth; vacation
Environmental influences	Natural disasters; political conflicts; violence in the community; exposure to war; temperature levels; noise levels; seasonal changes; abuse; diminished social support; socioeconomic status; poor housing conditions; pollution
Psychological determinants	Coping mechanisms; stress reactivity; behavioral inhibition; optimism; hostility; self-perception; resilience; intelligence
Physical factors	Illness; injuries; accidents; pain; pregnancy; heart disease; digestive problems; autoimmune disease; skin conditions

A brief list of normative and/or unexpected life events that can be considered stressful and may alter the body's homeostatic process.

Response-based phenomenon

Stress became part of our day-to-day conversations after having been used by engineers to explain forces that can put strain on a structure. For years, physics analyzed and designed solutions to environmental stressors that could allow man-made structures to withstand heavy loads. As physics talked about how stress affected buildings, the term progressively transitioned into the behavioral sciences. In 1936, Hans Selye became a pioneer in discussing stress from a physiological and medical perspective.[17] He borrowed the term and talked about stress as being a phenomenon representing the intersection of symptoms produced by a wide variety of harmful agents.[10] These agents would, in turn, produce physical changes in the body that were representative of a stress response (eg, enlargement of the adrenal gland, gastric ulceration).[11] Thus, this model portrays the concept of stress as a set of nonspecific responses of the body to any demand made on it.

Transactional model

The transactional model[18,19] suggests that stress entails a particular judgment about environmental or internal demands. In other words, a stress response is a result of the relationship between a person and the environment.[20] This model's basic assumption is that stress involves a balance between demands and psychological status. In short, it involves a cognitive appraisal process, whereby the definition of stress and the impact of such is purely subjective. The cognitive appraisal process itself entails a series of unconscious and conscious judgments (primary and secondary appraisals) that allow a person to either cope or succumb to these life demands.

Stimulus-based

The stimulus-based model was researched by Holmes and Rahe in 1967.[21] It defines stress as involving an event or life experience. This event might be unexpected (or necessary) and might require change in the ongoing life patterns of the individual. The model focuses on the stressor itself and its unique demands (eg, social, physical, psychological, and intellectual).[22] It also places an emphasis on how the stressor challenges a person's adaptive abilities. Adaptation and readjustment are perhaps the most investigated area of stress research (**Table 2**).[10]

THE BIOLOGICAL TRADITION

> **CLINICAL VIGNETTE: RITA**
>
> *During her appointment, Rita mentioned having noticed changes in the way she has been feeling. She complained of headaches, dizziness, tachycardia, chest pain, lightheadedness, indigestion, sweaty palms, frequent hand tremors, skin irritation, and rash. Furthermore, she mentioned that in the past 5 months she has not been able to lose any of the baby weight she gained during her pregnancy. In fact, she has gained 5 lb in the last 3 weeks. She added that 2 days ago, she began to feel a slight fever accompanied by minor body aches. Flustered and helpless, Rita cried out: "Of course this would happen to me... with all I have to do and I end up getting sick." Rita does not take any prescription medications, does not take over-the-counter supplements, and does not do drugs. Rita has no family history of heart disease. However, on evaluation her blood pressure reading was 122/80. Because of her complaints and slight elevation in blood pressure, her PCP gave her a task of monitoring her blood pressure every day for a week and report back to him. As agreed, Rita took her blood pressure every day after picking her son up from daycare, around 6:00 PM. Her blood pressure readings for the week read as follows: 117/80, 120/82, 125/80, 130/87, 122/81, 117/76, 121/80. During her follow-up, Rita had grown increasingly concerned and flustered about her health and inquired about the benefits of being evaluated by a medical specialist to rule out any significant condition. Because Rita was specifically restless about her cardiovascular health, she was referred to a cardiologist for further evaluation. An electrocardiogram (ECG) and echocardiogram were performed. There was no evidence of irregular heartbeats, structural abnormalities, or chemical imbalances in the ECG or echocardiogram. In fact, there was no significant physical finding and no physiological explanation for her cardiovascular complaints. Additional diagnostic tests were performed to further help Rita understand the probable causes of her ailments. A full blood panel and metabolic testing were completed. The most significant findings in Rita's lab tests were slight elevations in her low-density lipoprotein (LDL) cholesterol (132), fasting glucose levels (102), and white blood cells (4200).*

The biological tradition of measuring stress is linked to the response-based model of Selye.[23] It focuses on the activation of specific physiological systems that are influenced by both physiologically and physically demanding conditions.[24] This biological perspective characterizes stress as anything that activates the sympathetic nervous, endocrine, and immune system response. These systems represent measures of allostatic medicine.

The term allostasis was introduced in 1988 by Sterling and Eyer[25] to describe how the cardiovascular system adjusts to resting and active states of the body. The term implies that there is a need for preservation of a homeostatic process and adaptation even when there is change. It is therefore a theoretical construct and a measure of cumulative "wear and tear" on a psychological system caused by chronic stress.[26] At present there are assortments of biomarkers that can be used for measuring the components of an allostatic load. Biomarkers are cellular, biochemical, or molecular indicators of a disease process,[27] which serve to evaluate normal biological processes, pathogenic responses, or medication outcomes. Biomarkers thus provide information about a condition that can be measured reliably in tissues, cells, or fluids, and can be used to detect early changes in a patient's health (diagnosis and prognosis specific). In allostatic medicine biomarkers range from anthropometric, cardiovascular, and metabolic to inflammatory fluctuations. Changes in central nervous system (CNS) activity, renal and lung function, and bone density and adiposity are additional examples of physiological stress cues.[28]

Hypothalamic-Pituitary-Adrenocortical Axis

Stress has a domino effect on the endocrine system, which consists of specific glands that release hormones directly into the bloodstream.[29] The interpretation of a situation

Table 2
Conceptualizing models of stress

Approach	Researchers	Key Words	Conceptualization
Response-based	Hans Selye,[128] 1956	Systematic stress Psychobiological markers	Physiological: nonspecific response to a stimulus. Stress can cause wear and tear on the body. This process can contribute to illness, disease, and death
Transactional	Holroyd & Lazarus,[19] 1982	Cognitive psychology Cognitive appraisals and coping potential	Psychological: a threat, harm, or a challenge. Emotions, coping responses, and behaviors emerge from these cognitive appraisals. Stress occurs when situations exceed a person's resources
Stimulus-based	Holmes & Rahe,[21] 1967	Adaptation and readjustment Life charts, life changes, hassles, uplifts	Environmental: life events require coping strategies that restore the homeostatic process. These coping strategies result in adaptation and readjustment

The most influential stress theories, their corresponding traditions, and the most prominent figures in the stress field. Some of the information was adapted from Lyon's (2012)[17] work on stress, coping, and health outcomes as defined in stress theories.

as being stressful leads to the activation of the hypothalamic-pituitary-adrenocortical (HPA) axis, and to the subsequent secretion of cortisol and catecholamine in humans. It involves an ongoing process that can be defined by various steps. First, the hypothalamus stimulates the pituitary gland to secrete adrenocorticotropic hormone (ACTH; corticotropin). In turn, ACTH stimulates the adrenal glands. The outer layer of the adrenal glands, called the adrenal cortex, is the primary end point of the HPA-axis activation as it releases corticosteroids when stimulated in such a manner. These steroids include cortisol and cortisone, which boost resistance to stress, foster muscle development, and induce the liver to release glucose.[30] These functions help the organism respond to emergency situations and defend against threats. The release of corticosteroids is one particular reason why persistent stress may eventually lead to health problems.[31] Indeed, while short bursts of cortisol help the body to respond to stress, continuous secretion can also compromise the immune system by disrupting the production of antibodies. Ultimately chronicity increases a person's vulnerability and susceptibility to colds and other infectious diseases.[32]

Hypothalamic-pituitary-adrenocortical-axis activation
Research has shed light on HPA-axis activation and has demonstrated the feasibility of detecting stress using physiological measurements.[33] Specifically, hormone levels involved with glucocorticoids, corticotropin-releasing hormone, prolactin, ACTH, dehydroepiandrosterone, arginine, vasopressin, and catecholamine are parameters of adrenal activity.[28] These factors represent biomarkers for HPA-axis activation that can be easily measurable in blood, urine, excreta, and saliva. One particular study[34]

also presents the use of enzyme immunoassays (EIA) in analyzing hormone stress indicators in animals through fecal samples (**Table 3**).

Sympathetic-Adrenal-Medullary System

The HPA axis is involved in the long-term effects of both acute and chronic stress. Whereas the sympathetic-adrenal-medullary (SAM) axis is activated immediately during the stressor and shuts off after the removal of the stress, the HPA axis is slower in activation and continues to be activated long after the stressor has been removed.

The observation of a dissociated stress habituation pattern of the HPA axis compared with SAM parameters corroborates recent findings from this laboratory. A stress protocol such as the Stroop color-word interference test elicits SAM responses (eg, heart rate increase); however, it is insufficient for significant HPA-axis activation if performed in a one-on-one (one subject, one experimenter) setting. If the same task is performed in front of an evaluative audience, a significant increase in cortisol levels can also be observed.[35] These data are in line with findings from the Frankenhäuser laboratory. Frankenhäuser suggested that effort, distress, and control are the forces driving an endocrine stress response. Although effort without distress (as in the Stroop test) will result in an epinephrine response, only distress will lead to cortisol secretion in her model.[36]

Walter Cannon's work[8] on the fight-or-flight response sparked interest in measuring SAM activation in the body. Cannon's work proposed that the SAM system reacts to emergencies by secreting increased amounts of epinephrine (adrenaline) and norepinephrine (noradrenaline). These hormones are secreted by the inner layer of the adrenal glands, called the adrenal medulla. When an organism is threatened, these hormones are immediately activated to help the body prepare to fight or flee by accelerating the heart rate and stimulating the liver to release stored glucose. The acceleration experienced by an organism as a consequence of this body's response is known by many as an adrenaline rush.

Measurement of sympathetic-adrenal-medullary activation

As with HPA-axis activation, biomarkers can be used to assess the extent of change in the body resulting from variations in SAM activation. While cortisol is one common biomarker for HPA-axis activation, blood and urine samples for SAM activation assess the levels of catecholamines that the adrenal glands secrete (eg, adrenaline and noradrenaline). Additional assessment methods have been used to identify the indirect effects of SAM activation by the use of proxy autonomic measures.[33] Proxy autonomic measures assess autonomic arousal using electrical and mechanical equipment that take measurements of vital signs. These measures can be used in combination with biomarkers or as a substitute, for instance to evaluate salivary cortisol and salivary α-amylase when biomarkers are too expensive and time consuming.[35] Common biomarkers include blood pressure, heart rate, perspiration, and blood flow through peripheral vessels.

Blood pressure Blood pressure is a sympathetic parameter that assesses the force that pumped blood exerts on the walls of blood vessels.[36] Stress can affect blood pressure in both the short and long term. During the fight-or-flight response, for example, blood pressure can spike temporarily by causing the heart to beat faster and blood vessels to constrict. If repeated over time, spikes can cause damage to blood vessels and, although it does not directly cause hypertension, it can have an effect on its development. Furthermore, when elevations are coupled with other stress-induced habits or behaviors (eg, overeating, drinking alcohol, poor sleeping

Table 3
HPA-axis activation

Biomarker	Brief Description	Collection Method	Normal Ranges	Association with Disease
Prolactin	Secreted from the pituitary gland in response to eating, mating, estrogen treatment, ovulation, and nursing. It plays an essential role in metabolism, regulation of the immune system, and pancreatic development.	Blood	2–18 ng/mL for males 2–29 ng/mL for nonpregnant females 10–209 ng/mL for pregnant women	High levels affect behaviors and tend to lead to manifestations of hostility and low libido.
Cortisol	Released by the zona fasciculata of the adrenal cortex. Involved in energy production, conservation of carbohydrates, reduction of inflammation, among other functions.	Saliva, urine, & blood	5–23 µg/dL or 138–635 nmol/L in the morning 3–16 µg/dL or 83–441 nmol/L in the afternoon	Persistently high levels associated with depression, anxiety, and poor cognitive functioning. Higher levels of cortisol indicate greater reported psychological stress.
Catecholamine (norepinephrine)	Used by the nerve endings in the sympathetic nervous system. It is involved with maintaining normal body functions like heart rate, blood pressure and sugar levels. It also helps the body respond to perceived threats.	Urine & blood	15–80 µg in 24 h for urine 600 pg/mL for blood	Low levels of norepinephrine can depress cognitive functioning. On the other hand, high levels can lead to feelings of hyperarousal, which can cause a person to experience prolonged bouts of anxiety, restlessness and irritability.
Catecholamine (epinephrine)	Derived from tyrosine, it is involved with maintaining normal body functions like heart rate, blood pressure, sugar, breathing, increased blood flow, and other functions that enable the body to fight or run away when encountering a perceived threat.	Urine & blood	0.5–20 µg in 24 h for urine 900 pg/mL in blood	Low levels of epinephrine can decrease on cognitive functioning. On the other hand, high levels can lead to feelings of hyperarousal, which can cause a person to experience prolonged bouts of anxiety, restlessness and irritability.

List of some of the most common biomarkers used to measure the hypothalamic-pituitary-adrenocortical (HPA) axis activation under stress. The list provides a general overview of the collection methods and numeric ranges possibly seen after brief or prolonged exposure to stress. The reader can also refer to Konduru's work (2011)[27] and Piazza and colleagues (2010)[28] for detailed information regarding biomarkers of chronic stress.

patterns), the effect on blood pressure is multiplied.[37] Stress effects on health can be measured using a simple vital-signs monitor or a noninvasive sphygmomanometer.

Heart rate/pulse rate Negative emotions (eg, anxiety and irritability) alter heart rate variability (HRV). In fact, indices of autonomic nervous system activity are usually calculated using HRV. In general, the sympathetic activity leads to an increase in HRV, whereas parasympathetic activity induces a decrease in HRV. HRV is a relatively new method for assessing the effects of stress on the body.[24] Peripheral blood flow reflects autonomic nervous system activity, the latter being a known indicator of the level of mental stress.[38] Research evidence increasingly links high HRV to good health and a high level of fitness, whereas decreased HRV is linked to stress, fatigue, and even burnout.[39–47] The association between negative affect and reduced HRV may thus provide a potential mechanism linking chronic stress to disease outcomes (eg, risk of coronary heart disease).

Aside from HRV, finger pulse rate can also provide valuable information about stress levels. ECG and finger plethysmography (FPG) (eg, Finometer) are examples of useful tools in stress detection. Both are simple and noninvasive methods to monitor peripheral circulation, and can be used to detect vital changes in the body. In a study conducted in 2013, Minakuchi and colleagues[35] suggested that the presence of stress can be detected when finger pulse rate increases and pulse wave amplitude decreases. The variability signal usually becomes simpler and weaker as result of disease.[48,49]

Respiratory rate The respiratory rate (RR) refers to the rate or frequency of breathing, that is, the number of breaths taken within 1 minute. RRs may increase with fever, illness, medical conditions, and stress.[50] In terms of the latter, some studies suggest that emotional arousal and psychosocial stress decrease airway resistance to the degree that they are accompanied by sympathetic activation and/or parasympathetic withdrawal.[51] Other studies suggest that different emotional states, such as anxiety, anger, and joy, are equally capable of eliciting increases in airway resistance, especially in asthmatics.[52–54] Experimental tasks that demand an active coping response typically elicit autonomic adjustments and are therefore expected to decrease airway resistance. On the other hand, stressful situations that are unavoidable and require passive coping response may increase airway resistance.[55,56]

RR can be determined by watching a person's shoulders and chest. It can also be measured by using an electronic strain gauge or other sensory devices, including stethoscopes, pneumatographs, or spirographs, which are commonly implemented in monitoring the vital signs of a patient. Total respiratory resistance can also be measured by forced oscillations using the Siemens Siregnost FD5 with a fixed oscillation frequency of 10 Hz.[51]

Body temperature and galvanic skin response

Body temperature, a measure of the body's ability to generate and dissipate heat, can be measured in many locations in the body (eg, mouth, ear, armpit, rectum, and forehead). The galvanic skin response is also known as the skin conductance response or the electrodermal response. It is a phenomenon whereby the skin becomes an improved conductor of electricity when the system is activated because of either external or internal stimuli that are physiologically arousing.[27] Stress influences body temperatures in humans. In fact, body temperature is very sensitive to hormone levels and may be higher or lower depending on what occurs to an organism.[57]

Overall, body temperature can be easily measured using a thermometer. The link between body temperature and stress is based on the well-known fact that the electrodermal response is associated with stress-related sweat-gland activity. Because the sweat glands are controlled by the sympathetic nervous system, sweating causes changes in skin conductance. At the same time, this offers an indication of emotional excitement. To this end, a study conducted by Viqueira-Villarejo and colleagues[58] concluded that the more stressed a person feels, the more his or her hands will sweat, thus decreasing resistance and increasing output voltage in measures of physiological reaction. As a person relaxes, there is a decrease in the output voltage for that period of time. To this end, the body's signals increase or decrease depending on the effort or the mental situation of the individual. Constant or slight variations in the galvanic responses and temperatures can thus be measured and charted.

Measurement devices

A biofeedback (BF) device is an evidence-based assessment and treatment measure[59] that provides information about a person's response to stress. A BF device can detect changes in internal bodily functions with sensitivity and precision.[60] Through sensors, it measures muscle tension, skin temperature, heart rate, respiration, brain-wave activity, and flow of blood in the brain. In addition to providing information to the subject about a person's body, it also promotes awareness of stress responses. The polygraph, also a widely used measure of stress,[61] consists of a physiological recorder that assesses 3 indicators of autonomic arousal: cardiovascular activity (such as heart rate), respiration, and skin conductivity. Most examiners today use computerized recording systems. However, miniature polygraphs have been created that can be carried around for easy assessment of body changes and variations in response to a stressful event (**Table 4**).

Case Discussion

Now that relevant information in terms of physiological assessment of stress has been reviewed, Rita's case can now be discussed. During her PCP appointments, Rita presented with several physical complaints that slightly concerned her provider. Her chest pain and tachycardia, coupled with her elevated blood pressure readings, were among the symptoms that could have suggested the possibility of cardiovascular problems. However, her ECG and echocardiogram were normal and, although some of her blood pressure readings were high, overall they were within the normal range. The fluctuations in blood pressure alone could suggest the possibility of elevations or spikes triggered by stress. However, a full blood panel was ordered to rule out any possible medical problems. The most significant findings in Rita's lab tests were slight elevations in her LDL cholesterol and glucose levels, and a low white blood cell count. A closer look at these results is warranted.

A normal reading for fasting glucose is usually 70 to 100 mg/dL. However, for Rita her glucose was at 102 mg/dL. On further exploration, there is no family history of prediabetes or diabetes, and Rita has never had any abnormal blood sugar readings in the past. According to the stress research, Rita's results might be explained by alterations in hormones caused by the fight-or-flight response. Under stress, the body prepares itself to react by ensuring that enough energy is readily available. As the stress response begins, insulin levels decrease, glucagon and epinephrine (adrenaline) levels increase, and more glucose is released from the liver. At the same time growth hormone and cortisol levels increase, which cause body tissues to be less sensitive to insulin.[62] As a result, more glucose is available in the bloodstream. If it is not used, glucose is converted into triglycerides and is accumulated as fat tissue.[13] All of these determinants also affect daily glucose, cholesterol, and weight. In the case of Rita, her LDL or bad cholesterol was at 132 mg/dL, which is considered borderline high (130–159 mg/dL), and she had mentioned having gained 5 lb in the past 2 to 3 weeks. Notwithstanding, stress not only affects hormone production but also causes poor eating habits and poor food choices. Eating and exercise habits would thus need to be explored further with Rita. Likewise, research has documented the mechanisms throughout which stressful emotions alter the function of white blood cells.[63] Although stress might not necessarily impair the immune system, a weakened immune system may increase the susceptibility to many illnesses, including the common cold[64,65] and atopic dermatitis conditions. In fact, skin problems are found to be closely related to the degree of stress affecting a person.[66] These findings could potentially explain Rita's decreased white blood cell count and skin complaints.

Measurement Considerations

Strengths

There are several assessment measures that explore the relationship between stress and health and allow scientists to collect data about human behavior. In the quest to improve the medical and social sciences, several advances in using measures of physiological arousal to assess stress have been identified. Research has demonstrated the feasibility of detecting the bodily effects of emotions[67] and stress reactions from physiological measures. In considering this strength, one can also add that physiological measures are practical, objective, fairly reliable, and easily quantified. In addition, quantitative assessments using proxy measures are noninvasive, can be acquired with minimal discomfort for the subject, and can be obtained rapidly. Some of these techniques and assessment measures have also been shown to yield excellent performances in many applications and settings.[35]

Limitations

Although physiological measures afford health providers with a wide array of advantages in the assessment of stress, there are several limitations that need to be taken into consideration. Physiological markers and proxy autonomic measures may be expensive and may require extensive training on the part of the professional. In fact, depending on the methods of data collection, information needs to be analyzed by chemists using special procedures and equipment. The results of physiological measurement may be also affected by factors such as gender, weight, age, and activity before assessment; anxiety related to the tests themselves; and the use of psychoactive substances such as caffeine.[68,69] Physical responses can vary greatly from one person to the next,[70] thus limiting generalization. In addition, there are many determinants that can explain the neurobiological responses seen in laboratory tests and neuroimaging that do not necessarily correspond with stress. Other medical conditions or medication effects, for example, might have an impact on physiological stimulation. Thus, further evaluation is needed; in particular, a detailed medical and psychological history is in order when considering possible causes of a person's somatic complaints and autonomic responses. At the same time, there are several stress responses that do not imply physical changes/arousal that cannot be quantified through medical studies. For instance, not all stressors reliably elicit cortisol, inflammatory responses, or other autonomic changes. Positive life events, such as graduation or the start of a new job, may involve a certain degree of stress resulting from role changes and unpredictability. Physiological measures (and the results obtained from them) may be biased toward visually discernible effects and may not reflect the true stress status of a person.[33] In this sense, cost-effectiveness and reliability, in the long term, are 2 of the biggest challenges faced.

Table 4
SAM activation

Biomarker	Brief Description	Collection Method	Normal Ranges	Association with Disease
Cortisol	Released by zona fasciculata of adrenal cortex. Involved in energy production, conservation of carbohydrates, reduction of inflammation, among other functions	Saliva, urine, blood	5–23 μg/dL or 138–635 nmol/L in the morning 3–16 μg/dL or 83–441 nmol/L in the afternoon	Persistently high levels associated with depression, anxiety, and poor cognitive functioning. Higher levels of cortisol indicate greater reported psychological stress
Catecholamine (norepinephrine)	Used by the nerve endings in the sympathetic nervous system. Involved with maintaining normal body functions such as heart rate, blood pressure, and sugar levels. It also helps the body respond to perceived threats	Urine & blood	15–80 μg in 24 h for urine 600 pg/mL for blood	Low levels of norepinephrine can depress cognitive functioning. On the other hand, elevations can lead to feelings of hyperarousal, which can cause a person to experience prolonged bouts of anxiety, restlessness, and irritability
Catecholamine (epinephrine)	Derived from tyrosine. Involved with maintaining normal body functions such as heart rate, blood pressure, sugar, breathing, increased blood flow, and other functions that enable the body to fight or run away when encountering a perceived threat	Urine & blood	0.5–20 μg in 24 h for urine 900 pg/mL in blood	Low levels of epinephrine can depress cognitive functioning. On the other hand, elevations can lead to feelings of hyperarousal, which can cause a person to experience prolonged bouts of anxiety, restlessness, and irritability

Proxy Autonomic Measure

Measure	Description	Collection methods	Numeric ranges	Interpretation
Blood pressure	Systolic: peak arterial pressure during heartbeat. Diastolic: lowest arterial pressure between heartbeats. Both are indicators of cardiovascular health. Ensure delivery of oxygen to vital organs and skeletal muscles	Sphygmomanometers	120/80 depending slightly on age, conditions, and medication side effects	High levels indicate diastolic hypertension especially among younger adults, owing to poor lifestyle choices (eg, obesity, high fat and high sodium diet, and nicotine use). This places young adults at risk for myocardial infarction or other cardiovascular problems. Elevations indicate physiological symptoms associated with the body's stress response
Heart rate	Number of heartbeats per unit time. Indicator of cardiovascular health. Delivers blood flow and oxygen to skeletal muscle	Heart rate monitor, ECG, FPG, Finometer	70–99 beats/min at rest	High levels indicate hypertension. Elevations indicate physiological symptoms associated with the body's stress response. Finger pulse rate increased and pulse wave amplitude decreased as a sign of stress
Respiratory rate	Number of breaths taken within 1 min	Stethoscope, pneumatograph, spirograph	15 breaths/min in adults	Increase in breathing rate found to be associated with negative emotional states
Body temperature and galvanic skin response	Indication of emotional excitement via sweat gland activity and temperature	Thermometer, E-meter, biofeedback machines	37.0°C (98.6°F)	Increase in perspiration (galvanic skin response), drops in temperature ranging from 5° to 20°C, or temperature increase of <10°C associated with high levels of stress

List of some biomarkers and proxy autonomic measures that can provide information about SAM activation in response to stress. The list provides a general overview of the collection methods and numeric ranges possibly seen after brief or prolonged exposure to stress. The reader can also refer to Konduru's work (2011),[27] Piazza, and colleagues (2010),[28] and Solowiej and colleagues (2010)[71] for detailed information regarding biomarkers of chronic stress.

THE PSYCHOLOGICAL TRADITION

CLINICAL VIGNETTE: RITA

During her appointment, Rita admitted to feeling overwhelmed with her life and nervous about her health. Her PCP suspected that stress could be the cause of her health complaints, and thus recruited Rita to do a little bit of detective work with him. Because of her elevated blood pressures, her PCP encouraged her to keep a log of her blood pressures and also write down how she was feeling at the time of the reading. To help minimize her worry, he informed her that in the future, pharmacological treatment would be considered if needed. In the meantime, Rita's provider encouraged changes in her diet and lifestyle with the hope of implementing a holistic approach to improving her health. Her PCP also concluded that a conversation with a mental health provider could be helpful, and proceeded to explore Rita's thoughts on this possibility. Concerned about what this might mean and somewhat reluctant, Rita accepted and met with the clinic health behaviorist for a walk-in evaluation. During this visit, the health behaviorist administered several instruments that asked her about recent changes in her mood, coping skills, behaviors, thoughts, and general outlook on life. Specifically, the Beck Anxiety Inventory, Beck Helplessness Scale, Coping Strategies Inventory, and Symptom Checklist-90 Revised were used. Rita was feeling nervous, restless, worried, and increasingly concerned about her future; at times she felt sad and helpless. Rita exclaimed, "If I cannot handle this change in my life, then I can never be a successful partner at the firm." This verbalization led Rita and her behaviorist to ponder on several working hypotheses. For instance, they seemed to agree that Rita would frequently feel out of control of her life, which would lead to many self-defeating thoughts such as "I will never be able to manage." At work, she became easily distracted and noticed that it was becoming increasingly difficult for her to concentrate. She began to forget important tasks and was having trouble meeting deadlines. In addition, Rita was not sleeping or eating well, did not exercise, was drinking coffee 3 times a day, and had begun drinking 2 glasses of wine a night to calm herself down.

Stress Appraisal

Hans Selye was the first to define stress as a human response. However, there were several researchers who criticized Selye's theory of stress, particularly the notion that the determinants of stress response are nonspecific. John Mason (1960), for example, determined that the activation of a stress response depends on the interpretation the individual has about an event. He placed an emphasis on the organism's perception and evaluation of the potential harm posed by human experience.[72] After spending many years sustaining his theory and measuring stress hormone levels, he was able to describe 4 main psychological determinants that would induce a stress response in any individual exposed to them. For Mason, a stressor needs to be (1) novel; (2) unpredictable; (3) a threat to one's physical/emotional integrity; and (4) capable of inducing a feeling or sense that the person does not have control of the stressor.[11] This concept came to be known as the NUTS model.

In 1982 Holroyd and Lazarus[19] created their own stress model, which suggests that there are multiple cognitive responses to a stressor. This model states that the impact of stress depended on 2 dimensions: primary appraisal and secondary appraisal. A primary appraisal is a judgment by which a person determines whether a threat is real and if it has the potential for growth. A secondary appraisal, on the other hand, is determined by the person's subjective belief about whether he or she is able to cope with the perceived threat. It is, in a sense, a transaction between judgment, emotion, and behavior. As an overview, the primary and secondary appraisal process involves: (1) the person's belief about the experience; (2) thinking patterns about the experience and its relation to the future; (3) the person's feelings associated with the experience; (4) behaviors in response to a situation; and (5) a combination of all of the above. After appraising a stressor or evaluating it as a threat, a person will react, often with an emotional and behavioral response.

Cognitive response

The aforementioned questions led to the inclusion of other ideas that promoted the growth of cognitive psychology. Are certain things stressful or is it just because of how they are perceived? Individuals react differently to stress depending on their psychological ability to cope with it. A key mediator in the stress process is cognition, a primitive appraisal process whereby the social world is perceived and appraised by the individual.[2] The psychological tradition of measuring stress focuses on the individual's subjective evaluations of specific events. The way that an individual responds to a stressor (from the appraisal through the stress response) depends on various factors that may mediate or moderate the way in which an individual thinks and then responds to a stressor.[73–75] These primary appraisals include factors that can be external to the individual (eg, the imminence of being harmed, the magnitude or intensity, the duration, and the potential controllability) and/or internal to the individual (eg, beliefs, values, personality traits). Both internal and external determinants can lead to self-defeating thoughts, immature defense mechanisms, and ineffective cognitive coping styles. Examples include catastrophizing, rumination, magnification, generalization, and learned helplessness.[76] These determinants can also trigger neurological signs that range from forgetfulness, distractibility, and decreased productivity to problems with decision making and judgment, among others.

Emotional response

Psychological stress is best regarded as a subset of emotions. Stress carries a heavy toll on emotions and involves both positive and negative affect states. These states include happiness, joy, fear, and irritability, among others. However, anger, anxiety, guilt, shame, sadness, envy, jealousy, and disgust are commonly referred to as the stress emotions.[77] Often, stress is also linked to many troublesome psychological disorders and/or increased susceptibility for comorbidity. Anxiety is, essentially, one of the most common forms of psychological disorders associated with prolonged stress. Therefore, psychologists emphasize the perception of stress, particularly when prolonged, whereby the demands potentially exceed a person's ability to cope with them. It also focuses on a person's affective response[20] and his or her engagement and disengagement with life. When providers attempt to ascertain a person's emotional state, they typically ask the individual to describe the emotions being experienced. Verbal responses are important when exploring emotions. However, nonverbal indices are also crucial. In this sense, physiological processes to stress can lead to changes in coloration (eg, blushing), facial expression (eg, tired, confused), and other signs of emotion (eg, posture, hygiene).

Behavioral response

The behavioral aspect is also important. Emotions often motivate us to act out or express our feelings through the fight-or-flight response.[1] When a stimulus is appraised as requiring a coping response, individuals evaluate their resources to determine whether they can cope with a situation or not.[76] That is, individuals react in a way that either lessens or eliminates the threat of stress. Aside from lessening or eliminating stress, individuals might also try to adapt to stress by using coping strategies. These strategies allow a person to confront a stressor head-on and find ways in which to balance out the demands of daily life. In this sense, stress leads to expressing strong emotional responses in the form of behaviors. Common reactions might include crying, screaming, yelling, hitting, avoidance, exercising, dieting, prayer, and increased social support.[78] Tone of voice, posture, and other kinds of body language are additional common signals of emotion. This particular process is a secondary appraisal.

Psychological Assessment

Once the concept of stress was introduced and researched in psychology, it became part of the group of psychological concepts that can be measured.[79] Measures of perceived stress and negative affect help distinguish between the cognitive, emotional, and behavioral impact of stress. Therefore, when measuring the psychological response to stress, one wishes to specifically evaluate both external and internal factors in relation to a psychological experience and cognitive summation of all life stressors (eg, overall perceived stress). If a person understands that he or she has sufficient coping strategies, little or no stress occurs. If, on the other hand, the demands of the stressors surpass a person's resources, stress is experienced. To this end, measures were developed to assess a wide range of psychological signs and symptoms that can be induced by exposure to stressful events.[11] Specifically, psychological functions can be measured through self-reports, checklists, questionnaires, and objective/projective testing. Some of these assessment tools inquire about thoughts and beliefs about different stressors and the extent of their impact with regard to how well a person adapts to a situation. Other instrument responses are obtained by asking about the frequency and extent to which a person has been bothered by several symptoms within a specific time frame (usually 2–3 weeks). Using these instruments, patients are asked to evaluate their symptoms via rating scales that have specific cutoff points used to identify cases of mild, moderate, and severe symptoms. More elaborate measures of stress (eg, Rorschach Inkblot Test) might involve free association techniques that allow the individual to respond to ambiguous stimuli and reveal hidden emotions or internal conflicts. A list of psychological measures is presented in **Table 5**.

Case Discussion

Now it is known that Rita is in good health medically speaking, one can move on to conceptualizing her complaints within a psychological framework. During her psychologist's evaluation, Rita was able to talk and process her feelings about the changes that have happened in her life over the last year. At home, Rita is a working mother with little support from her husband. She feels that she does not have the emotional resources necessary to be successful in her new endeavors: in a word, helpless. Her work, marriage, and baby are a blessing for Rita, but balancing them all out is challenging. Thus she has grown nervous, restless, worried, and increasingly concerned about her future. She also feels sad at times. On a cognitive level, she feels out of control of her life and frequently tells herself that she will never be able to cope or have success again. She has also begun to take notice of her distractibility, lack of concentration, and forgetfulness, which reinforce her belief that she is a failure. Behaviorally she has also implemented poorer health practices, which include bad choices in terms of her eating habits, lack of physical activity, and increased caffeine and alcohol use. Overall, the sum of her verbal complaints, physical symptoms, and results from her checklists/questionnaires suggest that Rita was experiencing a significant amount of stress. Moreover, she is at increased risk of anxiety, depression, and alcohol abuse. Her PCP was thus accurate in predicting that stress was a culprit in her clinical presentation and encouraging her to reflect on how her life changes have been affecting her health.

Measurement Considerations

Strengths

Self-report, checklists, and questionnaires are popular for many reasons, but mostly because they represent an inexpensive way to obtain information from someone and can be easily implemented in large samples. These assessment methods are also used often because they elicit direct information from the responder, by asking for their opinion and perspective on their life situation or complaints. Similarly, there are also times when self-report measures are preferred because of their greater face validity and reliability.[80]

Limitations

Although it might sound contradictory, many of the so-called strengths of psychological measures of stress are also considered to be part of their limitations. Although there are measures that have great validity and reliability, the main disadvantage of self-reporting is that there are also several potential associated validity problems, which is particularly the case when evaluating ethnic minorities or culturally diverse individuals. To this day, many professionals are not strongly convinced of the value of patient-reported outcome measurements in the assessment of psychological symptoms and subsequent evaluation of treatment progress.[81] Probably one of the greatest challenges in the receptivity of self-report measures is its subjectivity. In other words, individuals differ in the expression of their symptoms, exhibiting between-person differences and endorsing variations in symptom expression from one culture to another. Therefore, measures using subjective stress ratings are confusing and do not provide a clear binary classification of stress.[82] Furthermore, their utility in research might be limited by the length of questionnaires and the time required to administer them. In fact, self-report measures place a significant time-response cost on the participant, making frequent collection of such measurements impractical.[33]

THE ENVIRONMENTAL TRADITION

CLINICAL VIGNETTE: RITA

Rita admitted to having been feeling stressed about being a new mom. Her husband works 60 hours a week, which means that she has had to take care of her son almost all on her own. Between preparing for depositions and a baby to take care of, she has not been able to sleep more than 2 consecutive hours in the last month. For Rita, a new baby, a new stage in her marriage, and a potentially promising career were considered burdens she felt too overwhelming to bear. While talking to her PCP and health behaviorist, she was made aware of the multiple changes she has faced in the last year. During her PCP and psychology appointments, she talked about her stressors and identified pregnancy, childbirth, maternity leave, and work changes as the most significant. She also talked about her work schedule, her son's day care, and about the messes she finds in her home at the end of the night. Her home and her bed are no longer her safe heavens but rather places in which to worry. Moreover, she talked about feeling overweight, having almost no time to be intimate with her partner, and worrying too much about her home and finances. Rita reflected on her life and verbalized that in the past she would have been able to manage with all of the day-to-day demands. However, now that she is a new mother, her schedule has changed so dramatically that she feels she cannot keep up. Stress, in short, was destroying her life.

Life Changes

Holmes and Rahe defined stress as something that involves a change. Most of the evidence available about the role of stress in human disease has come from research

Table 5
Psychological and environmental measures of stress

Instrument Name	Source	Rating System	Theoretical Underpinnings
Activities Checklist	Arbuckle, Gold, Chaikelson, & Lapidus, 1994	Respondent based	Behavioral
Beck Anxiety Inventory (BAI)	Beck, 1988	Respondent based	Emotional and somatic
Beck Hopelessness Scale (BHS)	Beck, Weissman, Lester, & Trexler, 1974; Beck & Steer, 1988	Respondent based	Cognitive
Blessed Memory Orientation (BMO)	Katzman, Brown, Fuld et al., 1983	Investigator based	Cognitive
Coping Strategies Inventory (CSI)	Tobin, 1984; 2001	Respondent based	Cognitive and behavioral
Daily Hassles and Uplift Scale	Lazarus & Folkman,[2] 1984	Respondent based	Environmental
Daily Stress Inventor	Brantley, Waggoner, Jones, & Rappaport, 1987	Respondent based	Environmental
General Anxiety Disorder-7 (GAD-7)	Spitzer, Williams, Kroenke et al, 1999	Respondent based	Behavioral, cognitive, and emotional
General Health Questionnaire (GHQ)	Goldberg, 1992	Respondent based	Behavioral, emotional, and somatic
Going Through Changes Questionnaire	Renner & Mackin, 1998	Respondent based	Environmental
Hammen Life Stress Interview	Adrian & Hammen, 1993; Rudolph & Hammen, 1999	Investigator based	Environmental
Hamilton Anxiety Rating Scale (HAM-A)	Hamilton, 1959	Respondent based	Behavioral, emotional, and somatic
Hopkins Symptom Checklist	Parloff, Kelman, and Frank, 1950; Derogatis, 2000	Respondent based	Behavioral, emotional, and somatic
Illness Cognitions Questionnaire (ICQ)	Evers & Kraaimaat, 1998	Respondent based	Cognitive
Impact of Event Scale (IES) and Impact of Events Scale Revised (IES-R)	Horowitz, Wilner, and Alvarez, 1979; Greenberg, 2013	Respondent based	Cognitive, behavioral, emotional, and somatic
Job Control Questionnaire	Karasek & Theorell, 1990	Respondent based	Cognitive and environmental
Kendler Life Stress Interview	Kendler (year unknown to author)	Investigator based	Environmental
Lesserman Stressful Life Events and Difficulties Interview	Lesserman (year unknown to author)	Investigator based	Environmental

Instrument	Reference	Type	Domains
List of Recent Experiences	Henderson, Byren, & Duncan-Jones, 1981	Respondent based	Cognitive, behavioral, and emotional
Maslach Burnout Inventory (MBI)	Maslach & Jackson, 1997	Investigator based	Cognitive
Mini Mental Status Examination (MMSE)	Folstein, Folstein, & McHugh, 1975	Respondent based	Emotional
Mood Adjective Checklist (MACL)	Nowlis & Green, 1957	Respondent based	Cognitive and emotional
Multiple Affect Adjective Checklist (MAACL)	Zuckerman & Lubin, 1965	Investigator based	Environmental
Munich Event List	Wittchen et al, 1989	Investigator based	Environmental
Paykel Brief Life Events List	Paykel, 1983	Investigator based	Environmental
Positive Affect and Negative Affect Schedule (PANAS)	Watson, Clark, & Tellegen, 1988	Respondent based	Emotional and environmental
Profile of Mood States (POMS)	McNair, Lorr, & Droppleman, 1971	Respondent based	Emotional
Psychological Stress Measure (PMS-9)	Lemyre & Tessier, 1988, 2002	Respondent based	Cognitive, emotional, and somatic
PTSD Checklist Civilian Version (PCL-C)	Weathers, Huska, & Keane, 1991; 1994	Respondent based	Behavioral, cognitive, emotional, and somatic
Symptom Checklist-90 Revised (SCL-90-R)	Derogatis, 1994; Derogatis & Savitz, 1999	Respondent based	Behavioral, cognitive, emotional, and somatic
Schedule of Recent Events	Holmes & Rahe,[21] 1967	Respondent based	Environmental
Standardized Event Rating System (SEPRATE)	Dohrenwend et al,[83] 1990	Investigator based	Environmental
State-Trait Anger Expression Inventory	Spielberger, 1988	Respondent based	Affective and behavioral
State-Trait Anxiety Inventory (STAI)	Spielberger, Groscuh, & Lushene, 1970	Respondent based	Cognitive and emotional
Stress Appraisal Measure (SAM)	Peacock & Wong, 1990	Respondent based	Cognitive and emotional
Stress/Arousal Adjective Checklist (SACL)	King, Burrows, & Stanely, 1983	Respondent based	Cognitive and emotional
Stressful Situations Questionnaire	Hodges & Felling, 1970	Respondent based	Environmental
Structured Life Events Inventory (SLI)	Wethington, Kessler, & Brown, 1993	Investigator based	Environmental
Survey of Recent Life Experiences	Kohn & Macdonald, 1992	Respondent based	Cognitive and environmental
The Changes in Outlook Questionnaire (CiOQ)	Joseph, Williams, & Yule, 1993	Respondent based	Cognitive and environmental

(continued on next page)

Table 5
(continued)

Instrument Name	Source	Rating System	Theoretical Underpinnings
The Emotional Stress Reaction Questionnaire (ESRQ)	Larsson, 1987	Respondent based	Emotional
The Detroit Couples Study Life Events Method	Kessler & Wethington, 1991	Investigator based	Environmental
The Differential Emotions Scale (DES)	Izard, Dougherty, Bloxom, & Kotsch, 1974	Respondent based	Emotional
The Glazer-Stress Control Lifestyle Questionnaire	Glazer, 1978	Respondent based	Behavioral
The Job Content Questionnaire (JCQ)	Karasek, Brisson, Kawakami, Houtman, & Bongers, 1998	Respondent based	Cognitive, emotional, and environmental
The Kessler Psychological Distress Scale (K10)	Kessler, 1992	Respondent based	Emotional
The Life Events and Difficulties Schedule (LEDS)	Brown & Harris,[86] 1989	Investigator based	Environmental
The Life Orientation Test	Scheier & Carver, 1985	Respondent based	Cognitive and emotional
The Perceived Benefits Scale	McMillen & Fisher, 1998	Respondent based	Behavioral, cognitive, and emotional
The Perceived Stress Scale (PSS)	Cohen, Jamarck, & Mermelstein, 1983	Investigator based	Cognitive, emotional, and environmental
The Posttraumatic Growth Inventory (PTGI)	Tedeschi & Calhoun, 1996	Respondent based	
The Profile of Mood States (POMS)	McNair, Lorr, & Droppleman, 1971	Respondent based	Cognitive and emotional
The Stress-Related Growth Scale (SRGS)	Park, Cohen, & Murch, 1996	Respondent based	Behavioral, cognitive, and emotional
The Social Readjustment Rating Scale	Holmes & Rahe,[21] 1967	Respondent based	Environmental
Trier Inventory for the Assessment of Chronic Stress	Schulz & Schlotz, 1999	Respondent based	Environmental
Ways of Coping Questionnaire	Folkman & Lazarus, 1988	Respondent based	Cognitive, behavioral, and emotional

This table is a compilation of most widely used checklist, questionnaires, and interviews available for the measurement of stress. Instruments are listed with their original sources, rating methods, and corresponding assessment area (eg, somatic, cognitive, behavioral, and emotional). Most of these instruments have copyrights and thus cannot be published within the contents of this article.

exploring the impact of the environment and quantifying life changes or life events. Changes come from both positive events (eg, the birth of a child) and negative events (eg, the loss of a loved one). Research has shown that people who experience a greater number of life changes are more likely to suffer from maladjustment, abnormal behavior, and physical health problems.[83] To this end, the importance of the environment (eg, stimulus-based model) is its focus on the unique demands (eg, social, physical, psychological, and intellectual) placed by the environment, and the subsequent need for readjustment and adaptation.

Measurement

Adolfo Meyer (1930) was among the pioneers in exploring life changes during medical examinations and in promoting the use of life charts. He believed that exploring life events could help providers understand the etiology of important physical ailments and illness.[72] His idea was highly influential and gave rise to continued work in the conceptualization of stress. New ideas were consistent with the definition of stress described in physics, and thus some investigators focused on stress as a stimulus. For instance, epidemiologists define stress as an objective observable stressful event that: (1) requires changes or adaptations; (2) might have a negative impact on a person; and (3) demands more than what the person can control or cope with. To this end, stress involves events that are new or unexpected, and require a significant change in the ongoing life pattern of the individual.[21] The environment, and the stimuli a person is exposed to on a daily basis, is thereby seen as a source of conflict. According to these stimulus theories, distinct types of stimuli lead to unique and predictable patterns of stress responses. Thus, the environmental tradition of measuring stress focuses on the assessment of environmental events or experiences that are normatively (objectively) associated with substantial adaptive demands.[24]

In 1957 an important contribution to the environmental assessment came from Hawkins and his collaborators. In an effort to standardize Meyer's life charts, researchers developed the Schedule of Recent Experiences (SRE), which is one example of many respondent-based assessment measures available for use. Over the decades Hawkins' investigation was used by several researchers, who made modifications to the SRE, The most notable among researchers using this approach were Holmes and Rahe (1967), who devised a list of major life events known as the Social Readjustment Rating Scale, which became the most widely used scale of life events.[84] The scale was made by constructing a list of events or life-change units derived from clinical experience. Examples of these life changes include taking a vacation, death of a loved one, or an illness or injury.

The Daily Hassles Scale (DHS) was also developed as an alternative to the assessment of stressful major life event inventories. The DHS was designed by Richard Lazarus and his associates. This scale tries to evaluate whether minor stressors and pleasures of everyday life might have a more significant effect on health than the big events (taking into account the cumulative nature of stress).[85] These events are called hassles. Examples include concerns about weight, health of a family member, rising prices of common goods, home maintenance, too many things to do, misplacing or losing things, outside home maintenance, property/investment/taxes, crime, and physical appearance. In addition to the hassles scale, The Daily Uplifts Scale (DUS) was also created by Lazarus (a list of additional environmental measures is provided in **Table 5**). The DUS measures the good events in life that allow people to endure their daily hassles. Examples include relating well to spouse or lover, relating well with friends, completing a task, feeling healthy, getting enough sleep, eating out, meeting your responsibilities, visiting, phoning, or writing to someone, spending time with family, and being in a pleasant home.

In the 1970s, a newer generation of researchers began to challenge the basic assumptions involved in the construction of these inventories. Among the most drastic changes was the creation of life-event interviews as an adjunct to the rating scales. This interview-based rating (IBR) or investigator-based assessment (IBA) was an attempt to estimate the impact of an event in a specific context by avoiding individual subjective reactions. IBA and IBR are different from self-reports in the sense that they check on respondent bias and attempt to eliminate the respondent's subjective report/response. The Life Events and Difficulties Schedule (LEDS)[86] is considered to be the gold standard of IBA of life stress.[87] The LED systematically inquires about potential stressors in 10 domains of life functioning (eg, education, work, reproduction, housing, finance, crime/legal, health, martial/partner relationship, other relationships, and death/miscellaneous) and creates a life-stress profile. What is most important about IBA/IBR is that after the administration/interview and ratings are completed, there is a consensus process with a panel of independent reviewers, further helping to eliminate interviewer bias. In this way the interviewer reaction to the narrative provided by the respondent can be minimized (**Table 6**).

Case Discussion

The physiological changes that Rita and her provider have noticed include somatic complaints, in addition to activation of specific biomarkers identified through laboratory testing. In addition to her biological changes, Rita and her health behaviorist have also identified how stress has affected her psychological well-being and has contributed to behavioral changes. However, yet to be discussed are the environmental stressors that have contributed to the causes of Rita's clinical presentation.

Rita is a 32-year-old woman in the prime of her life. Not only is she in a new and exciting stage in her marriage, she is also a new mother, and has high hopes of becoming a partner at her law firm. However, she feels unable to cope with all of the demands that these changes have brought on her. Although her new baby was identified to be a blessing, she feels overwhelmed with all the other responsibilities that come with it, including having to leave work early to pick her son up from daycare, coming home to an empty home with toys all over the floor, having to cook, and bathing her child all by herself. Her home is no longer a place of joy but rather a place of stress, and her bed is the place where she has to worry about the next day. For Rita, these new changes represent challenges in terms of dealing with her personal and professional life. She is concerned not only about her time constraints but also

Table 6
Environmental assessment methods

Respondent-Based Assessment	Investigator-Based Assessment
Self-report checklists	Semistructured interview
Standardized process	Flexible process
Emotional reaction and subjecting rating	Contextual rating and objective data
Respondent is responsible for rating	Investigator is responsible for rating
No training needed	Training required
Low implementation cost	High cost of implementation

Overview of the differences between respondent based assessment and investigator-based assessment.

about her excess baby weight, her physical appearance, economic pressures, and home upkeep. All of these hassles contributed to the etiology and/or exacerbation of her stress levels.

Rita's case is not unusual. A change in one's life, no matter how delightful, can lead to significant stress and strain on a person's well-being. Life demands, day-to-day problems, and job pressures can all contribute to the onset of stress. To top it off, feeling alone in the midst of her changes has highlighted the reality of her current stress load. To this end, research has established that social relationships play an important and pivotal role in almost every aspect of stress and coping. Moreover, levels of satisfaction and disappointment with how much others are involved or disengaged in stressful situations affect well-being.[88] It has been estimated that people with greater social support experience fewer exacerbations in health conditions than those who rely almost exclusively on their own coping abilities and defense mechanisms.[89]

Measurement Considerations

Strengths
Because life changes, human experiences, and environmental cues are known to correlate with stress and health outcomes, assessment of stated determinants is highly important. Use of these measures allows identification of the environmental sources of stress in a manner that is uncompounded by an individual's reactions or coping styles. Understanding these determinants not only provides information about the unique demands the individual faces but also provides data about the challenges to the person's ability to adapt and readjust. All of this information guides the clinician into forming a real and genuine understanding of the human being, and provides a guide for adequate treatment planning. In an effort to assess these environmental demands, years of research has also provided clinicians with diverse methods of assessment, including respondent-based and investigator-based methods, both of which provide direct information from the respondent about his or her stressors and the extent of the impact on human suffering. However, IBA/IBR further allows for greater precision in the definition of the types of stressors in addition to precision in identifying the timing of exposure and outcome. In fact, McQuaid and colleagues[90] found that 62% of checklists identified stressors that were found to be discrepant with those identified by the IBA/IBR measures (eg, LEDS).[91]

Limitations
One of the most salient disadvantages of environmental assessment is that of reliability. Thinking about life events can be a challenge for most, and requires an accurate recollection of those stressors that have required adaptation and readjustment on the part of the individual. In addition, the longer the length of time that has passed since the stressor occurred, the greater the likelihood of errors in remembering how the event was appraised. In fact, the reliability of life-event checklists has been suspected to be low,[92] owing to the effect time has on how well people remember and report on what allegedly caused them stress. If one looks at both the respondent-based and investigator-based models, association between life stress and illness has been modest with self-report measures. However, stronger associations have been documented with investigator-based models.[72] Notwithstanding, although investigator-based assessments allow for greater precision in the definition of types of stressors, training is necessary, and it therefore takes more time and effort for the professional.

Furthermore, even though research has provided valuable evidence linking stress with various disease end points, many problems have been identified with this methodology. Foremost among these is the limited content of items contained in stress inventories. Concerns have been raised about scales not including an adequate, representative sample of all the major life events and hassles that may occur in a person's life. For example, culturally specific events (eg, exposure to war, political uprising) might not be contemplated as possible stressors. The complexity of items on stress and health questionnaires, the questionable methods used for assigning weights in scaling the impact of life events, and the generally low reliability and validity of the instruments themselves[93] are other concerns. Moreover, checklists have demonstrated poor test-retest reliability. In one study conducted by McQuaid and colleagues,[90] in 60% of checklists events reported at time 1 were inconsistent with events for the same period reported at time 2 (6 weeks later). In this sense, self-reported measures are surprisingly subjective and unreliable. People differ in their thresholds for defining the presence or absence of events, and are also unreliable in reporting event timing and duration. Measures are also costly and require extensive training on the part of the professional to ensure proper administration and interpretation of results. Thus, there is a burden in terms of time and effort for administration for both the professional and the respondent.

STRESS AND HEALTH: CONNECTING THE MIND AND BODY

Stress is widely recognized as a major factor in a wide range of physical illnesses[94] as it alters physiological functioning and leads to disease pathways.[64,95–97] It has been estimated that as many as 3 out of 4 visits to physicians are due to stress-related problems.[98–100] In fact, research of health care utilization has demonstrated that 30% to 80% of all medical visits are for illness experiences that are not disease-based, with stress as the common contributor.[101,102] It is also important that stress was once implicated in more than half of human morbidity and mortality rates.[103,104] Stress affects tissues and impairs the body's defenses against disease. It may lead to permanent structural changes of pathogenic significance, elevated markers of biological aging, higher cortisol levels, changes in growth hormone and prolactin levels, suppressed immune function, increases in proinflammatory cytokines, slower wound healing, greater risk of infectious disease, and higher levels of prostate-specific antigen.[6,66] Stress is also directly implicated in cardiovascular disease,[103,105–108] and in injuries, suicides, and homicides.[103] Indirectly it is associated with cancer,[103,109–111] upper respiratory infections and colds,[51,103,112–115] wound healing and skin disorders,[116] arthritis,[15,117,118] and diabetes.[115,118–121]

Stress also changes behaviors. It has been hypothesized that exposure to stress and negative life events is related to poor health outcomes[100,122,123] as it alters adherence to medical regimens and increases care seeking. In fact, the effect of stress on lifestyle choices and health practices is one of the leading contributors to early death.[6] Cigarette smoking, excessive drinking, poor diet, and/or lack of exercise, for example, are among the most common stress-related behaviors. Beyond a certain point, stress can also trigger the onset of serious mental health problems. There is strong evidence of the risk of mental disorders associated with prolonged stress. Since the 1970s, interest in biological bases of psychiatric disorders has linked HPA-axis activation with depression. Studies have found that cortisol secretion is more frequent and of longer duration among depressed patients than among other psychiatric patients (**Table 7**).[124,125]

It was Descartes (1596–1650) who first talked about a separation between mind and body (dualism). Although the mind and body were separate domains (once upon a time), a countless number of scientific works have suggested a greater appreciation

Table 7
Integrative assessment of stress

Assessment	Signs and Symptoms	Stress Effects on Health
Physiological	Pressure or constriction in chest, choking feelings, sighing, dyspnea, pressure or constriction in chest, tachycardia, palpitations, pain, throbbing of vessels, fainting feelings, missing beat, blurry vision, dilated pupils, difficulty in swallowing, abdominal pain, burning sensations, abdominal fullness, nausea, vomiting, looseness of bowels, loss of weight, constipation, pain, soreness, muscle tension, premenstrual irregularities, erectile dysfunction, decreased libido, debilitating general fatigue, chronic fatigue, inflammation, skin irritation, sweaty palms, hair loss, frequent colds, increased body fat, sudden weight loss, dizziness, light-headedness, headaches	Common cold Influenza Allergies Ulcers and colitis Asthma Diabetes Hypertension Cancer Tension headaches Migraine headaches Temporomandibular joint dysfunction Chronic fatigue syndrome Hypothyroidism Fibromyalgia Irritable bowel syndrome Obesity Rheumatoid arthritis Coronary heart disease
Behavioral	Psychomotor agitation, stooped posture, anger outbursts, short temper, impulsivity, complaining, nagging, negative statements, suicidal or parasuicidal behaviors, hostility, withdrawal, increased alcohol intake, drug abuse, tobacco use, increased caffeine use, anorexia or increased eating, nail biting, pacing, procrastination, overscheduling, restlessness, nervousness, avoidance, changes in health practices, changes in adherence to medical advice	Adjustment disorder Anxiety Posttraumatic stress disorder Conduct disorder Depression Anorexia nervosa Obsessive Compulsive Disorder Panic disorder Medication seeking Drug abuse Alcohol use disorder Physician visits
Emotional	Apparent sadness, anger, poor frustration tolerance, irritability, daydreaming, mood changes, liability, decreased self-esteem, helplessness, hopelessness, unhappiness, avolia	
Cognitive	Forgetfulness, difficulty concentrating, distractibility, lack of attention to details, poor judgment and insight, decreased problem-solving skills, constant worrying, mental slowness, confusion, self-harm ideas, cynicism, fears and frequent concerns, unrealistic expectations	

Integration of cognitive, emotional, behavioral, and physiological manifestations of stress that can serve as potential cues in the assessment and measurement of stress. All signs and symptoms can also be integrated within a heuristic model that provides insight into the effects of stress on health and disease.

for the interconnection between mental states and physical responses. As a consequence, the effects of stress bring into discussion the debate about the relationships between mind and body. Today, scientists recognize the interconnection between the two and examine the role of stress in both mental and physical well-being. The influence of stress on all aspects of health and understanding the complex interaction of the mind and body has become increasingly important. Identifying individual stress levels is thus the first step in moving toward primary prevention of stress-related illness and disease. In a sense, stress has taken on great importance for humans in the modern world.

SUMMARY

The overall purpose of this article is to offer information on stress and explore assessment measures that provide a greater understanding of the human experience. Overall, 3 influential stress theories stand out: the psychoimmunological, psychological, and environmental perspectives. Each one provides a particular approach and explanation of stress. Nevertheless, adopting a unifying model of the stress process or stress response, as opposed to one particular explanation, is important. A comprehensive and integrative understanding of these models can sustain the ongoing need for health research as it proposes changes to how the human experience is understood. This unifying and comprehensive conceptualization highlights that mind and body merge at different stages of the stress response.[6] Therefore, both need to be recognized in the conceptualization of illness and health.[59] Understanding the role of perceived stress and the relationship between biological and psychosocial dimensions of stress can also expand the potential for effective health care interventions.[20] In this way, the best measures of stress should capture how social environments or psychological states affect a person's biology and psyche.

Signs and symptoms play a major role in the presentation, detection, and management of stress. Stress is a broad topic and can therefore be measured in several ways. For this reason, physiological methods of assessment have emerged. However, assessment strategies do not have to be exclusively focused on symptoms. Rather, the use of specific measures also depends on several additional psychosocial factors that capture the overall essence of the human experience. Such factors include environmental demands, sustained social conflict, social and role loss, social rejection, psychological distress, perceived control, positive affect, and social support.[6] Other determinants play a pivotal role in the manifestation of stress. Of all these other factors, culture is the most salient. Culture affects the way people perceive life and how they suffer. Thus, cultural considerations are essential, and questions should be raised about the sensitivity and appropriateness of any measure being used with a particular person, including ethnic minorities.[20,24] Unfortunately, there is no particular test or instrument that will be appropriate, or even standardized, for all populations across cultures and subcultures.

IMPLICATIONS FOR CLINICAL PRACTICE AND FUTURE CONSIDERATIONS

Opportunities to contribute to stress and health exist, and there is still enough room for growth in both the medical and psychological fields. For instance, research has further explored the body's response to stressors and has shed light on additional biomarkers that can provide useful data on how individuals react and adapt under stressful conditions. Longitudinal studies can explore which biomarkers are most predictive of specific health outcomes, which measures of allostatic load show most promise, and how these are vulnerable to different types of psychosocial stressors. The topic of diversity should also be considered, and exploration of how allostatic profiles of load expression differ by ethnicity and gender might prove useful. Specifically, research should focus on how individual differences account for variability in the stress response. The use of questionnaires and checklists also need to be contextually appropriate so as to understand the full domain of the life experience of stress,[126,127] with the capacity to extrapolate findings. In this sense, it is important to consider the effects of culture, socioeconomic status, and other individual differences (beliefs, values, personality traits) that can allow measures to be used in several countries and contexts. On a broader level, further research that focuses on how individual differences and personality traits account for the way people perceive stress and the impact stress has on health and quality of life is needed. One important contribution would be to examine stress thoroughly via longitudinal studies as a determinant on subjective distress and health outcomes and compare results across cultures. Finally, emphasizing the positive impact of stress as opposed to only focusing on the detrimental effects on health is also important. Although stressful events have been studied primarily as risk factors for disease, it is also known that stressful events can lead to positive outcomes, including personal growth, reprioritizations of life goals, increased feelings of self-esteem and self-efficacy, and strengthening of social networks.[72] A greater emphasis on the benefits of stress and the role of resilience would likely broaden our understanding of the stress process.

Assessments that include measures of environmental challenge, psychological factors (cognitive and affective responses), and biological indices have the greatest potential for success within a field. To this effect, studying, conceptualizing, and measuring stress within a holistic/heuristic approach is relevant. The benefits and rewards in working within this approach are 3-fold. First, it provides a comprehensive understanding of the human experience and can genuinely help understand the complexities of human resilience and suffering. Second, it can promote a greater understanding of the mind-body connection as it relates to increased risk of physical and psychiatric disease; this would encourage intercollaborative work between medicine and behavioral health fields. Third, it provides the foundation for planning appropriate interventions, implementing them, and evaluating their effectiveness and outcomes.

REFERENCES

1. Lazarus RS. Psychological stress and the coping process. New York: McGraw-Hill; 1966.
2. Lazarus RS, Folkman S. Stress, appraisal, and coping. New York: Springer; 1984.
3. Chrousos GP, Gold PW. The concepts of stress and stress system disorders: overview of physical and behavioral homeostasis. Journal of the American Medical Association 1992;267(9):1244–52.
4. Yehuda R, McEwen BS. Biobehavioral stress response: protective and damaging effects of the biobehavioral stress response. International Society of Psychoneuroendocrinology, Academy of Sciences. 34th Annual ISPNE Conference. New York, October 29, 2004.
5. Nevid JS, Rathus SA, Greene B. Stress, psychological factors and health. Chapter 5. In: Nevid JS, Rathus SA, Greene B, editors. Abnormal psychology in a changing world. 6th edition. New Jersey: Pearson Prentice Hall; 2010. p. 140–69.

6. National Institute on Aging, Division of Behavioral and Social Research. Stress measurement meeting. San Francisco (CA): University of California; 2011.

7. Szabo S, Tache Y, Somogyi A. The legacy of Hans Selye and the origins of stress research: a retrospective 75 years after his landmark brief "letter" to the editor of Nature. Stress 2012;15(5):472–8.

8. Cannon WG. The wisdom of the body. New York: W.W. Norton; 1932.

9. Ellis BJ, Jackson JJ, Boyce WT. The stress response systems: universality and adaptive individual differences. Dev Rev 2006;26:175–212.

10. Hill-Rice V. Theories of stress and its relationship to health. Chapter 2. In: Hill-Rice V, editor. Handbook of stress, coping, and health: implications for nursing research, theory, practice. 2nd edition. Detroit (MI): Sage Publications, Inc; 2012. p. 22–42.

11. Centre for Studies on Human Stress. How to measure stress in humans. Quebec (Canada): Fernand- Seguin Research Center; Lafontaine Hospital; 2007. Available at: http://www.stresshumain.ca/documents/pdf/Mesures%20physiologiques/CESH_howMesureStress-MB.pdf. Accessed September 20, 2014.

12. Davis M, Eshelman E, McKay M. The relaxation and stress reduction workbook. Oakland (CA): New Harbinger Publications; 2000.

13. Björntorp P. Do stress reactions cause abdominal obesity and comorbidities? Obes Rev 2001;2(2):73–86.

14. American Psychological Association. Stress survey. Stress: a major health problem in the U.S. 2007. Available at: http://www.apahelpcenter.org/articles/article.php?id=165.

15. Cohen S, Janicki-Deverts D, Miller GE. Psychological stress and disease. Journal of the American Medical Association 2007;298(14):1685–7.

16. Krohne HW. Stress and coping theories. 2002. Available at: http://userpage.fu-berlin.de/schuez/folien/Krohne_Stress.pdf.

17. Lyon BL. Stress, coping, and health. Chapter 1. In: Hill-Rice V, editor. Handbook of stress, coping, and health: implications for nursing research, theory, practice. 2nd edition. Detroit (MI): Sage Publications, Inc; 2012. p. 2–20.

18. Mackay C, Cox T, Burrows G. An inventory for the measurement of self-reported stress and arousal. Br J Soc Clin Psychol 1978;17(3):283–4.

19. Holroyd K, Lazarus R. Stress, coping, and somatic adaptation. In: Goldberger L, Breznitz S, editors. Handbook of stress: theoretical and clinical aspects. New York: The Free Press; 1982. p. 21–35.

20. Cohen JI. Stress and mental health: a bio-behavioral perspective. Issues Ment Health Nurs 2000;21:185–202.

21. Holmes TH, Rahe RH. The social readjustment rating scale. J Psychosom Res 1967;11:213–8.

22. Weiner IB, Nezu AM, Nezu CM, et al. Handbook of psychology. In: Weiner I, editor. Health Psychol, vol. 9. 2nd edition. Hoboken (NJ): John Wiley & Sons, Inc; 2012. p. 5–98.

23. Selye H. Stress without distress. Philadelphia: J.B. Lippincott; 1974.

24. MacArthur J, MacArthur C. Measures of psychological stress. 2000. Available at: http://www.macses.ucsf.edu/research/psychosocial/stress.php.

25. Sterling P, Eyer J. Allostasis: a new paradigm to explain arousal pathology. In: Fisher S, Reason JT, editors. Handbook of life stress, cognition, and health. New York: Wiley; 1988. p. 629–49.

26. National Institute on Aging. Behavioral and social research program. NIA Exploratory Workshop on Allostatic Load. Washington, DC, November 29-30, 2007.

27. Konduru L. Thesis: biomarkers of chronic stress. University of Pittsburgh; Graduate School of Public Health; November 4, 2011. Available at: http://d-scholarship.pitt.edu/10858/1/Laalithya_Thesis_Revised_(2).pdf.

28. Piazza JR, Almeida DM, Dimitrieva NO, et al. Frontiers in the use of biomarkers of health in research on stress and aging. J Gerontol B Psychol Sci Soc Sci 2010;65(5):513–25.

29. Hiller-Sturmhöfel S, Bartke A. The endocrine system: an overview. Alcohol Health Res World 1998;22(3):153–64.

30. Jerjes WK, Peters TJ, Taylor NF, et al. Diurnal excretion of urinary cortisol, cortisone, and cortisol metabolites in chronic fatigue syndrome. J Psychosom Res 2006;60(2):145–53.

31. Kunz-Ebrecht SR, Mohamed-Ali V, Feldman PJ, et al. Cortisol responses to mild psychological stress are inversely associated with proinflammatory cytokines. Brain Behav Immun 2003;17:373–83.

32. Takai N, Yamaguchi M, Aragaki T, et al. Effect of psychological stress on the salivary cortisol and amylase levels in healthy young adults. Arch Oral Biol 2004;49: 963–8.

33. Shi Y, Nguyen MH, Blitz P, et al. Personalized stress detection from physiological measurements. 2008. Available at: http://www.ca.cs.cmu.edu/projects/stress_detect/stress_detect.pdf.

34. Mostl E, Palme R. Hormones as indicators of stress. Domest Anim Endocrinol 2002;23:67–74.

35. Minakuchi E, Ohnishi E, Ohnishi J, et al. Evaluation of mental stress by physiological indices derived from finger plethysmography. J Physiol Anthropol 2013; 32(17):1–11.

36. National Institute for Health and Clinical Excellence. Quick reference guide: clinical management of primary hypertension in adults. 2011. Available at: http://www.nice.org.uk/nicemedia/live/13561/56015/56015.pdf.

37. Kulkarn S, O'Farrell I, Erasi M, et al. Stress and hypertension. Wis Med J 1998; 97(11):34–8.

38. Akselrod S, Gordon D, Ubel S, et al. Power spectrum analysis of heart rate fluctuation: a quantitate probe of beat-to-beat cardiovascular control. Science 1981;213:220–2.

39. Karim N, Ara-Hasan J, Sanowar S. Heart rate variability - A review. J Basic Appl Sci 2011;7(1):71–7.

40. Kawachi I, Sparrow D, Vokonas PS, et al. Decreased heart rate variability in men with phobic anxiety. Am J Cardiol 1995;75:882–5.

41. Offerhaus RE. Heart rate variability in psychiatry. In: Kitney RJ, Rompelman O, editors. The study of heart rate variability. Oxford (United Kingdom): Oxford University Press; 1980. p. 225–38.

42. Yeragani VK, Balon R, Pohl R, et al. Decreased R-R variance in panic disorder patients. Acta Psychiatr Scand 1990;81:554–9.

43. Yeragani VK, Pohl R, Berger R, et al. Decreased heart rate variability in panic disorder patients: a study of power-spectral analysis of heart rate. J Psychiatr Res 1993;1(46):89–103.

44. Haines AP, Imeson JD, Meade TW. Phobic anxiety and ischemic heart disease. BMJ 1987;295:297–9.

45. Kawachi I, Sparrow D, Vokonas PS, et al. Symptoms of anxiety and risk of coronary heart disease: the normative aging study. Circulation 1994;90:2225–9.

46. Mittleman MA, Maclure M, Sherwood JB, et al. Triggering of acute myocardial infarction onset by episodes of anger. Circulation 1995;92:1720–5.

47. Sloan RP, Shapiro PA, Bigger T, et al. Cardiac autonomic control and hostility in healthy subjects. Am J Cardiol 1994;74:298–300.
48. Sumida T, Anmitu Y, Tahara T, et al. Mental conditions reflected by the chaos of pulsation in capillary vessels. Int J Bifurcat Chaos 2000;2000:2245–55.
49. Fujimoto Y, Yamaguchi T. Evaluation of mental stress by analyzing accelerated plethysmogram applied chaos theory and examination of welfare space installed user's vital sign. In Proceedings of the 17th World Congress. The International Federation of Automatic Control. 2008. Available at: http://www.nt.ntnu.no/users/skoge/prost/proceedings/ifac2008/data/papers/4157.pdf.
50. Suess WM, Alexander B, Smith DD, et al. The effects of psychological stress on respiration: a preliminary study of anxiety and hyperventilation. Psychophysiology 1980;17(6):535–40.
51. Ritz T, Steptoe A, DeWilde S, et al. Emotions and stress increase respiratory resistance in asthma. Psychosom Med 2000;62(3):401–12.
52. Smith MM, Colebatch HJ, Clarke PS. Increase and decrease in pulmonary resistance with hypnotic suggestion in asthma. Am Rev Respir Dis 1970;102:236–42.
53. Tal A, Miklich DR. Emotionally induced decreases in pulmonary flow rates in asthmatic children. Psychosom Med 1976;38:190–200.
54. Florin I, Freudenberg G, Hollaender J. Facial expressions of emotion and physiologic reactions in children with bronchial asthma. Psychosom Med 1985;47:382–94.
55. Lehrer PM, Hochron S, Carr R, et al. Behavioral task-induced bronchodilation in asthma during active and passive tasks: a possible cholinergic link to psychologically induced airway changes. Psychosom Med 1996;58:413–22.
56. Fuller GD. Biofeedback methods & procedures in clinical practice. San Francisco (CA): Biofeedback Press; 1977.
57. Vinkers CH, Penning R, Hellhammer J, et al. The effects of stress on core and peripheral body temperature in humans. Stress 2013;16(5):520–30.
58. Viqueira-Villarejo M, García-Zapirain B, Méndez-Zorrilla A. A Stress sensor based on galvanic skin response (GSR) controlled by ZigBee. Sensors (Basel) 2012;12:6075–101.
59. Moss D. Biofeedback, mind-body medicine, and the higher limits of human nature. In: Moss D, editor. Humanistic and transpersonal psychology: a historical and biographical sourcebook. Westport (CT): Greenwood; 1998. p. 145–61.
60. Giggins OM, Persson U, Caulfield B. Biofeedback in rehabilitation. J Neuroeng Rehabil 2013;10(60):1–11.
61. The British Psychological Association. A review of the current scientific status and fields of application of polygraphic deception detection. Final report from the BPS Working Party. 2004. Available at: http://www.bps.org.uk/sites/default/files/documents/polygraphic_deception_detection_-_a_review_of_the_current_scientific_status_and_fields_of_application.pdf. Accessed September 20, 2014.
62. Trovato GM, Catalano D, Martines GF, et al. Psychological stress measures in type 2 diabetes. Eur Rev Med Pharmacol Sci 2006;10:69–74.
63. Marsland AL, Bachen EA, Cohen S, et al. Stress, immune reactivity and susceptibility to infectious disease. Physiol Behav 2002;77:711–6.
64. Cohen S, Tyrrell DA, Smith AP. Psychological stress and susceptibility to the common cold. N Engl J Med 1991;325:606–12.
65. Cohen S, Doyle WJ, Skoner DP, et al. Types of stressors that increase susceptibility to the common cold in healthy adults. Health Psychol 1998;17:214–23.
66. Littrell J. The mind-body connection: not just a theory anymore. Soc Work Health Care 2008;46(4):17–38.

67. Kim KH, Bang SW, Kim SR. Emotion recognition system using short- term monitoring of physiological signals. Med Biol Eng Comput 2004;42:419–27.
68. Carter-Snell C, Hegadoren K. Stress disorders and gender; implications for theory and research. Can J Nurs Res 2003;35(2):34–55.
69. Geary DC, Flinn MV. Sex differences in behavioral and hormonal response to social threat; commentary on Taylor et al. (2000). Psychol Rev 2002;109(4):745–50.
70. Williamon A, Aufegger L, Wasley D, et al. Complexity of physiological responses decreases in high-stress musical performance. J R Soc Interface 2013;10(89): 20130719.
71. Solowiej K, Mason V, Upton D. Psychological stress and pain in wound care, Part2: A review of pain and stress assessment tools. J Wound Care 2010; 19(3):110–5.
72. Cohen S, Kessler R, Underwood Gordon L. Strategies for measuring stress in studies of psychiatric and physical disorders. In: Cohen S, Kessler R, Underwood Gordon L, editors. Measuring stress. New York: Oxford University Press; 1995. p. 2–26.
73. McEwen BS, Sapolsky RM. Stress and cognitive function. Curr Opin Neurobiol 1995;5(2):205–16.
74. Mendl M. Performing under pressure: stress and cognitive function. Appl Anim Behav Sci 1999;65:221–44.
75. Duke S, Stoebber J. Test anxiety, working memory, and cognitive performance. Cogn Emot 2001;15:381–9.
76. Cohen S, Evans GW, Stokols D, et al. Stress process and the cost of coping. Chapter 1. In: Cohen S, Evans GW, Stokols D, editors. Behavior, health, and environmental stress. New York: Plenum Press; 1986. p. 1–23.
77. Lazarus RS. From psychological stress to the emotions: a history of changing outlooks. Annu Rev Psychol 1993;44:1–21.
78. Humara M. The relationship between anxiety and performance: a cognitive-behavioral perspective. Athl Insight 2002;2:1–11.
79. Lazarus RS. Theory based stress measurement. Psychol Inq 1990;1:3–13.
80. Bourne LE, Yaraoush RA. Final report. Stress and cognition: a cognitive psychological perspective. National Aeronautics and Space Administration; 2003. Available at: http://humansystems.arc.nasa.gov/eas/download/non_EAS/Stress_and_ Cognition.pdf.
81. APA Presidential Task Force on Evidence-Based Practice. Evidence-based practice in psychology. Am Psychol 2006;61(4):271–85.
82. Plarre K, Raij A, Monowar-Hossain S, et al. Continuous interference of psychological stress form sensory measurements collected in the natural environment. 2011. Available at: http://pie.eng.usf.edu/wp-content/uploads/2011/12/plarre-ipsn20111.pdf.
83. Dohrenwend BP, Link BG, Kern R, et al. Measuring life events: the problem of variability within event categories. Stress Med 1990;6(3):179–87.
84. Scully JA, Tosi H, Banning K. Life event checklists: revisiting the social readjustment rating scale after 30 years. Educ Psychol Meas 2000;60(6):864–76.
85. Kanner AD, Coyne JC, Schaefer C, et al. Comparison of two modes of stress measurement: daily hassles and uplifts versus major life events. J Behav Med 1981;4(1):1–39.
86. Brown GW, Harris TO. Life events and illness. New York: Guildford Press; 1989.
87. Bulmash E, Harkness KL, Stewart JG. Personality, stressful life events, and treatment response in major depression. J Consult Clin Psychol 2009;77(6):1067–77.
88. DeLongis A, Holtzman S. Coping in context: the role of stress, social support, and personality in coping. J Pers 2005;73(6):1633–56.

89. Mohr DC, Pelletier D. A temporal framework for understanding the effects of stressful life events on inflammation in patients with multiple sclerosis. Brain Behav Immun 2006;20:27–36.
90. McQuaid JR, Monroe SM, Roberts JR, et al. Toward the standardization of life stress assessments: definitional discrepancies and inconsistencies in methods. Stress Med 1992;8:47–56.
91. McQuaid JR, Roberts JE, Monroe SM, et al. A comparison of two life stress assessment approaches: prospective prediction of treatment outcome in recurrent depression. J Abnorm Psychol 2000;109(4):787–91.
92. Turner RJ, Wheaton B. Checklist measurement of stressful life events. In: Cohen S, Kessler R, Underwood-Gordon L, editors. Measuring stress: a guide for health and social scientist. New York: Oxford University Press; 1995. p. 29–58.
93. Zimmerman M. Methodological issues in the assessment of life events: a review of issues and research. Clin Psychol Rev 1989;3:339–70.
94. Artemiadis AK, Anagnostouli MC, Alexopoulus EC. Stress as a risk factor for multiple sclerosis onsets or relapse: a systematic review. Neuroepidemiology 2011;36:109–20.
95. Cohen S, Tyrrell DA, Smith AP. Negative life events, perceived stress, negative affect, and susceptibility to the common cold. J Pers Soc Psychol 1993;64:131–40.
96. Herbert TB, Cohen S. Measurement issues in research on psychological stress. In: Kaplan HB, editor. Psychosocial stress: perspectives on structure, theory, life course, and methods. New York: Academic Press Inc; 1996. p. 295–332.
97. Jemmot JB, Locke SE. Psychosocial factors, immunologic mediation, and human susceptibility to infectious disease: how much do we know? Psychol Bull 1984;95:78–108.
98. Charlesworth EA, Nathan RG. Stress management: a comprehensive guide to wellness. New York: Ballantine Books; 1984.
99. Centers for Disease Control and Prevention. Costs of chronic disease. 2003. Available at: http://www.cdc.gov/nccdphp/overview.htm.
100. American Psychological Association. Mind/Body health: for a healthy mind and body, talk to a psychologist. 2012. Available at: http://www.drrodneytimbrook.com/about/for_a_healthy_mind_and_body-talk_to_a_psychologist.pdf. Accessed September 20, 2014.
101. Cummings NA, Vandenbos GR. The twenty year Kaiser-Permanente experience with psychotherapy and medical utilization: implications for national health policy and national health insurance. Health Policy Q 1981;1:159–75.
102. National Institute for Occupational Safety and Health. Stress at work. 2010. Available at: http://www.cdc.gov/niosh/topics/stress/.
103. Campbell-Quick J. Introduction to the measurement of stress at work. J Occup Health Psychol 1998;3(4):291–3.
104. World Health Organization. World health statistics annual. Geneva (Switzerland): 1994. Available at: http://www.who.int/occupational_health/publications/declaration/en/.
105. Jain D. Mental stress, a powerful provocateur of myocardial ischemia: diagnostic, prognostic, and therapeutic implications. J Nucl Cardiol 2008;15:491–3.
106. Lippi G, Montagnana M, Favaloro FJ, et al. Mental depression and cardiovascular disease: a multifaceted, bidirectional association. Semin Thromb Hemost 2009;35:325–36.
107. Nemeroff CB, Goldschmidt-Clermont PJ. Heartache and heartbreak - the link between depression and cardiovascular disease. Nat Rev Cardiol 2012;9:526–39.

108. Rozanski A, Kubzansky LD. Psychological functioning and physical health: a paradigm of flexibility. Psychosom Med 2005;67(1):S47–53.
109. Cohen S, Rabin BS. Psychological stress, immunity, and cancer. J Natl Cancer Inst 1998;90:30–6.
110. Siegel B. Love, medicine, and miracles. New York: Harper & Row; 1986.
111. Antonova L, Mueller CR. Hydrocortisone down-regulates the tumor suppressor gene BRAC1 in mammary cells: a possible molecular link between stress and breast cancer. Genes Chromosomes Cancer 2008;47(4):341–52.
112. Cohen S, Doyle WJ, Skoner DP, et al. State and trait negative affect as predictors of objective and subjective symptoms of respiratory viral infections. J Pers Soc Psychol 1995;62(1):159–69.
113. Wright RJ, Rodriguez M, Cohen S. Review of psychosocial stress and asthma: an integrated bio-psychosocial approach. Thorax 1998;53(12):1066–74.
114. Nielson NR, Kristensen TS, Schonohr P, et al. Perceived stress and cause specific mortality among men and women: results from a prospective study. Am J Epidemiol 2008;168(5):481–91.
115. Fitzgerald PJ. Is elevated noradrenaline an etiological factor in a number of diseases? Auton Autacoid Pharmacol 2009;29(4):143–56.
116. Lebwohl M, Tan MH. Psoriasis and stress. Lancet 1998;351:82.
117. Crofford LJ, Jacobson J, Young E. Modeling the involvement of the hypothalamic-pituitary-adrenal and hypothalamic-pituitary gonadal axes in autoimmune and stress-related rheumatic syndromes in women. J Womens Health 1999;8(2):203–15.
118. Straub RJ, Dhabhar FS, Bijlsma JW, et al. How psychological stress via hormones and never fibers may exacerbate rheumatoid arthritis. Arthritis Rheum 2005;52(1):16–26.
119. Inui JA, Kitaoka H, Majima M, et al. Effects of the Kobe earthquake on stress and glycemic control in patients with diabetes mellitus. Arch Intern Med 1998;158(3):274–8.
120. Cox DM, Gonder-Frederick L. Major developments in behavioral diabetes research. J Consult Clin Psychol 1992;60:628–38.
121. Surwit RS, Schneider MS, Feinglos MN. Stress and diabetes. Diabetes Care 1992;15:1413–22.
122. Australian Psychology Association. Stress and wellbeing in Australians survey. 2013. Available at: http://www.psychology.org.au/inpsych/2013/december/npw/. Accessed September 20, 2014.
123. Lantz PM, House JS, Mero RP, et al. Stress, life events, and socioeconomic disparities in health: results from the American's changing lives study. J Health Soc Behav 2005;46:274–88.
124. Lewinsohn PM, Rohde P, Seeley JR, et al. Age cohort changes in the lifetime occurrence of depression and other mental disorders. J Abnorm Psychol 1993;102(1):110–20.
125. Stansfeld SA, Shipley MJ, Head J, et al. Repeated job strain and the risk of depression: longitudinal analyses from the Whitehall II study. Am J Public Health 2012;102:2360–6.
126. Cortes T, Lee A, Boal J, et al. Using focus groups to identify asthma care and education issues for elderly urban-dwelling minority individuals. Appl Nurs Res 2004;17(3):207–12.
127. Ruiz J, Fullerton J, Guerrero LC, et al. Development of a culturally sensitive stress instrument for pregnant Hispanic women. Hisp Health Care Int 2006;4(1):27–33.
128. Selye H. The stress of life. New York: McGraw-Hill; 1956.

Stress and Anxiety
Counterpart Elements of the Stress/ Anxiety Complex

Alexander Bystritsky, MD, PhD[a],*, David Kronemyer, MA[b]

KEYWORDS

- Stress • Anxiety • Nonlinear dynamical psychiatry • Cognitive behavioral therapy
- Belief revision • Escape/avoidance • Exposure/response prevention • A-B-C model

KEY POINTS

- Stress and anxiety are complementary aspects of an entire stress/anxiety complex, with environmental, physiological, psychological, and behavioral components.
- At our current level of knowledge, categorical definitions of stress and anxiety are not helpful. Rather than creating artificial distinctions between them, a transdiagnostic approach better describes their overlapping phenomenology and processes.
- When stress and anxiety are introduced into an organism's learning history, they can become conditioned responses to environmental stimuli.
- From a neurobiological standpoint, stress and anxiety involve autonomic protective alarm responses arising primarily from the sympathetic nervous system, and neurohumoral responses arising primarily from the hypothalamic-pituitary-adrenal axis.
- Stress and anxiety are evolutionary adaptations that deal with challenging circumstances an organism confronts in its environment. When overextended, the stress/anxiety complex has the potential to cause allostatic overload as the body attempts to regain homeostasis.
- When stress and anxiety exceed a person's adaptive capacity, or coping strategies are inadequate, a variety of physical and mental conditions can emerge or worsen. Anxiety disorders are the paradigm case of this phenomenon.
- The nature, degree, and persistence of stress are particularly important in anxiety disorders and other related psychiatric conditions. Catastrophic stress can produce posttraumatic stress disorder, even in genetically healthy people. Persons who are genetically predisposed can develop anxiety syndromes, even with a lower degree of stress. The degree and persistence of stress should become an important part of case conceptualization in anxiety and related disorders.

Continued

Disclosures: The authors have nothing to disclose.
[a] UCLA Anxiety and Related Disorders Program, Department of Psychiatry and Biobehavioral Sciences, Semel Institute for Neuroscience and Human Behavior, David Geffen School of Medicine, University of California, Los Angeles, 300 UCLA Medical Plaza, Room 2335, Los Angeles, CA 90095-6968, USA; [b] UCLA Anxiety and Related Disorders Program, Department of Psychiatry and Biobehavioral Sciences, Semel Institute for Neuroscience and Human Behavior, David Geffen School of Medicine, University of California, Los Angeles, 300 UCLA Medical Plaza, Room 2330, Los Angeles, CA 90095-6968, USA
* Corresponding author.
E-mail addresses: abystritsky@mednet.ucla.edu; abystritsky@sbcglobal.net

Psychiatr Clin N Am 37 (2014) 489–518
http://dx.doi.org/10.1016/j.psc.2014.08.002
0193-953X/14/$ – see front matter © 2014 Elsevier Inc. All rights reserved.

Continued

- Stress and anxiety can be reconceptualized as components of a nonlinear dynamic brain process.
- This approach clarifies the relationships between environmental triggers, physiological alarms, cognitive appraisals, and resulting coping strategies.

Abbreviations	
A-B-C model	Alarms-Beliefs-Coping Strategies model
CR	Conditioned response
CRF	Corticotropin-releasing factor
CS	Conditioned stimulus
dACC/dmPFC	Dorsal anterior cingulate cortex/dorsomedial prefrontal cortex
DSM-5	*Diagnostic and Statistical Manual of Mental Disorders* (Fifth Edition)
DSM-IV-TR	*Diagnostic and Statistical Manual of Mental Disorders* (Fourth Edition, Text Revision)
GAD	Generalized anxiety disorder
GAS	General adaptation syndrome
HPA	Hypothalamic-pituitary-adrenal
MDD	Major depressive disorder
mPFC	Medial prefrontal cortex
OCD	Obsessive-compulsive disorder
PTSD	Posttraumatic stress disorder
SAD	Social anxiety disorder
SOD	Superoxide dismutase
UR	Unconditioned response
US	Unconditioned stimulus

The terms stress and anxiety are ambiguous, and this has led to confusion from semantic, physiological, psychiatric, and behavioral perspectives. In this article the authors advocate that they are counterpart elements of an entire stress/anxiety complex. Because they occur on a spectrum or continuum, it makes more sense to regard them as variations of what essentially is the same phenomenon and components of the same response. This article reviews some of the common features of stress and anxiety, and conceptualizes them as intertwined dynamical brain processes. Dynamic implies not only that each strand unfolds longitudinally in time but also that they mutually influence and often exaggerate each other. The article concludes with a discussion of several intervention strategies, and suggestions for further research.

Each year the American Psychological Association conducts an annual survey, "Stress in America."[1] In 2013, 42% of adults reported their stress level had increased over the past 5 years; 36% reported it had not diminished. Whereas 61% of adults reported that managing stress was extremely or very important, only 35% reported they were doing an excellent or very good job at it. Forty-four percent of adults reported they were not doing enough or were not sure whether they were doing enough to manage their stress; 19% reported they never engage in stress-management activities. Money (71%), work (69%), and the economy (59%) were the most commonly reported sources of stress. Concurrently, in the United States anxiety disorders as a group are the most prevalent form of psychiatric disorder, affecting approximately 40 million adults in a given year, for a prevalence rate of approximately 18%.[2] These disconcerting statistics suggest that the overview of the relationships between stress and anxiety presented herein is both appropriate and timely.

DEFINITIONS OF STRESS AND ANXIETY
Stress

The Austrian neurologist Hans Selye was one of the first to establish a relationship between aversive environmental stimuli and physiological responses. Together with Walter Cannon, he initiated the era of stress.[3] Selye's early writings primarily were concerned with endocrinological responses to strenuous circumstances. Later, he invented the phrase "general adaptation syndrome" (GAS) to characterize the body's responses to stress. Over time, Selye's concept of stress underwent morphological transition and began to refer to environmental stimuli, such as challenging life circumstances, rather than to a set of adaptive responses. Goodnite traces the etymology of stress, concluding that it has 3 dynamic elements: "(1) the application of tension, force, or pressure (an environmental stimulus); (2) the appraisal of the stimulus as overwhelming, that is, one perceives one is unable to meet the challenge; (3) a measurable response to the stimulus."[4(p72)]

At present, both the scientific community and the lay public literature use the term stress interchangeably to describe both a source of threat, and an adaptive response to it. Our environment presents us with numerous challenges, triggers, and potentially noxious stimuli, ranging from the mundane to the catastrophic. Stress is an automatic, autonomic state of mental or emotional strain or tension resulting from adverse or demanding environmental circumstances, particularly when resources are limited. One might be working too hard and not have enough time. One might be hedged in by sociocultural restrictions and circumstances, or be in the midst of family or social conflict. One might be too hot, or too cold, or physically restrained. Stress also can be caused by the mental reconstruction of traumatic events or experiences, as is typical with posttraumatic stress disorder (PTSD). Like many other psychophysiological responses, stress is based on a transactional relationship between a person and his or her environment. It has evolved to maintain homeostasis and facilitate self-preservation, and is a response to challenges arising from the environment that triggers adaptive processes over several body systems.[5,6]

People respond differently to stressful circumstances, depending on their physiological, cognitive, and affective resources. Pathological reactions to severe or prolonged stressful stimuli are harmful. By altering mental processes, stress has the potential to cause serious mental illness. By altering physiological processes, it has the potential to cause serious physical illness.[7] Psychiatrists and psychologists long have recognized associations between both.

Anxiety

Anxiety describes a set of narrower and more psychological or mental responses or states. It is fear-based, usually requiring cognitive appraisal and recognition of an environmental stimulus as a threat. One can, however, be anxious even if one is unable to identify the precise nature of the threat causing the fear, such as with generalized anxiety disorder (GAD). Anxiety typically is about an imminent event or something with an uncertain outcome. Like Selye's stress response, it is in the nature of a reaction to threat. It is accompanied by feelings such as nervousness, worry, unease, anticipation, or mental tension, together with physiological and bodily responses preparing one to either avoid or fight the threat causing the fear. Within these definitions, anxiety can be viewed as a variant of GAS adaptation. It significantly overlaps with stress both in phenotypical presentation and psychophysiological-biological characteristics.

Organisms Versus Humans

The authors would like to clarify that any organism can be stressed or threatened using stimulus provocation. A recent article by Fossat and colleagues,[8] for example, concluded that even crayfish exhibit what might be characterized as a fear-based stress response. Nobody contends, however, that crayfish have the cognitive capacity to perceive it as such. Although there is no bright-line test, research suggests that vertebrates are the lowest subphylum that can experience primal emotional feelings.[9,10] Rather, the focus in this article is on humans. **Table 1** identifies the various elements of the stress/anxiety complex as conceptualized by the authors.

DSM-5 DEFINITION OF STRESS

The *Diagnostic and Statistical Manual of Mental Disorders* (Fifth Edition) (DSM-5), published by the American Psychiatric Association, defines stress as follows.

Exposure to actual or threatened death, serious injury, or sexual violence in 1 (or more) of the following ways:

1. Directly experiencing the traumatic event(s)
2. Witnessing, in person, the event(s) as it occurred to others
3. Learning that the traumatic event(s) occurred to a close family member or close friend. In cases of actual or threatened death of a family member or friend, the event(s) must have been violent or accidental
4. Experiencing repeated or extreme exposure to aversive details of the traumatic event(s) (eg, first responders collecting human remains; police officers repeatedly exposed to details of child abuse)[11]

Stress, in other words, is caused by catastrophic stimuli resulting in psychiatric adaptation breakdowns or mental disorders. DSM-5 specifies 2 disorders for which stress is the primary etiological factor: PTSD at §309.81, and acute stress disorder at §308.3. Stress disorders in DSM-5 now comprise a separate diagnostic category, whereas formerly in *Diagnostic and Statistical Manual of Mental Disorders* (Fourth Edition, Text Revision) (DSM-IV-TR) they were in the same category with all other anxiety disorders.

As with many others in DSM-5, its definition of stress is disappointing and has been widely criticized.[12–15] Contrary to Selye, it does not describe disorders arising from the stress response. A more accurate definition would provide that GAS is caused by or results from abnormal or catastrophic levels of environmental stimuli. There are numerous ways whereby a person can experience stress, and whereby stress can materially contribute to psychopathology, other than those set forth at criteria (1) to (4).[16] In fact, DSM-5's predecessor, DSM-IV-TR,[17] had an entire Axis IV for psychosocial stressors, which DSM-5 has eliminated completely.

Furthermore, by establishing narrow categories of what counts as stress rather than adopting more of a dimensional approach of symptoms that occur in response to stress (including responses that clearly are adaptive), DSM-5 artificially limits the depth, breadth, and scope of contexts in which stress may be a precipitating or contributing factor. The categorical approach of DSM-5 requires one to meet a specified set of criteria, such as (1) to (4), to qualify for a diagnosis of a stress or anxiety

Table 1
Some similarities and differences between stress and anxiety

	Stress	Anxiety
Symptoms	Increased arousal; strain and tension; part of GAS	Apprehension and worry; vigilance and expectation of threat; mostly fear-based
Autonomic nervous system	Heart rate increase; blood pressure increase; faster breathing; muscle tension	Irregular breathing; heart palpitations; blood pressure increase; muscle tension
Central nervous system	Anterior hypothalamus; anterior insula/orbitofrontal cortex; rostral parts of the dorsal anterior cingulate cortex/dorsomedial prefrontal cortex; somatomotor cortex	Amygdala; limbic system; ventromedial prefrontal cortex; anterior cingulate cortex; basal ganglia, including striatum and globus pallidus; insula and orbitofrontal cortex
Neurotransmitters	Adrenaline, noradrenaline, cortisol, glucocorticoids	γ-Aminobutyric acid; serotonin; adrenaline; noradrenaline to a lesser extent
Cognitive neuroscience	Starting as an automatic adaptation to the environment, stress eventually becomes 1 element of a cognitive, whole-brain response to prompting events or triggers, appraising them and reacting to them with behavioral adjustments	Stress pushes the default mode network into a highly activated, unstable state. This is interpreted as anxiety when it results in intense physiological alarms, dysfunctional beliefs, dysregulated emotions, or maladaptive coping strategies
Behavior	Fear-related stress response following stimulus provocation	Stress combines with cognitive, affective and environmental variables, and is interpreted as anxiety. Behavioral experiments accumulate evidence, which then affect stress response, belief revision, and future behavior
Triggers	Mostly environmental	Mostly internal representations or conditioned environmental triggers
Alarms	Mostly HPA axis and sympathetic nervous system activation	Alarm directed to threat; limbic system and threat information processing system activation
Beliefs and thoughts	Difficult to elicit; only enter into the picture when stress is cognitively appraised	Prominent and related to possible negative or catastrophic outcomes, leading to anxiety disorders
Coping	Mostly related to automatic adjustment of autonomic, physiological, or immune functions; when strain is recognized; adjustments are possible	Includes safety rituals and avoidance behavior aimed at escaping the threat-maintaining anxiety, in case of system breakdown

To a large extent these divisions are artificial because stress and anxiety largely overlap and enhance each other.

Abbreviations: GAS, general adaptation syndrome; HPA, hypothalamic-pituitary-adrenal.

disorder. A dimensional approach, on the other hand, evaluates a continuum of different symptoms, syndromes, and cognitive phenotypes.[18] Symptoms are particular features of a disorder, which can be ascertained from subjective self-reports and clinical judgments of behavior. Symptoms tend to co-occur in clusters, which are syndromes. Symptoms and syndromes are components of higher-order constructs or cognitive phenotypes, such as anxiety. For example, if social anxiety is the syndrome, fear of a negative evaluation arising out of social situations is a symptom and a dysfunctional belief hierarchy is a cognitive phenotype.[19] Symptoms occur along a continuum, and there is no necessary relationship between how a disorder is classified and its clinical presentation.

This approach makes complete sense for something as ubiquitous as stress. Even though not recognized by DSM-5, different DSM-5 diagnoses present with different levels and degrees of stress. Temporally stress may be single, episodic, persistent, or chronic. From the standpoint of acuity it may be mild, moderate, severe, or catastrophic. From the standpoint of the nature of the stressor it may be a single factor, several factors, or multiple factors. In principle, every DSM-5 diagnosis should be accompanied by a unique stress specifier that would situate it along a diagnostic continuum. Panic disorder (DSM-5 §300.01), for example, might be classifiable as episodic-severe-single factor if it was the result, say, of a severe car accident. It might be classifiable as multiple-factor if it was the result of persistent childhood abuse or neglect, as with the case of complex PTSD. It even could be a syndrome occurring in the offspring of a person who has panic disorder.

CLINICAL VIGNETTE

At the UCLA Anxiety and Related Disorders Clinic, the authors recently treated a 29-year-old female patient for panic disorder with agoraphobia. She presented with classic panic attack symptoms such as shortness of breath, racing heart, and a sensation of chest compression. After a year of therapy, she finally trusted her physicians enough to reveal that her panic attacks started after she was raped in college. She also revealed that she had nightmares, and avoided numerous other reminders of the traumatic event. Her underlying psychopathology was PTSD, DSM-5 §309.81, even though she presented with symptoms of panic disorder, DSM-5 §300.01. Her case illustrates how symptoms are not necessarily associated with categorical definitions of psychopathology, emphasizing the need for a transdiagnostic case conceptualization and intervention strategy using a unified protocol.

RELATIONSHIP OF STRESS TO ANXIETY

As the foregoing makes clear, stress and anxiety are a combination of (1) environmental threat; (2) physiological arousal; (3) cognitive appraisal; and (4) one's behavior in response to it. As described next, any of these junctures can be an appropriate intervention point depending on the patient's clinical presentation.

There is a reciprocal relationship between stress and anxiety. Different persons have different levels of resilience and vulnerability.[20] It is possible for a person to experience more stress with less anxiety. For example, a worker under pressure to complete a task under time, scheduling, and resource constraints will be able to do so with less anxiety if he or she is skilled in the performance of the task.[21] When perceived as unmanageable or excessive, stress has the potential to become a threat. The worker's anxiety level will increase. Conversely, a person can experience more anxiety with less stress. An obsessive worker performing a mundane task that is not stressful under ordinary circumstances might develop considerable anxiety about whether he or she is performing the task correctly. This person's slow or repetitive behavior could be driven by an overly granular information-processing style, even without stress induction.[22] Stress may enter the picture later, for example, when a supervisor evaluates the worker's performance. Under such circumstances, persistent fear and anxiety have the potential to become another stressor.

Stress and anxiety are dynamically related. Just as stress has the potential to produce anxiety, so anxiety can inaugurate another cycle of stress. Extreme anxiety makes a person more vulnerable to any kind of stress. This type of cumulative stress is even more intractable, because it imports all of the problematic cognitive, affective, and behavioral processing that accompanies anxiety. The interaction effect between stress and anxiety is one of the main diagnostic features of chronic stress, such as that caused by worry, a characteristic feature of GAD and social anxiety disorder (SAD). The more these repetitive factors come into play, the less stress is required to create anxiety. It becomes a self-reinforcing, continuously reacting process, as conceptualized in **Fig. 1**.

Temporally, stress typically emphasizes either a past or present strain or threat. Anxiety, on the other hand, typically emphasizes either one that is imminent or one that is anticipated to occur later, sometimes in the distant future. In both cases, however, one focuses on the event as if it were occurring in the present moment. There are numerous interesting uses of language to characterize stress and anxiety, which merit their own investigation. For example, one might report that one is "stressing out" in the present moment, even though what one is worried about is an event that is expected to occur in the future. The Cambridge philosopher Ludwig Wittgenstein emphasized that the meaning of a word only could be discerned from the context of its use, not some internal mental or emotional state.[23] The scientific and common literature tends to use stress and anxiety interchangeably. If nothing else, this emphasizes the lack of clarity surrounding these concepts.

Specific stressors typically are associated with specific types of anxiety, although this may vary. A phobia, for example, typically is aroused by the direct sensory point-in-time perception of the feared object. Response to it typically is initiated by

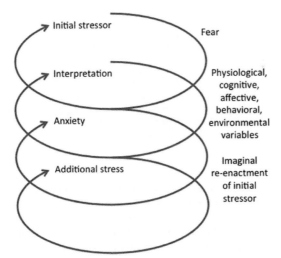

Fig. 1. Conceptualization of the stress cycle. Initial stressor triggers fear. Based on a variety of idiographic variables, including cognitive, affective, behavioral, and environmental processing, stress is interpreted as anxiety. The initial stressor then is cued or primed for imaginal reenactment, leading to additional stress.

a fear-conditioning paradigm (see later discussion). Pathological stress enters the picture only when phobic avoidance persists and interferes with adaptive coping. With PTSD, the stress response is not as straightforward. As DSM-5 §309.81 makes clear, PTSD initially is prompted by some kind of a traumatic real-world act, transaction, event, or occurrence (or a series of them, in the case of complex PTSD). Subsequent intrusive recollections, however, may be stimulated by mental reconstructions of them, in lieu of their actual recurrence (or the actual recurrence of something in the world sufficiently similar to them).[24] Eventually secondary adversities (such as lost jobs, compromised relationships, missed developmental stages) add to stress, draining resources, perpetuating further stress and anxiety, and leading to the development of additional psychiatric syndromes. This downward spiral is characteristic of chronic PTSD.[25]

When one isolates the stress component of PTSD in this manner, there may be no discernible relationship between the nature of the stressor and any subsequent disordered cognitions or behavior. In many instances it is difficult to identify stressors that are uniquely associated with the obsessive thoughts motivating compulsive behavior, as in obsessive-compulsive disorder (OCD), as opposed to more generalized preoccupations.[26] The diffuse profile of GAD, whereby the person may live more or less constantly on edge as a result of continuous stimulation and persistent worry about stressful life events, is even more amorphous and less specific.[27]

One can have more than 1 anxiety disorder at a time, and their symptoms may overlap or be completely different. Compulsive behavior, for example, may be the action-expression of beliefs associated with trauma, rather than coupled with obsessional thinking, as might be seen in social anxiety.[28] Under such circumstances, it is misleading to designate OCD, SAD, and PTSD as separate diagnostic categories. In cases like these, canonical relationships between symptoms and classifications are not explanatory, and potentially could lead to misdiagnosis of the underlying psychopathology.

CLINICAL VIGNETTE

The UCLA Anxiety and Related Disorders Clinic has a 6-week intensive outpatient program for persons with OCD, DSM-5 §300.3. In about one-third of cases, the onset of OCD symptoms can be traced to an underlying traumatic event. For example, a 36-year-old former air traffic controller almost caused a serious motor vehicle accident. He then developed severe "just right" thinking, accompanied by checking rituals. Psychologically he had established a cause-effect relationship between his checking rituals and the prevention of further catastrophes. He also developed co-occurrent severe SAD, DSM-5 §300.23. His main SAD symptoms were inability to talk over the telephone or to eat out in public. He lost his job and eventually was unable to even leave his house. His case illustrates that patients presenting with OCD could have underlying PTSD etiology. Later, they also could develop secondary social avoidance that turns into SAD, resulting in functional deterioration and depression.

Although detailed review is beyond the scope of this article, stress also is a major contributor to depression, which may result in loss of adaptive capability. A recent meta-analysis by Ionescu and colleagues[29] examined a subtype of major depressive disorder (MDD), which the investigators labeled as "anxious depression." Drawing on structural neuroimaging, electroencephalographic, genetic, and neuropsychiatric studies, the investigators identified numerous differences between anxious depression and MDD. A recent study by Wang and colleagues[30] examined the behavioral responses of mice exposed to stress. Twenty-two percent of the mice displayed "learned helplessness," a depression-like phenotype whereby the mouse gives up attempting to escape from electric foot shocks; the rest were resilient. Helplessness was associated with enhanced excitatory synaptic transmission onto neurons in the medial prefrontal cortex (mPFC), whereas resiliency was associated with reduced synaptic transmission. By enhancing the activity of the mPFC neurons in the resilient mice, the researchers were able to convert approximately 25% of them into helpless mice. These results were somewhat consistent with human studies showing that inhibiting neuronal activity in the mPFC (eg, using deep brain stimulation) was effective in reducing depression symptoms.

Looking at diagnostic evolution over time is an important issue because best-practices case conceptualization of psychiatric disorders now uses a transdiagnostic approach, and recommends treatment of them using a unified protocol.[31–33] Simultaneously, recent emphasis is on personalized medicine in psychiatry, rather than a "one-size-fits-all" type of approach.[34] At our current level of knowledge, categorical diagnoses do not capture many phenomena that should be inclined to be situated on the stress/anxiety continuum. The transdiagnostic method, on the other hand, is more sensitive to overlapping categories and processes, including semantic, neurobiological, phenomenological, and even genetic. The development of dynamic, interactive models of diagnoses will further improve our understanding of mental illness.

SUBJECTIVE PHENOMENOLOGY OF STRESS AND ANXIETY

The experience of stress and anxiety can be disconcerting. Imagine you are a member of a nomadic tribe of hunter-gatherers, living somewhere in North America during the Pleistocene epoch. You're out pursuing bison, or perhaps a wild moose. Suddenly, a sabre-tooth tiger jumps in your path—a threatening environmental stimulus. Among other consequences, the hunter's experience of the sabre-tooth tiger will be perceptually exaggerated. It might appear to be taller or closer than it actually is. The experience of confronting it might seem to be temporally elongated, and certainly more intense than ordinary, normative interactions with the environment.[35] Do you fight? Do you flee? Do you freeze? The safest thing to do is to get out of there as quickly as possible, or else the sabre-tooth tiger will eat you instead of the other way around, the so-called fight-or-flight response, which for years has been the cornerstone of anxiety theories.[36]

Under some circumstances, it might not even be necessary for the sabre-tooth tiger to actually appear if one is under the continuous apprehension of imminent predator attack. Nomadic tribes also faced longer-term stressors arising out of their environment, for example, the lack of natural resources (such as food) or predation by other tribes. These competitive pressures undoubtedly created a pervasive atmosphere of anxiety and fear, further disrupting their efforts to respond to the affordances offered by their environment and come to some form of accommodation with it.

Contemporary theorizing about this scenario starts with William James and Carl Lange,[37,38] who hypothesized that perception and interpretation of an environmental stimulus creates physiological arousal (eg, faster heart contractions). In turn these precipitate behavior, which results in the experience of an emotion (such as stress and anxiety or fear).[39] When the hunter runs from the sabre-tooth tiger, it is not because he is afraid of it; rather, he is afraid of it because he runs from it. Walter Cannon and Philip Bard bifurcated this process, holding that both physiological arousal and the experience of stress and anxiety are separate, independent, and co-occurrent processes.[40] Stanley Schachter and Jerome Singer introduced further modifications to the James-Lange and Cannon-Bard models. Schachter and Singer held that experiencing stress and anxiety requires both physiological arousal and cognitive appraisal to identify and label it correctly in the environmental context where it occurs.[41] **Fig. 2** conceptualizes each of these 3 models.

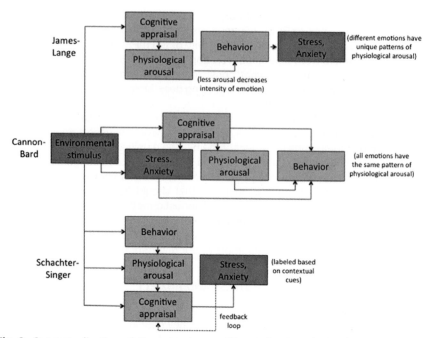

Fig. 2. Conceptualization of the James-Lange, Cannon-Bard, and Schachter-Singer models of emotion.

As James-Lange, Cannon-Bard, and Schachter-Singer hypothesized, emotions such as stress or fear responses and anxiety are evolutionarily adaptive reactions to dangerous or threatening objects or situations.[42,43] Normal stress/anxiety is useful, and high levels of stress/anxiety might occasionally be required for optimal performance and survival. The fight-or-flight response is a self-preservation mechanism. By enhancing the flow of blood carrying essential resources (such as oxygen and glucose), it prevents the predator from becoming prey. Without stress and anxiety as signaling mechanisms, life would be chaotic and dangerous, because one accidentally might not be able react to a hazardous situation.[44,45] It only is when stress/anxiety become excessive that they have the potential to become pathological, leading to maladaptive coping strategies and transformation into anxiety disorders.

Damasio[46] reinterpreted these precedents and advocated what he called a somatic marker hypothesis, conceptualized in **Fig. 3**. Perception of an environmental stimulus results in recording states of physiological arousal ("somatic markers"). Over time one learns how to interpret them and use them to predict outcomes associated with counterpart behavior. If as a result of one's learning history a somatic marker has been paired or coupled with a positive response outcome, this is a signal that it is safe or beneficial to engage in the behavior. Conversely, if the somatic marker has been paired or coupled with a negative response outcome, the associated behavior should be escaped or avoided. Although Damasio does not deal with it, presumably there is some risk of false positives and false negatives under either scenario. Damasio refers to this progression of events as the "body loop." One need not, however, experience the environmental stimulus in vivo to stimulate the somatic marker. A mental reconstruction of it also may be sufficient to activate it, precipitating the same sequence: what Damasio refers to as the "as if loop." The experience of an emotion comprises this entire complex of somatic markers, interpretations, and learned outcome

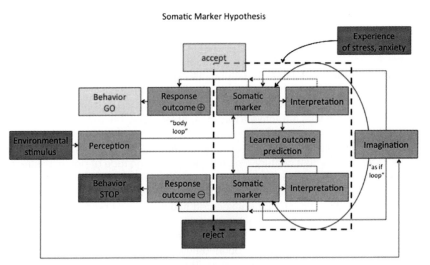

Fig. 3. Conceptualization of the somatic marker hypothesis.

predictions. Example: confronting a sabre-tooth tiger creates physiological arousal consistent with an emotion such as anxiety or fear, because one's environment consistently has delivered evidence that such a scenario is potentially dangerous; this activates a fight-or-flight response. Even worse, just thinking about a sabre-tooth tiger (having a mental image of one) might provoke physiological arousal and an action urge toward the same behavioral output channel. This notion (among other things) accounts for defensive behaviors such as hypervigilance and anticipatory readiness, when out hunting in sabre-tooth tiger territory.[47] A recent article by Chika-zoe and colleagues[48] suggests that, contrary to the somatic marker hypothesis, positive response outcomes and negative response outcomes both are encoded across sensory modalities in the same brain regions (the orbitofrontal cortices).

Other recent dual-process theorists include Stanovich and West[49] ("System 1" is fast, intuitive emotional; "System 2" is slower, deliberative, cognitive) and Daniel Kahneman and Amos Tversky[50] ("thinking fast" vs "thinking slow"). Broadly speaking, System 1 is associated with the amygdala and the rest of the limbic system, whereas System 2 is associated with the prefrontal cortex. While of course occurring along a spectrum within the stress/anxiety complex, System 1 and thinking fast are more characteristic of stress, whereas System 2 and thinking slow are more characteristic of anxiety. The more one cognitively appraises physiological arousals, the more one will veer toward a System 2 response. A System 2 response, on the other hand, is a more appropriate way to cognitively reregulate the physiological arousal and emotional stress caused by System 1. If one assumes that at any moment one can draw on a limited inventory of physiological, cognitive, and affective resources, cognitive appraisal thus has the potential to act as a regulator or governor of the intensity of stress response (and, consequently, make it more amenable to cognitive interventions).[51,52] Emotion regulation strategies are particularly effective in the treatment of stress-based and anxiety disorders.[53] Recent research by Todd and colleagues[54] suggests that affective biasing of attention, the predisposition to attend to certain categories of affectively salient stimuli over others, is another important emotional regulation technique. The cognitive-affective distinction "represents some real aspects of neuromental existence." It is not just "a fictional parsing of neuropsychological space."[55(p4)]

Stress and anxiety also have evolutionary disadvantages. For example, hormones such as hydrocortisone and medications such as yohimbine produce noradrenaline. Schwabe and colleagues[56] concluded that noradrenaline reduces activity in the orbitofrontal and mPFC, both associated with goal-directed behavior. As a result, brain regions such as the dorsolateral striatum, associated with habitual, routine-driven behavior, were prioritized. In another study, Rantala and colleagues[57] concluded that men with higher levels of cortisol were more likely to have lower testosterone levels, making them less attractive to women, presumably decreasing their chances for reproduction.

Transplant the sabre-tooth tiger or lack of resources scenarios to the second decade of the twenty-first century. The number and magnitude of potential stressors has proliferated,[58,59] but we still have the same basic tools as our hunter-gatherer ancestors to cope with them. Modern man has evolved little over the past 50,000 years.[60] We are still surprised by unexpected situations, and process information in the same way. The problem is that our social world is much more different now than it was thousands of years ago. Social environment is one of the main contributors to stress.[61,62] There is a mismatch, though, between stressful events, on the one hand, and what one can do about it on the other. The nature of the threat now primarily is psychological rather than bodily safety. Concomitantly, our repertoire of potential behavioral responses has contracted; some that formerly were effective no longer work. For example, one cannot take a cave-person club and start banging on the head of someone who is annoying. Not only is it socially unacceptable, it also is maladaptive (you will likely go to jail).

At the same time the pace of modern society has sped up. The result is a proliferation of mental illness, a peculiar kind of "American mania."[63] As a matter of evolutionary psychopathology, one might wonder why the mind is not designed better than it is; evolution is "constrained by previous design feature, the importance of tradeoffs between advantages and disadvantages of different traits [and] the way social dilemmas and conflicts have shaped the evolution of human motivational systems."[64(p353)]

Regardless of their different emphases, all of these theorists agree that stress and anxiety are hybrid mind-body transactions between person and environment.[65] Furthermore, as discussed next, each stage of the model represents a possible point for clinical intervention. Physiological arousal can be reduced using distress tolerance techniques or crisis survival strategies such as distraction, focusing on physical sensations, or use of guided imagery and other relaxation techniques. Cognitive appraisals can be made more realistic by revising beliefs to align them with evidence derived from behavioral hypotheses about how one's environment might respond, given certain contingencies. Emotions can be reregulated by developing a richer vocabulary to observe and describe them, reducing one's vulnerability, building positive experiences, and engaging in pleasurable activities. Problematic behavior can be reformulated by engaging in progressive exposure/response prevention. Techniques such as these are particularly important and useful, given the way the stress/anxiety complex straddles both the mental and physical milieus.

NEUROBIOLOGICAL PROCESSES ASSOCIATED WITH STRESS AND ANXIETY

Stress and anxiety have distinct but overlapping neurobiological signatures. As delineated by Selye, GAS proceeds in 3 stages: alarm, resistance, and exhaustion. Alarm is associated with exaggerated sympathetic nervous system response. Resistance is associated with discharge of hormones from the hypothalamic-pituitary-adrenal

(HPA) axis. This cascade starts with corticotropin-releasing factor (CRF) secretion from the suprahypothalamic nuclei, which activates corticotropin, which then mobilizes hydrocortisone from the suprarenal glands. The end products of this cascade are cortisol, epinephrine, and norepinephrine, which enable the body to maintain arousal and also activate the immune system.[66] Exhaustion is what happens when these systems break down, resulting in the emergence of illnesses caused by a reduced ability to fight them.

Subsequent research has continued to refine the dynamic elements of this process. The Swedish physiologist Björn Folkow studied the relationship between environmental arousal and physiological response.[67,68] He found that challenging psychosocial stimuli activate the anterior hypothalamus, triggering sympathetic nervous system reactions such as the release of adrenaline, vasoconstriction in the cardiovascular system, and vasodilation in skeletal muscles. Physiological assets such as blood flow and oxygen are redeployed from passive processes (such as digestion) to active ones (such as spear-throwing or running). It now is recognized that stress and anxiety disorders involve a variety of functionally interconnected neuroendocrine, neurotransmitter, and neuroanatomical disruptions,[69–71] a contributor to the semantic and phenomenological confusion described earlier.

From a neurological perspective, both stress and anxiety are associated with the activation of the anterior insula/orbitofrontal cortex and rostral parts of the dorsal anterior cingulate cortex/dorsomedial prefrontal cortex (dACC/dmPFC).[72,73] The right anterior insular/opercular region and the somatomotor and cingulate cortices also are involved.[74] Although reports conflict, stress literature places more emphasis on hormonal influences and dysregulation of the HPA axis[75,76] and the sympathetic nervous system,[77] as suggested by Selye in his description of GAS.

Too much stress leads to allostatic overload as the body attempts to regain homeostasis. Hormones such as cortisol, adrenaline, and noradrenaline have the potential to result in physiological changes such as organ deterioration and critical illness.[78,79] As Selye initially discovered, CRF regulates the HPA axis, and the production and release of neurotransmitters such as norepinephrine.

In addition to HPA-axis effects, chronic stress also results in glucocorticoid receptor resistance, which is associated with compromised immune system response.[80] Chronic stress recruits bone marrow-derived monocytes, which in turn promote anxiety-like behavior in knockout mice.[81] It causes dendritic pruning in *Caenorhabditis elegans*[82] and acts as a trigger for plaque rupture and thrombogenesis, resulting in an increased risk of myocardial infarction.[83] As this research shows, the cascade of changes in homeostasis caused by stress affects multiple body systems.

It must be emphasized that the neurobiology and neurocircuitry of anxiety and stress overlap, particularly so for disorders such as PTSD. If there is a difference between the two, the anxiety literature places more emphasis on fear circuitry involving the amygdala and other limbic nuclei.[84] These circuits are responsible for threat recognition and forming rapid, conditioned responses (CRs) to the threatening stimuli. Neuroanatomical involvement of primitive information-processing systems such as the striatum and corticothalamic circuits are involved in disorders such as OCD, but are rarely are considered in the stress literature. Norepinephrine and serotonin play an important role in regulating the biological mechanisms of alarm system disorders such as panic.

DIATHESIS-STRESS

Another important contributor to the relationship between stress and anxiety is the concept of diathesis-stress. As stated in a recent review by Lucassen and colleagues[66(p109)] on what they describe as the "neuropathology of stress," "environmental challenges are part of daily life for any individual. In fact, stress appears to be increasingly present in our modern, and demanding, industrialized society. Virtually every aspect of our body and brain can be influenced by stress." Diathesis-stress means that an individual has a genetic disposition or proclivity toward a particular psychiatric disorder (diathesis), which then becomes activated by an environmental stimulus (stress).[85,86]

Although originally associated primarily with psychotic disorders, diathesis-stress now has been applied to almost every type of psychological problem, including anxiety disorders. Anxiety disorders are highly inheritable (30%–67%). Molecular genetic association studies have implicated multiple anxiety-vulnerability genes, often with distinct clinical presentations.[87,88] Family studies and large-registry genetic studies conducted in anxiety disorders also typically produce genetic overlap between anxiety, depression, and substance abuse.[89] Genetic vulnerability has an inverse relationship with the amount of stress required to produce the disorder. The greater the genetic loading, the less environmental stimulus is required to initiate a stress cycle.

Anxiety disorders also frequently result from epigenetic factors regulating gene expression, such as gene/genotype environmental interactions and developmental plasticity.[90] A recent meta-analysis by Hunter and McEwen[91] concluded that "stress has a direct impact on epigenetic markers at all life history stages" and reciprocally that "epigenetic mechanisms play a role in altering stress responsiveness, anxiety and brain plasticity across the lifespan and beyond to succeeding generations."[91(p177)] When these genetic and environmental factors interact, it creates diathesis-stress.

CLINICAL VIGNETTE

The cases observed at the UCLA Anxiety and Related Disorders Clinic tend to have high genetic loading. If several first-degree relatives have anxiety, depression, or OCD, the patient's anxiety disorder has a tendency to occur early (as early as before adolescence); the course and progression of illness is more severe; and the disorder is less treatment responsive. These patients seem to require less stress, or even no traceable stress, to provoke the onset of the disorder. This situation occurred in the case of a patient who had been diagnosed with SAD and OCD in middle school. Several siblings and a parent were affected by a fairly similar condition. The patient started having difficulties in college, and had to withdraw. The authors saw him at age 20, still living with his parents, working occasionally at a job much below his intellectual level. His disorder was progressing to the point where he had become incapacitated by it. His 2 siblings also developed symptoms later in life when they went to college, and were somewhat more functional in that they were able to obtain their degrees and find employment. This vignette illustrates another major point about the relationship between stress and anxiety. Once the anxiety disorder is expressed, resulting functional impairments can perpetuate by themselves further developments and worsening condition of the patient.

CONDITIONING PARADIGM

Another way of looking at the relationship between stress and anxiety is to consider the role stress plays in conditioning and extinction paradigms. GAS is more than just a generalized reaction to stressful stimuli, and anxiety is more than just a generalized reaction to threat. A person's environment can shape one up so that both become ingrained, habitual responses. In the classical Pavlovian conditioning scenario, an unconditioned stimulus (US) initially provokes an unconditioned response (UR), which happens because the relationship between US and UR is a natural feature of the organism. As a result of repeated pairings, the organism couples the US with a neutral stimulus, transforming it into a conditioned stimulus (CS). The relationship between US and CS is not a natural feature of the organism, but rather arises solely as a result of this association process. The CS then results in a CR, which has physiological, cognitive, and affective features similar to those of the UR before coupling. Because of neural plasticity, fear conditioning even has the capability to effect changes in the brain's behavioral and physiological stress response systems.[92] **Fig. 4** conceptualizes this process.

Stress is a visceral, instinctive, and adaptive reaction in response to aversive environmental stimulation (US). If recognized as a threat, it provokes anxiety (UR), in a manner similar to fear conditioning.[93] As already discussed, much of anxiety is based on fear. A person might be afraid of an object (eg, in the case of a phobia) or something arising out of the environment (eg, in the case of SAD), or the consequences of response to threat (eg, in the case of panic disorder). Persons might be afraid of correlative physiological alarms and interoceptive sensations, and their consequences; they also might have thoughts or feelings associated with a previous aversive event, which now acts as an imaginal trigger.

This sequence particularly is clear in the case of PTSD, which is the paradigmatic case of a fear-based stress disorder.[94] PTSD is "the only major mental disorder for which a cause is considered to be known: that is, an event that involves threat to the physical integrity of oneself or others and induces a response of intense fear, helplessness or horror."[95(p769)] Its basic template is as follows: the traumatic incident(s) underlying PTSD (US) creates an initial fear memory (UR). Subsequent cues or primes based on features of the traumatic incident(s) (CS) then engage reexperiencing of symptoms, avoidance, and hyperarousal (CR).[96] PTSD is also similar to fear

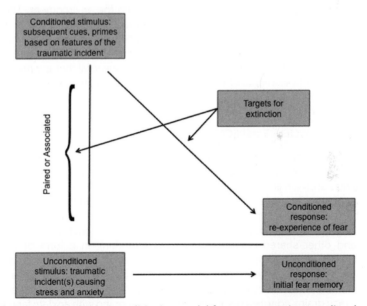

Fig. 4. Basic Pavlovian classical conditioning model for posttraumatic stress disorder. A traumatic incident causes stress (unconditioned stimulus). Stress precipitates or triggers an initial fear memory (unconditioned response). Subsequent cues or primes based on the traumatic incident (conditioned stimulus) activate a reexperience of the fear (conditioned response), with corollary symptoms such as avoidance, isolation, impulsivity, anger, vigilance, and hyperarousal.

processing from a neurological standpoint, associated with excessive amygdala and insula reactivity and dysregulation of the dorsal anterior cingulate and medial prefrontal regions.[97] Given its mechanism of action, it might make more sense to regard "posttraumatic stress disorder" as a "posttraumatic stressor" or "threat-trigger disorder," which more accurately characterizes the precursors initiating its onset.

There is considerable evidence to support this scenario. Stress triggers anxiety symptoms such as anger, isolation, and impulsivity. Rather than remaining neutral toward incoming perceptual data, one's sensitivity to physiological alarms skews one toward having an exaggerated autonomic arousal. In turn, this creates overattention and vigilance toward threat.[98] One starts engaging in excessively detailed, granular information processing, which leads to signal prediction errors and impaired conflict monitoring.[99] Moreover, it leads to dysfunctional thought patterns; for example, assuming something is frightening when it is not (a false positive), or assuming something is not frightening when it is (a false negative). One builds anxiety up to a level where it is uncomfortable, maybe even distressful, and starts enacting maladaptive behaviors to contend with it. In effect, one becomes fear conditioned.[100]

Fear can be extinguished by using an appropriate behavioral paradigm such as exposure/response prevention, activating a reverse inhibitory learning process, and allowing for more adaptive control of the CR by forming a consolidated extinction memory.[101] Learning-related synaptic plasticity plays an important role in this process.[102] Fear extinction is a powerful intervention strategy that is effective against multiple anxiety disorders.[103,104] Conversely, fear can be restored as a result of spontaneous recovery, context renewal, reinstatement, or reacquisition.[105]

Both stress and anxiety can be addressed by therapeutic intervention. For example, a worker experiencing a stressful environment, such as timed performance tasks, can reduce the amount of stress experienced by modifying the environment. The worker can either reduce the number of tasks to be performed within a given time frame, or expand the time frame to accommodate the completion of a designated number of tasks. A program of cognitive therapy for anxiety might reframe the worker's relationship to the environment and the tasks. A program of behavioral therapy might deconstruct the component elements of task performance and examine what was inhibiting their timely and efficient completion.

COGNITIVE NEUROSCIENCE ASPECTS

The relationship between stress and anxiety also can be conceptualized from the standpoint of cognitive neuroscience. The basic premise of cognitive neuroscience is that the human brain is a sophisticated information-processing system, comprising functionally dependent networks of interconnected brain regions, which together are responsible for cognitive and affective activity. Each component of the dynamical system competes with all others for physiological assets (such as blood flow and oxygen) and other shared resources (such as attention), in a form of winnerless competition whereby the alteration of one element automatically provokes adjustment throughout the entire system. Winnerless competition means that if assets and resources are purposed for one component, the amount available for others is reduced. Extreme stress drains adaptive resources and makes coping with anxiety far more difficult. Initially the concept of winnerless competition is based on simple Lotka-Volterra models of predator-prey interaction, corresponding to the intuition that one can attend only to a single thing at a time. Thus, for example, if one's focus is on reducing interoceptive alarms (such as panic), fewer resources are available for belief revision or behavior modification. It is difficult to process information when having a panic attack.

On the other hand, compulsive behavior (characteristic of OCD) tends to defuse the obsessive beliefs. Depressive beliefs, in turn, drive out behavioral activation.

Under normative conditions the brain is awaiting activation in what has become characterized as the default mode network. Different areas in the brain are activated/connected if they show synchronized variations while the brain is at rest. Stress and its associated external sensory stimulation interact with baseline conditions, initiating network modulations such as switching between or selecting among different networks, or otherwise "pushing" the applicable network into an alternative, activated state. Initially the system is itinerant and highly unstable; however, it self-organizes as it develops hypotheses, conducts behavioral experiments, and receives evidentiary outcome data from the environment. It then evaluates this evidence, which either confirms or disconfirms the hypotheses, changing various subsets of the system's parameters. If there is no evidence, it takes steps to consequate to the environment by establishing behavioral contingencies. If the evidence is ambiguous, it continues to refine the hypotheses until it locks into an informative feedback loop. It constructs a series of transient pathways from equilibrium to the attractor.[106] The pathways are linked by heteroclinic channels into a series of metastable states. Metastable states are coordinated interactions between perceptual, affective, and cognitive processes resulting in different spatiotemporal patterns of brain activity, functionally organized within a phase space to implement specific mental events, which can be measured by various control parameters. With attentional control, different sensory modalities such as vision, audition, and tactility cooperate, resulting in heteroclinic binding. As it coalesces at various metastable states, it results in a single output channel of behavior. It then initiates another cycle using the same operations, building on the learning history that is the result of previous cognitive-affective-environmental interactions.[107]

Psychopathology occurs when these networks are disrupted, creating unstable and unpredictable conditions, analogous to noise versus signal. Noise is characteristic of many psychiatric disorders and anxiety disorders in particular. Encountering a feared situation initially triggers panic-type alarms, resulting in transient chaos. One attends vigilantly to perceived stimuli. Focused attention heightens self-monitoring, resulting in greater interoceptive sensitivity to and perception of the resulting physiological alarms.[108,109] Attending to something also converges intentional orientation toward it. This process not only maintains a pathogenic belief structure but also cognitively prioritizes the pursuit of behaviors designed to reduce the resulting cognitive distress. The resulting trajectories exhibit greater oscillation in the heteroclinic channel.[110]

A-B-C MODEL

It follows that the purpose of therapeutic intervention is to restore homeostasis in the default mode network by modulating neurobiological activity.[111] From a clinical standpoint, this procedure is operationalized through a variation on cognitive-behavioral therapy developed by the authors, called the A-B-C model[112]: "A" stands for alarms; "B" stands for beliefs; and "C" stands for coping strategies. Its premise is that because the process of anxiety disorders is nonlinear, dynamic, and interactive, their clinical presentation may become accentuated or pathologized at any point within the anxiety-producing system.

Initially alarms are precipitated by triggers, which are unavoidable real-world events, or mental reconstructions of them. Alarms are somatic, physiological, bodily based, or emotional responses to triggers.[113] Examples are: palpitations, pounding heart, or accelerated heart rate (tachycardia); sweating (diaphoresis); trembling or shaking; sensations of shortness of breath or smothering (dyspnea); feelings of choking; chest pain or discomfort; nausea or abdominal distress; feeling dizzy, unsteady, light-headed, or faint (disequilibrium); chills or heat sensations; numbness or tingling sensations (paresthesias); temporary loss of sensation (hypoesthesia); feelings of unreality (derealizations) or being detached from oneself (depersonalization); fear of losing control or "going crazy;" or even fear of dying (thanatophobia). Persons experience these alarms as unpleasant or aversive, and sometimes are even incapacitated by them.

Beliefs are the resulting thoughts and cognitions: the cognitive or psychological component of the equation. Beliefs underlie, explain, and contextualize one's underlying construction of a situation and one's behavioral response to it. In the case of stress, these cognitions primarily are associated with ascriptive predicates such as frustration, nervousness, fear, unease, or worry, all of which are classified under the general heading of anxiety. Beliefs typically are framed as the hypotheses, some with better evidentiary support than others.[114] For example, "If I participate at a meeting, then I will look foolish and people will think I'm stupid." Seen this way, beliefs engender evidentiary data points that support one's theory about the cause and effect of the stress. Competing beliefs resolve into a single output action-channel of behavior, which provides evidence that either supports or disconfirms the belief hypotheses. Revised hypotheses then modulate alarm sensitivity and attenuate subsequent behavioral enactments. Beliefs also frequently are accompanied by emotions (happy, sad), although affective states may involve the suspension of cognitive ones.[115–117]

Coping strategies are behaviors, which can be broadly classified as either escape/avoidant or exposure/response-preventive. Escape/avoidant occurs when one is presented with a feared stimulus but then flees from it to seek comfort, safety, or refuge.[118] Such safety behaviors are "covert and overt actions adopted by the individual to prevent feared outcomes and maintain a sense of safety."[119(p226)] These behaviors maintain a state of emotional vulnerability and alarm sensitivity, a type of contrast avoidance.[120] For example, one does not go to an office party (overt avoidance); or, once there, leaves immediately rather than spending time with colleagues (overt escape); or, once there, disassociates (covert avoidance). Pathological escape/avoidance is characterized by interpersonal, employment, legal, and other similar difficulties and, in extreme cases, is expressed as substance abuse, self-harm, suicidal ideation, anger, or self-isolation, all of which not only are personally distressful but also socially maladaptive. It becomes a form of conditioned behavior in response to any kind of fear or threat, however benign.

The key feature of escape/avoidant coping strategies is that, over the medium to long term, they are ineffective in downregulating alarm intensity or providing evidence to reformulate beliefs. The reason why is because one thinks one has handled the problem, but in reality has not. One simply has deferred dealing with it. As a result, interoceptive arousal leads to defensive responses as cognitive and physiological assets are recruited by and redeployed to other processes such as the autonomic nervous system.[121,122]

Exposure/response prevention techniques are the tools that help to disrupt pathological A-B-C cycles. Using this technique, a person slowly is exposed to fearful stimuli while maladaptive escape/avoidance behavior is actively prevented. Exposure/response preventive coping strategies maximize the likelihood of timely and informative environmental feedback. In its most primitive form, adaptive coping is the ability to take care of basic personal needs such as food, clothing, and shelter. At higher levels of functioning it is the capacity to navigate social norms and comply with cultural expectations, yet still remain sufficiently flexible to contend with unexpected adversity.

The intuition behind it is that one achieves behavioral flexibility in the face of a feared stimulus. Rather than letting it take control, one confronts and opposes it,[123,124] thereby extinguishing or unlearning the relationship between CS and CR. Exposure/ response prevention introduces variability and dissonance into one's knowledge base, a form of "antifragility,"[125] decreasing habituation and resulting in a lower subjective probability evaluation that the feared outcome will actually occur. To continue with the office party example, a better strategy would be to remain engaged, gradually acclimate to the environment, take tentative steps to mingle with colleagues, realize you haven't done anything foolish, then engage in normative interactions. **Table 2** illustrates the application of the A-B-C model for panic, the symptoms of which are a key feature of most anxiety disorders.

The focus of contemporary behavioral therapy is to reduce alarm intensity through just this kind of exposure/response prevention. The theory is that doing so reciprocally inhibits or disrupts the connection between trigger/alarm and escape/avoidance behavior. Although of course they are interrelated,[115,117] it is important to emphasize that exposure/response prevention only will be successful when accompanied by an acceptable belief revision.

Because it reformulates psychological problems such as anxiety as a throughput process, unfolding longitudinally in time, the A-B-C model improves both case conceptualization and corollary intervention strategies using both cognitive and behavioral techniques.[126] For example, by increasing awareness of environment-body interactions, greater interoceptive sensitivity should downregulate the trigger-alarm relationship, reducing the intensity of alarm-related distress. Fear of reexperiencing interoceptive sensations often results in increased vigilance for threat and exacerbating sensitivity to triggers, thus increasing the likelihood of their recurrence and correlative perception of alarm intensity. Reduced experience of alarms in turn should reduce the incidence of dysfunctional beliefs and lessen reliance on escape-avoidant coping strategies that interfere with facile, robust functioning. Alarms exacerbate dysfunctional beliefs and point toward ineffective coping strategies designed primarily for distress tolerance rather than comprehensive anxiety reduction. More effective coping strategies reciprocally should downregulate alarm intensity and provide evidence supporting the generation of more adaptive, flexible beliefs. **Fig. 5** depicts the component elements of this cycle.

People with high interoceptive sensitivity require a different case conceptualization/ intervention than those whose main focus is on maintaining a repertoire of workable coping strategies. Because they are so discombobulated, their symptomatology is haphazard as they are buffeted by immediate, attention-grabbing stimuli. If one has an elaborate belief structure, it may be easier to recognize the evidence supporting them and cluster them into belief subsets. Conversely one may have a more detailed, granular information-processing style, tending to get stuck on insignificant details, resulting in behavioral deactivation. As already described, stress and anxiety are intimately intertwined. Unveiling a person's A-B-C patterns will suggest pathways for better management of the stress/anxiety complex. Following case conceptualization using the A-B-C method one can use specific, step-wise tools, including psychopharmacology, mindfulness, cognitive restructuring, and exposure/response prevention, among others.

Mindfulness is particularly useful in reducing stress and anxiety. A recent study by Rose and colleagues[127] found that an intervention group using a computer/Web-based program of self-guided stress management training based on the A-B-C approach showed significant stress reduction in comparison with a control group using videos and published materials. Bullis and colleagues[128] found that persons

Table 2
Application of the A-B-C model for panic, a key feature of most anxiety disorders

Typical Triggers	Typical Alarms	Typical Beliefs	Typical Coping Strategies
Separation from one to whom the person is attached (DSM-5 §309.21); interaction with phobic object (DSM-5 §300.2x); social situations (DSM-5 §300.23); being in an enclosed space (DSM-5 §300.22); intrusive recollections (DSM-5 §309.81); anxiety and fear of recurrent symptoms itself may become a stressor (see **Fig. 1**)	Palpitations, pounding heart, or accelerated heart rate; sweating; trembling or shaking; sensations of shortness of breath or smothering; feelings of choking; chest pain or discomfort; nausea or abdominal stress; feeling dizzy, unsteady, light-headed, or faint; chills or heat sensations; numbness or tingling sensations (DSM-5, §300.01)	"I'm going crazy"; "I might lose control"; "I might die"; "I can't handle these sensations"; "These sensations will keep recurring"; "I'll be disabled"; "I won't be able to work/stay in school"; "I might end up being destitute"	Effective ⊕: exercise; relaxation; mindfulness; volunteering; pleasurable activities; taking up a hobby Maladaptive ⊖: substance abuse; self-harm; impulsivity; isolation; anger

Stress is a combination of triggers and alarms; anxiety is a combination of stress overlaid with fear-based cognitive appraisals (beliefs) and coping strategies (behavior). Effective coping strategies are those that downregulate the frequency, intensity, and duration of alarms, and the incidence of dysfunctional beliefs. Ineffective or maladaptive coping strategies not only are intrinsically harmful but also ineffective in accomplishing the same outcome; they actually even may be worse than doing nothing, because one thinks or contended with associated alarms and beliefs, when in fact one simply has deferred dealing with them, further animating them on their inevitable recurrence.

Abbreviation: DSM-5, *Diagnostic and Statistical Manual of Mental Disorders*, 5th edition.

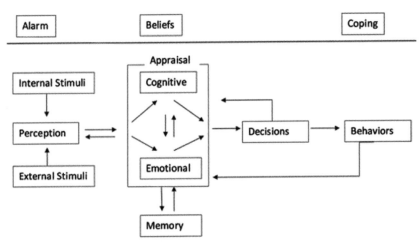

Fig. 5. The A-B-C (Alarm-Beliefs-Coping) model. (*From* Bystritsky A, Nierenberg AA, Feusner JD, et al. Computational nonlinear dynamical psychiatry: a new methodological paradigm for diagnosis and course of illness. J Psychiatr Res 2012;46(4):430. http://dx.doi.org/10.1016/j. jpsychires.2011.10.013; with permission.)

using habitual trait-based emotion regulation and distress tolerance strategies (such as mindfulness) were able to suppress stress more effectively than controls. Kasala and colleagues[129] found that mindfulness also reduced stress-mediated depression by raising levels of monoamines, increasing parasympathetic activity, reducing oxidative stress, enhancing levels of endogenous antioxidants (such as glutathione), and increasing the transcriptional expression of antioxidative enzymes such as glutathione S-transferase, Cu-Zn superoxide dismutase (SOD), Mn SOD, glutathione peroxidase, and catalase. Mindfulness training need not be extensive or complex; Creswell and colleagues[130] recently found that 25-minute sessions over 3 days had a significant clinical effect.

The exact mechanism of action of mindfulness on stress reduction requires further investigation. Hölzel and colleagues[131] proposed a taxonomy of (1) attention regulation; (2) body awareness; (3) emotion regulation (including reappraisal and exposure, extinction, and reconsolidation); and (4) change in perspective on the self. Goyal and colleagues,[132] on the other hand, found only moderate evidence that mindfulness meditation programs reduced anxiety, and evidence of no effect or insufficient evidence of any effect on similar outcome variables. Mindfulness interferes with all 3 components of the stress/anxiety complex. It reduces the frequency, intensity, and duration of alarms, and teaches observe-and-describe skills in lieu of escape/avoidance, thus resulting in behavioral, cognitive, and affective changes.

SUMMARY

Stress and anxiety are 2 distinct processes. Stress primarily involves strain of resources in one's environment, in the manner Selye described for GAS. Anxiety primarily is a fear-based response to threat. Most (if not all) of the time these processes intertwine, and it is difficult to distinguish between them. Stress and anxiety are component parts of an inseparable stress/anxiety complex reaction. When it persists, it has the potential to produce specific anxiety disorders, depending on triggers and the environmental context in which they arise, and on adaptive behaviors enacted to contend with them. Because the A-B-C protocol views anxiety disorders as dynamical and transdiagnostic, this protocol improves both case conceptualization and intervention strategies. In A-B-C terms, the stress/anxiety complex is a combination of all 3 elements: alarms, beliefs, and coping strategies. Initially it is triggered by a real-world (or mental) event, coupled with interoceptive sensations of resulting somatic/physiological responses. Although it may be distressful, the trigger-alarm combination is not the same entity as stress or anxiety; properly construed, it is more of an unfiltered sympathetic nervous system response. It must be interpreted by the belief-generating system, which produces (among other cognitions) a set of hypotheses about the environment (the causes of the triggers-alarms) and one's relationship to it. The trigger-alarm relationship can be imagined as a kind of envelope comprising the attack, sustain, decay, and release of alarm-like symptoms.

Stress disrupts information processing, belief retrieval, and one's ability to respond to new environmental contingencies. Once information processing is perturbed, stress disrupts normative belief production and becomes associated with anxiety. At a deeper level, stress affects one's self-sufficiency and ability to cope. This latter failure is particularly insidious because then one must contend not only with the original trigger-alarm-belief complex but also with the subsequent consequences of a coping strategy not performing as expected to contend with anxiety-related distress. The A-B-C model emphasizes that although one might not be able to reduce the frequency, intensity, onset or duration of triggers, one can achieve mastery over them through a combination of cognitive and behavioral interventions at each step of the anxiety-producing equation.

Scientists need to recognize that stress and anxiety are part of a general adaptive response to noxious environmental stimuli, and can be difficult to distinguish because similar neurobiological mechanisms are involved. Further research should concentrate on developing dynamical models tracing the course and progression of stress and anxiety responses over time (from the initial stress response to development of a stress-related disorder). Clinicians should start applying a "degree of stress" scale (ranging from mild to catastrophic) for every DSM-5 diagnosis. It is an important etiological factor that is important for assessing the maintenance and perpetuation of symptoms. Experiencing symptoms itself, and even carrying a diagnosis of a psychological disorder or mental illness, is stressful. A degree of stress scale also would enable the clinician to evaluate the adaptive quality of coping, and thus the likelihood or potential of relapse once stress and anxiety have been controlled. Precise psychophysiological tests should be developed to measure degrees of stress, and the patient's adaptive capacity from initiation through maintenance to conclusion of illness. Future treatments of anxiety disorders should incorporate more stress-reduction strategies such as relaxation, time management, and others that presently are being neglected in favor of strict exposure/response-prevention treatments.

REFERENCES

1. American Psychological Association. Stress in America. 2013. Available at: http://www.apa.org/news/press/releases/stress/2013/highlights.aspx. Accessed July 20, 2014.
2. National Institutes of Mental Health. Anxiety disorders. 2014. Available at: http://www.nimh.nih.gov/health/topics/anxiety-disorders/index.shtml. Accessed July 20, 2014.
3. Selye H. Stress and disease. Science 1955;122(3171):625–31. http://dx.doi.org/10.1126/science.122.3171.625.

4. Goodnite PM. Stress: a concept analysis. Nurs Forum 2014;49(1):71–4. http://dx.doi.org/10.1111/nuf.12044.
5. Karatsoreos IN, McEwen BS. Psychobiological allostasis: resistance, resilience and vulnerability. Trends Cogn Sci 2011;15(12):576–84. http://dx.doi.org/10.1016/j.tics.2011.10.005.
6. McEwen BS, Wingfield JC. What is in a name? Integrating homeostasis, allostasis and stress. Horm Behav 2010;57:105–11. http://dx.doi.org/10.1016/j.yhbeh.2009.09.011.
7. McEwen BS. Central effects of stress hormones in health and disease: understanding the protective and damaging effects of stress and stress mediators. Eur J Pharmacol 2008;583:174–85. http://dx.doi.org/10.1016/j.ejphar.2007.11.071.
8. Fossat P, Bacqué-Cazenave J, De Deurwaerdère P, et al. Anxiety-like behavior in crayfish is controlled by serotonin. Science 2014;344(6189):1293–7. http://dx.doi.org/10.1126/science.1248811.
9. de Wall FB. What is an animal emotion? Ann N Y Acad Sci 2011;1224:191–206. http://dx.doi.org/10.1111/j.1749-6632.2010.05912.x.
10. Panksepp J. The basic emotional circuits of mammalian brains: do animals have affective lives? Neurosci Biobehav Rev 2011;35(9):1791–804. http://dx.doi.org/10.1016/j.neubiorev.2011.08.003.
11. American Psychiatric Association. Diagnostic and statistical manual of mental disorders. 5th edition. Arlington (VA): American Psychiatric Association; 2013.
12. Bryant RA, Friedman MJ, Spiegel D, et al. A review of acute stress disorder in DSM-5. Focus 2011;9(3):335–50. http://dx.doi.org/10.1002/da.20737.
13. O'Donnell ML, Alkemade N, Nickerson A, et al. Impact of the diagnostic changes to post-traumatic stress disorder for DSM-5 and the proposed changes to ICD-11. Br J Psychiatry 2014. http://dx.doi.org/10.1192/bjp.bp.113.135285.
14. Spitzer RL, First MB, Wakefield JC. Saving PTSD from itself in DSM-V. J Anxiety Disord 2007;21(2):233–41. http://dx.doi.org/10.1016/j.janxdis.2006.09.006.
15. Weathers FW, Marx BP, Friedman MJ, et al. Posttraumatic stress disorder in DSM-5: new criteria, new measures, and implications for assessment. Psychol Inj Law 2014. http://dx.doi.org/10.1007/s12207-014-9191-1.
16. Nutt D, Miguel BG, Davies SJ. Phenomenology of anxiety disorders. In: Blanchard RJ, Blanchard DC, Griebel G, et al, editors. Handbook of anxiety and fear, vol. 17. Amsterdam (NL): Elsevier; 2008. p. 365–93. http://dx.doi.org/10.1016/S1569-7339(07)00017-3.
17. American Psychiatric Association. Diagnostic and statistical manual of mental disorders. 4th edition text revision (DSM-IV-TR). Washington, DC: Author; 2000.
18. Helzer JE, Kraemer HC, Krueger RF. The feasibility and need for dimensional psychiatric diagnoses. Psychol Med 2006;36(12):1671–80. http://dx.doi.org/10.1017/S003329170600821X.
19. Bilder RM, Howe A, Novak N, et al. The genetics of cognitive impairment in schizophrenia: a phenomic perspective. Trends Cogn Sci 2011;15(9):428–35. http://dx.doi.org/10.1016/j.tics.2011.07.002.
20. Franklin TB, Saab BJ, Mansuy IM. Neural mechanisms of stress resilience and vulnerability. Neuron 2012;75:747–61. http://dx.doi.org/10.1016/j.neuron.2012.08.016.
21. Poolton JW, Wilson MR, Malhotra N, et al. A comparison of evaluation, time pressure, and multitasking as stressors of psychomotor operative performance. Surgery 2011;149(6):776–82. http://dx.doi.org/10.1016/j.surg.2010.12.005.

22. Feusner JD, Moody T, Hembacher E, et al. Abnormalities of visual processing and frontostriatal systems in body dysmorphic disorder. Arch Gen Psychiatry 2010;67(2):197–205. http://dx.doi.org/10.1001/archgenpsychiatry.2009.190.

23. Wittgenstein L. Philosophical investigations. Anscombe GEM, trans. 2nd edition. New York: Macmillan Co; 1958.

24. Pearson DG, Deeprose C, Wallace-Hadrill SM, et al. Assessing mental imagery in clinical psychology: a review of imagery measures and a guiding framework. Clin Psychol Rev 2013;33(1):1–23. http://dx.doi.org/10.1016/j.cpr.2012.09.001.

25. Resick PA, Bovin MJ, Calloway AL, et al. A critical evaluation of the complex PTSD literature: implications for DSM-5. J Trauma Stress 2012;25(3):241–51. http://dx.doi.org/10.1002/jts.21699.

26. Rosso G, Albert U, Asinari GF, et al. Stressful life events and obsessive-compulsive disorder: clinical features and symptom dimensions. Psychiatry Res 2012;197(3):259–64. http://dx.doi.org/10.1016/j.psychres.2011.10.005.

27. Francis JL, Moitra E, Dyck I, et al. The impact of stressful life events on relapse of generalized anxiety disorder. Depress Anxiety 2012;29(5):386–91. http://dx.doi.org/10.1002/da.20919.

28. Fostick L, Nacasch N, Zohar JO. Acute obsessive compulsive disorder (OCD) in veterans with posttraumatic stress disorder (PTSD). World J Biol Psychiatry 2012;13(4):312–5. http://dx.doi.org/10.3109/15622975.2011.607848.

29. Ionescu DF, Niciu MJ, Mathews DC, et al. Neurobiology of anxious depression: a review. Depress Anxiety 2013;30(4):374–85. http://dx.doi.org/10.1002/da.22095.

30. Wang M, Perova Z, Arenkiel BR, et al. Synaptic modifications in the medial prefrontal cortex in susceptibility and resilience to stress. J Neurosci 2014; 34(22):7485–92. http://dx.doi.org/10.1523/jneurosci.5294-13.2014.

31. Clark DA. Cognitive behavioral therapy for anxiety and depression: possibilities and limitations of a transdiagnostic perspective. Cogn Behav Ther 2009; 38(Suppl 1):29–34. http://dx.doi.org/10.1080/16506070902980745.

32. Dudley R, Kuyken W, Padesky CA. Disorder specific and trans-diagnostic case conceptualization. Clin Psychol Rev 2011;31(2):213–24. http://dx.doi.org/10. 1016/j.cpr.2010.07.005.

33. Norton PJ, Barrera TL. Transdiagnostic versus diagnosis-specific CBT for anxiety disorders: a preliminary randomized controlled noninferiority trial. Depress Anxiety 2012;29(10):874–82. http://dx.doi.org/10.1002/da.21974.

34. Costa e Silva JA. Personalized medicine in psychiatry: new technologies and approaches. Metabolism 2013;62(Suppl 1):S40–4. http://dx.doi.org/10.1016/j. metabol.2012.08.017.

35. Harber KD, Yeung D, Iacovelli A. Psychosocial resources, threat, and the perception of distance and height: support for the resources and perception model. Emotion 2011;1080–90. http://dx.doi.org/10.1037/a0023995.

36. Fuller MD, Emrick MA, Sadilek M, et al. Molecular mechanism of calcium channel regulation in the fight-or-flight response. Sci Signal 2010;3(141):ra70. http://dx.doi.org/10.1126/scisignal.2001152.

37. Fink G. Stress: definition and history. In: Fink G, editor. Stress science: neuroendocrinology. San Diego (CA): Academic Press; 2010. p. 3–9.

38. Friedman BH. Feelings and the body: the Jamesian perspective on autonomic specificity of emotion. Biol Psychol 2010;84(3):383–93. http://dx.doi.org/10. 1016/j.biopsycho.2009.10.006.

39. James W. What is an emotion? Mind 1884;9:188–205.

40. Cannon WB. Bodily changes in pain, hunger, fear and rage. New York: D. Appleton & Co; 1927.

41. Schachter S, Singer J. Cognitive, social and physiological determinants of emotional state. Psychol Rev 1962;69(5):379–99. http://dx.doi.org/10.1037/h0046234.
42. Marks IM, Nesse RM. Fear and fitness: an evolutionary analysis of anxiety disorders. Ethol Sociobiol 1994;15:247–61.
43. Price JS. Evolutionary aspects of anxiety disorders. Dialogues Clin Neurosci 2003;5(3):223–36.
44. Darwin CR. The expression of emotion in man and animals. New York: Penguin Classics; 1872/2009.
45. Nesse RM, Bhatnagar S, Young EA. Evolutionary origins and functions of the stress response. In: Fink G, editor. Encyclopedia of stress. 2nd edition. Waltham (MA): Academic Press; 2007. p. 79–83.
46. Damasio AR. Descartes' error: emotion, reason, and the human brain. New York: Avon Books; 1994.
47. Dunn BD, Dalgleish T, Lawrence AD. The somatic marker hypothesis: a critical evaluation. Neurosci Biobehav Rev 2006;30(2):239–71. http://dx.doi.org/10.1016/j.neubiorev.2005.07.001.
48. Chikazoe J, Lee DH, Kriegeskorte N, et al. Population coding of affect across stimuli, modalities and individuals. Nat Neurosci 2013. http://dx.doi.org/10.1038/nn.3749.
49. Stanovich KE, West RF. Individual differences in reasoning: implications for the rationality debate? Behav Brain Sci 2000;23(5):665–726.
50. Kahneman D. Thinking fast and slow. New York: Farrar, Straus & Giroux; 2011.
51. Quirk GJ. Prefrontal-amygdala interactions in the regulation of fear. In: Gross JJ, editor. Handbook of emotion regulation. New York: Guilford Press; 2007. p. 27–46.
52. Gross JJ. Emotion regulation. In: Lewis M, Haviland-Jones JM, Barrett LF, editors. Handbook of emotions. 3rd edition. New York: Guilford Press; 2008. p. 497–512.
53. Campbell-Sills L, Barlow DH. Incorporating emotion regulation into conceptualizations and treatments of anxiety and mood disorders. In: Gross JJ, editor. Handbook of emotion regulation. New York: Guilford Press; 2007. p. 542–59.
54. Todd RM, Cunningham WA, Anderson AK, et al. Affect-based attention as emotion regulation. Trends Cogn Sci 2012;16(7):365–72. http://dx.doi.org/10.1016/j.tics.2012.06.003.
55. Panksepp J. At the interface of the affective, behavioral, and cognitive neurosciences: decoding the emotional feelings of the brain. Brain Cogn 2003;52(1):4–14. http://dx.doi.org/10.1016/S0278-2626(03)00003-4.
56. Schwabe L, Tegenthoff M, Höffken O, et al. Simultaneous glucocorticoid and noradrenergic activity disrupts the neural basis of goal-directed action in the human brain. J Neurosci 2012;32(30):10146–55. http://dx.doi.org/10.1523/jneurosci.1304-12-2012.
57. Rantala MJ, Moore FR, Skrinda I, et al. Evidence for the stress-linked immunocompetence handicap hypothesis in humans. Nat Commun 2012;3:694. http://dx.doi.org/10.1038/ncomms1696.
58. Sapolsky RM. Why zebras don't get ulcers. 3rd edition. New York: Holt Paperbacks; 2004.
59. Cantor D, Ramsden E. Introduction. In: Cantor D, Ramsden E, editors. Stress, shock, and adaptation in the twentieth century. Rochester (NY): University of Rochester Press; 2014. p. 1–18.
60. Eriksson A, Betti L, Friend AD, et al. Late Pleistocene climate change and the global expansion of anatomically modern humans. Proc Natl Acad Sci U S A 2012. http://dx.doi.org/10.1073/pnas.1209494109.

61. McEwen BS. Brain on stress: how the social environment gets under the skin. Proc Natl Acad Sci U S A 2012;109(Suppl 2):17180–5. http://dx.doi.org/10.1073/pnas.1121254109.

62. McEwen BS, Gianaros PJ. Central role of the brain in stress and adaptation: links to socioeconomic status, health, and disease. Ann N Y Acad Sci 2010; 1186:190–222. http://dx.doi.org/10.1111/j.1749-6632.2009.05331.x.

63. Whybrow PC. American mania: when more is not enough. New York: W.W. Norton & Co., Inc; 2005.

64. Gilbert P. Evolutionary psychopathology: why isn't the mind designed better than it is? Br J Med Psychol 1998;71(Pt 4):353–73.

65. Campbell J, Ehlert U. Acute psychosocial stress: does the emotional stress response correspond with physiological responses? Psychoneuroendocrinology 2012;37:1111–34. http://dx.doi.org/10.1016/j.psyneuen.2011.12.010.

66. Lucassen PJ, Pruessner J, Sousa N, et al. Neuropathology of stress. Acta Neuropathol 2014;127(1):109–35. http://dx.doi.org/10.1007/s00401-013-1223-5.

67. Folkow B. Psychosocial and central nervous influences in primary hypertension. Circulation 1987;76(Suppl I):1–10.

68. Folkow B. Mental "stress" and hypertension: evidence from animal and experimental studies. Integr Physiol Behav Sci 1991;26(4):305–8.

69. Wynne O, Sarkar DK. Stress and neuroendocrine-immune interaction. In: Kusnecov AW, Anisman H, editors. The Wiley-Blackwell handbook of psychoneuroimmunology. Hoboken (NJ): John Wiley & Sons; 2013. p. 198–211.

70. Greenberg J. Stress psychophysiology. In: Greenberg J, editor. Comprehensive stress management. 13th edition. New York: McGraw-Hill; 2013. p. 25–42.

71. Martin EI, Ressler KJ, Binder E, et al. The neurobiology of anxiety disorders: brain imaging, genetics, and psychoneuroendocrinology. Psychiatr Clin North Am 2009;32(3):549–75. http://dx.doi.org/10.1016/j.psc.2009.05.004.

72. Etkin A, Egner T, Kalisch R. Emotional processing in anterior cingulate and medial prefrontal cortex. Trends Cogn Sci 2011;15(2):85–93. http://dx.doi.org/10.1016/j.tics.2010.11.004.

73. Stein MB, Simmons AN, Feinstein JS, et al. Increased amygdala and insula activation during emotion processing in anxiety-prone subjects. Am J Psychiatry 2007;164(2):318–27.

74. Domschke K, Stevens S, Pfleiderer B, et al. Interoceptive sensitivity in anxiety and anxiety disorders: an overview and integration of neurobiological findings. Clin Psychol Rev 2010;30(1):1–11. http://dx.doi.org/10.1016/j.cpr.2009.08.008.

75. Hou R, Baldwin D. A neuroimmunological perspective on anxiety disorders. Hum Psychopharmacol 2012;27(1):6–14. http://dx.doi.org/10.1002/hup.1259.

76. Smitherman TA, Kolivas ED, Bailey JR. Panic disorder and migraine: comorbidity, mechanisms, and clinical implications. Headache 2013;53(1):23–45. http://dx.doi.org/10.1111/head.12004.

77. Simmons WK, Avery JA, Barcalow JC, et al. Keeping the body in mind: Insula functional organization and functional connectivity integrate interoceptive, exteroceptive, and emotional awareness. Hum Brain Mapp 2012. http://dx.doi.org/10.1002/hbm.22113.

78. Juster RP, McEwen BS, Lupien SJ. Allostatic load biomarkers of chronic stress and impact on health and cognition. Neurosci Biobehav Rev 2010;35:2–16. http://dx.doi.org/10.1016/j.neubiorev.2009.10.002.

79. Cuesta JM, Singer M. The stress response and critical illness: a review. Crit Care Med 2012;40(12):3283–9. http://dx.doi.org/10.1097/CCM.0b013e31826567eb.

80. Cohen S, Janicki-Deverts D, Doyle WJ, et al. Chronic stress, glucocorticoid receptor resistance, inflammation, and disease risk. Proc Natl Acad Sci U S A 2012. http://dx.doi.org/10.1073/pnas.1118355109.

81. Wohleb ES, Powell ND, Godbout JP, et al. Stress-induced recruitment of bone marrow-derived monocytes to the brain promotes anxiety-like behavior. J Neurosci 2013;33(34):13820–33. http://dx.doi.org/10.1523/jneurosci.1671-13. 2013.

82. Schroeder NE, Androwski RJ, Rashid A, et al. Dauer-specific dendrite arborization in *C. elegans* is regulated by KPC-1/Furin. Curr Biol 2013;23(16):1527–35. http://dx.doi.org/10.1016/j.cub. 2013.06.058.

83. Lanter BB, Sauer K, Davies DG. Bacteria present in carotid arterial plaques are found as biofilm deposits which may contribute to enhanced risk of plaque rupture. MBio 2014;5(3):e01206–14. http://dx.doi.org/10.1128/mBio.01206-14.

84. Rosen JB. The neurobiology of conditioned and unconditioned far: a neurobehavioral system analysis of the amygdala. Behav Cogn Neurosci Rev 2004; 3(1):23–41. http://dx.doi.org/10.1177/1534582304265945.

85. Nugent NR, Tyrka AR, Carpenter LL, et al. Gene-environment interactions: early life stress and risk for depressive and anxiety disorders. Psychopharmacology (Berl) 2011;214(1):176–96. http://dx.doi.org/10.1007/s00213-010-2151-x.

86. Rietschel L, Zhu G, Kirschbaum C, et al. Perceived stress has genetic influences distinct from neuroticism and depression. Behav Genet 2013. http://dx. doi.org/10.1007/s10519-013-9636-4.

87. Domschke K, Maron E. Genetic factors in anxiety disorders. In: Baldwin DS, Leonard BE, editors. Anxiety disorders. Basel (CH): Karger; 2013. p. 24–46. http://dx.doi.org/10.1159/000351932.

88. Maron E, Hettema JM, Shlik J. The genetics of human anxiety disorders. In: Blanchard RJ, Blanchard DC, Griebel G, et al, editors. Handbook of anxiety and fear, vol. 17. Amsterdam: Elsevier; 2008. p. 475–510. http://dx.doi.org/10. 1016/S1569-7339(07)00022-7.

89. Kendler KS, Eaves LJ, Loken EK, et al. The impact of environmental experiences on symptoms of anxiety and depression across the life span. Psychol Sci 2011; 22(10):1343–52. http://dx.doi.org/10.1177/0956797611417255.

90. Merikangas KR, Pine D. Genetic and other vulnerability factors for anxiety and stress disorders. In: Davis KL, Charney D, Coyle JT, et al, editors. Neuropsychopharmacology: the fifth generation of progress. Philadelphia: Lippincott Williams & Wilkins; 2002. p. 867–82.

91. Hunter RG, McEwen BS. Stress and anxiety across the lifespan: structural plasticity and epigenetic regulation. Epigenomics 2013;5(2):177–94. http://dx. doi.org/10.2217/epi.13.8.

92. McEwen BS, Gianaros PJ. Stress- and allostasis-induced brain plasticity. Annu Rev Med 2011;62:431–45. http://dx.doi.org/10.1146/annurev-med-052209-100430.

93. Shin LM, Liberzon I. The neurocircuitry of fear, stress, and anxiety disorders. Neuropsychopharmacology 2010;35(1):169–91. http://dx.doi.org/10.1038/npp. 2009.83.

94. Difede J, Olden M, Cukor J. Evidence-based treatment of post-traumatic stress disorder. Annu Rev Med 2014;65:319–32. http://dx.doi.org/10.1146/annurev-med-051812-145438.

95. Pitman RK, Rasmusson AM, Koenen KC, et al. Biological studies of post-traumatic stress disorder. Nat Rev Neurosci 2012;13:769–87. http://dx.doi.org/ 10.1038/nrn3339.

96. Morrison FG, Ressler KJ. From the neurobiology of extinction to improved clinical treatments. Depress Anxiety 2014;31(4):279–90. http://dx.doi.org/10.1002/da.22214.

97. Etkin A. Neurobiology of anxiety: from neural circuits to novel solutions? Depress Anxiety 2012;29(5):355–8. http://dx.doi.org/10.1002/da.21957.

98. Thibodeau MA, Gómez-Pérez L, Asmundson GJ. Objective and perceived arousal during performance of tasks with elements of social threat: the influence of anxiety sensitivity. J Behav Ther Exp Psychiatry 2012;43(3):967–74. http://dx.doi.org/10.1016/j.jbtep.2012.03.001.

99. Bateson M, Brilot B, Nettle D. Anxiety: an evolutionary approach. Can J Psychiatry 2011;56(12):707–15.

100. Samanez-Larkin GR, Hollon NG, Carstensen LL, et al. Individual differences in insular sensitivity during loss anticipation predict avoidance learning. Psychol Sci 2008;19(4):320–3. http://dx.doi.org/10.111/j.1467-9280.2008.02087.x.

101. Herry C, Ferraguti F, Singewald N, et al. Neuronal circuits of fear extinction. Eur J Neurosci 2010;31(4):599–612. http://dx.doi.org/10.1111/j.1460-9568.2010.07101.x.

102. Bredy TW, Sun YE, Kobor MS. How the epigenome contributes to the development of psychiatric disorders. Dev Psychobiol 2010;52(4):331–42. http://dx.doi.org/10.1002/dev.20424.

103. Graham BM, Milad MR. The study of fear extinction: implications for anxiety disorders. Am J Psychiatry 2011;168(12):1255–65. http://dx.doi.org/10.1176/appi.ajp.2011.11040557.

104. Hermans D, Craske MG, Mineka S, et al. Extinction in human fear conditioning. Biol Psychiatry 2006;60(4):361–8. http://dx.doi.org/10.1016/j.biopsych.2005.10.006.

105. Craske MG, Vervliet B. Extinction learning and its retrieval. In: Hermans D, Rimé B, Mesquita I, editors. Changing emotions. New York: Psychology Press; 2013. p. 53–9.

106. Wang Z, Chen LM, Négyessy L, et al. The relationship of anatomical and functional connectivity to resting-state connectivity in primate somatosensory cortex. Neuron 2013;78(6):1116–26. http://dx.doi.org/10.1016/j.neuron.2013.04.023.

107. Rabinovich MI, Muezzinoglu MK, Strigo I, et al. Dynamical principles of emotion-cognition interaction: mathematical images of mental disorders. PLoS One 2010;5(9):e12547. http://dx.doi.org/10.1371/journal.pone.0012547.

108. Simmons A, Strigo I, Matthews SC, et al. Anticipation of aversive visual stimuli is associated with increased insula activation in anxiety-prone subjects. Biol Psychiatry 2006;60(4):402–9. http://dx.doi.org/10.1016/j.biopsych.2006.04.038.

109. Woody SR, Nosen E. Psychological models of phobic disorders and panic. In: Anthony MM, Stein MB, editors. Oxford handbook of anxiety and related disorders. Oxford (United Kingdom): Oxford University Press; 2009. p. 209–24.

110. Schultz LT, Heimberg RG. Attentional focus in social anxiety disorder: potential for interactive processes. Clin Psychol Rev 2008;28(7):1206–21. http://dx.doi.org/10.1016/j.cpr.2008.04.003.

111. Miskovic V, Schmidt LA. Social fearfulness in the human brain. Neurosci Biobehav Rev 2012;36(1):459–78. http://dx.doi.org/10.1016/j.neubiorev.2011.08.002.

112. Bystritsky A, Khalsa SS, Cameron ME, et al. Current diagnosis and treatment of anxiety disorders. P T 2013;38(1):30–57.

113. Khalsa SS, Rudrauf D, Feinstein JS, et al. The pathways of interoceptive awareness. Nat Neurosci 2009;12(12):1494–6. http://dx.doi.org/10.1038/nn.2411.

114. Kronemyer D, Bystritsky A. A non-linear dynamical approach to belief revision in cognitive behavioral therapy. Front Comput Neurosci 2014;8:55. http://dx.doi.org/10.3389/fncom.2014.00055.

115. Ochsner KN, Gross JJ. Cognitive emotion regulation: insights from social cognitive and affective neuroscience. Curr Dir Psychol Sci 2008;17(2):153–8.

116. Ortony A, Clore GL, Collins A. The cognitive structure of emotions. Cambridge (United Kingdom): Cambridge University Press; 1990.

117. Pessoa L. On the relationship between emotion and cognition. Nat Rev Neurosci 2008;9(2):148–58. http://dx.doi.org/10.1038/nrn2317.

118. Plasencia ML, Alden LE, Taylor CT. Differential effects of safety behaviour subtypes in social anxiety disorder. Behav Res Ther 2011;49(10):665–75. http://dx.doi.org/10.1016/j.brat.2011.07.005.

119. Taylor CT, Alden LE. Safety behaviors and judgmental biases in social anxiety disorder. Behav Res Ther 2010;48(3):226–37. http://dx.doi.org/10.1016/j.brat.2009.11.005.

120. Newman MG, Llera SJ. A novel theory of experiential avoidance in generalized anxiety disorder: a review and synthesis of research supporting a contrast avoidance model of worry. Clin Psychol Rev 2011;31(3):371–82. http://dx.doi.org/10.1016/j.cpr.2011.01.008.

121. Olthius JV, Stewart SH, Watt MC, et al. Anxiety sensitivity and negative interpretation biases: their shared and unique associations with anxiety disorders. J Psychopathol Behav Assess 2012;34(3):332–42. http://dx.doi.org/10.1007/s10862-012-9286-5.

122. Smits JA, Berry AC, Tart CD, et al. The efficacy of cognitive-behavioral interventions for reducing anxiety sensitivity: a meta-analytic review. Behav Res Ther 2008;46(9):1047–54. http://dx.doi.org/10.1016/j.brat.2008.06.010.

123. Craske MG, Barlow DH, O'Leary TA. Mastery of your anxiety and worry. San Antonio (TX): Harcourt Brace/Graywind; 1992.

124. Zalta AK, Foa EB. Exposure therapy: promoting emotional processing of pathological anxiety. In: O'Donohue WT, Fisher JE, editors. Cognitive behavioral therapy: core principles for practice. New York: John Wiley & Sons; 2012. p. 75–104.

125. Taleb NN. Antifragile–things that gain from disorder. New York: Random House; 2012.

126. Bystritsky A, Nierenberg AA, Feusner JD, et al. Computational non-linear dynamical psychiatry: a new methodological paradigm for diagnosis and course of illness. J Psychiatr Res 2012;46(4):428–35. http://dx.doi.org/10.1016/j.psychires.2011.10.013.

127. Rose RD, Buckey JC Jr, Zbozinek TD, et al. A randomized controlled trial of a self-guided, multimedia, stress management and resilience training program. Behav Res Ther 2013;51(2):106–12. http://dx.doi.org/10.1016/j.brat.2012.11.003.

128. Bullis JR, Bøe HJ, Asnaani A, et al. The benefits of being mindful: trait mindfulness predicts less reactivity to suppression. J Behav Ther Exp Psychiatry 2014; 45(1):57–66. http://dx.doi.org/10.1016/j.jbtep.2013.07.006.

129. Kasala ER, Bodduluru LN, Maneti Y, et al. Effect of meditation on neurophysiological changes in stress mediated depression. Complement Ther Clin Pract 2014;20(1):74–80. http://dx.doi.org/10.1016/j.ctcp.2013.10.001.

130. Creswell JD, Pacilio LE, Lindsay EK, et al. Brief mindfulness meditation training alters psychological and neuroendocrine responses to social evaluative stress. Psychoneuroendocrinology 2014;44:1–12. http://dx.doi.org/10.1016/j.psyneuen.2014.02.007.

131. Hölzel BK, Lazar SW, Gard T, et al. How does mindfulness meditation work? Proposing mechanisms of action from a conceptual and neural perspective. Perspect Psychol Sci 2011;6(6):53759. http://dx.doi.org/10.1177/1745691611 419671.

132. Goyal M, Singh S, Sibinga EM, et al. Meditation programs for psychological stress and well-being: a systematic review and meta-analysis. JAMA Intern Med 2014; 174(3):357–68. http://dx.doi.org/10.1001/jamainternmed.2013.13018.

The Effect of Severe Stress on Early Brain Development, Attachment, and Emotions

A Psychoanatomical Formulation

Ricardo M. Vela, MD

KEYWORDS

- Child abuse • Child neglect • Limbic system development • Emotions • Attachment
- Amygdala • Psychoanatomical formulation

KEY POINTS

- Child abuse and neglect are the most severe forms of stress experienced by children and adolescents.
- Child abuse and neglect has severe developmental consequences to the development of the amygdala, septal nucleus, and anterior cingulate gyrus, which are rapidly developing, especially in very early infancy.
- The basic emotions of joy, surprise, sadness, anger, and fear develop in the first 6 months of life. Embarrassment, envy, empathy, pride, shame, and guilt (which requires self-consciousness) develop by 3 years of age.
- Synaptic modification and consolidation is very vulnerable during the experience-expectant, sensitive developmental periods. Child maltreatment may have severe consequences, resulting in maladaptive cell assemblies and synaptic connections.
- The psychoanatomical formulation is a theoretically based explanation used to conceptualize a clinical case by correlating the disturbed neuroanatomy with behavioral and emotional symptom expression. It provides the clinician with an added dimension in understanding a clinical case.

Child neglect and abuse are the most extreme forms of stress in children, with severe effects on social, emotional, interpersonal, and neuronal development. According to the US Department of Health and Human Services, from data submitted by 49 states, the District of Columbia, and the Commonwealth of Puerto Rico, there were 3,184,000 children who received child protective services in 2012. Overall, four-fifths (78.3%) of victims were neglected, 18.3% were physically abused, 9.3% were sexually abused,

Disclosures: The author does not have any commercial conflicts to disclose.
Child and Family Services, North Suffolk Mental Health Association, Massachusetts General Hospital, 301 Broadway, Chelsea, MA 02150, USA
E-mail address: rvela@mgh.harvard.edu

Psychiatr Clin N Am 37 (2014) 519–534
http://dx.doi.org/10.1016/j.psc.2014.08.005
0193-953X/14/$ – see front matter © 2014 Elsevier Inc. All rights reserved.

Abbreviations	
DSM-IV	Diagnostic and Statistical Manual of Mental Disorders, Fourth Edition
DSM-V	Diagnostic and Statistical Manual of Mental Disorders, Fifth Edition
EBS	Electrical brain stimulation
LTP	Long-term potentiation
NIMH	National Institute of Mental Health
PAG	Periaqueductal gray matter
PTSD	Posttraumatic stress disorder

and 8.5% were psychologically maltreated.[1] Child neglect is associated with adverse psychological and educational outcomes and it is hypothesized that these outcomes may be caused by adverse brain development.[2] Early life trauma is associated with persistent developmental brain changes that mediate the increased diathesis not only to mood and anxiety disorders but also to depression, posttraumatic stress disorder (PTSD), schizophrenia, and bipolar disorder.[3]

Animal and human studies have expanded knowledge of the emotional or limbic system, and provided insight into how normal and abnormal development unfolds. This article introduces the concept of the psychoanatomical formulation, developed by the author and defined as a theoretically based explanation used to conceptualize a clinical case by correlating the disturbed neuroanatomy with behavioral and emotional symptom expression. Following the vignette of a neglected 2.5-year-old child, the development and function of limbic structures involved in emotions and attachment is discussed, with emphasis on the first year of life. Next, the emergence of basic emotions in children from birth to 3 years is reviewed, followed by a discussion of basic principles of neural and synaptic development and their implications for child abuse and neglect. In addition, the developmental neuroanatomy of child neglect is brought together in the context of the psychoanatomical formulation of the case vignette.

CLINICAL VIGNETTE: A 2.5-YEAR-OLD GIRL WITH DISINHIBITED SOCIAL ENGAGEMENT DISORDER

Amy was 2.5 years old when her adoptive parents brought her to the child psychiatry clinic for evaluation and treatment of her emotional and behavioral problems, after requesting a referral from the pediatrician. The child appeared to be oblivious of danger and very accident prone. She would fall a lot; bump into furniture and walls; scream inconsolably, sometimes for an hour; and fight with her 4-year-old and 5-year-old adoptive brothers. Amy showed difficult behavior and frequent temper tantrums at the Head Start program she attended. She had out-of-control episodes, being aggressive, biting other children and, overall, being unpredictable. Her adoptive parents were appropriately concerned because Amy often went to strangers and was very friendly with them. On several occasions, she tried to leave the house with strangers who came to the door. She did not seem to show any wariness of unfamiliar people.

Past history revealed that Amy was born to Latino parents with no perinatal complications. Her biological father had been in jail since before Amy was born. Early history revealed disruptive, unstable, and chaotic child rearing. She was under the care of her biological mother from birth until 5 months of age. During that time her mother neglected taking care of her and failed to provide basic emotional needs for affection and reliable mother-child interactions. Her mother left her with multiple caregivers. She was moved consecutively to different homes of a relative and a friend before the Department of Social Services got involved when Amy was 20 months old. She was then placed with the current adoptive parents.

Medical evaluation did not show signs of physical or sexual abuse. There was no history of sexualized play. However, because language was delayed, knowing fewer than 50 intelligible words, she was referred for early intervention services. In a short period of time her speech showed improvement. She started putting 2-word phrases together and repeated phrases. She looked at people when they called her name, was affectionate with loved ones, and liked to be held often. She played appropriately with toys. However, she had trouble adjusting to change and continued to be aggressive toward other children, often hitting or biting them. She continued to have no sense of danger, banging into objects and falling from furniture she climbed, even though gross motor coordination was age appropriate. She continued to go up to unknown people indiscriminately, in spite of repeated warnings by her adoptive mother and father.

EMOTIONS, ATTACHMENT, LIMBIC NUCLEI DEVELOPMENT AND FUNCTIONS, AND TRANSITION PERIODS DURING EARLY INFANCY

In spite of controversies and open criticism by some neuroscientists,[4,5] the term limbic system, which MacLean[6] used to replace the old term rhinencephalon, has persisted in the neurologic, psychiatric, and neurobiological literature, to denote the structures that participate in generating emotions. The limbic system has become synonymous with the emotional system.[7] Five limbic structures have been posited to play a principal role in emotional expression and attachment behavior in the first year of life: hypothalamus, amygdala, septal nuclei, anterior cingulate gyrus, and hippocampus.[8] These structures form a circuit involved in the hierarchical control of emotions, with the anterior cingulate playing the role of an integrative cortical suprastructure, whereas, at the lower end, the hypothalamus (and periaqueductal gray matter [PAG]) act as a funnel through which all limbic-generated emotions are eventually expressed.[9] We argue later that child neglect and/or abuse lead to abnormal limbic development and, consequently, to severe psychological disorder. Concepts and evidence discussed here are used to provide a theoretic framework for the case using the psychoanatomical formulation.

According to Kagan and Baird[10] there are some correspondences between brain maturation and the ontogeny of human psychological competencies from birth to puberty, with significant maturational transitions that occur at specific ages. The first maturational transition period occurs at 2 to 3 months of postnatal life and is characterized by the disappearance of newborn reflexes, secondary to cortical inhibition of brain stem neurons and appearance of new synaptic contacts. There is a growth of inhibitory interneurons in the spinal cord that corresponds with the disappearance of these reflexes. There is a concomitant reduction in crying and an increase in social smiling that can probably be attributed to cortical inhibition of brain stem nuclei that mediate crying, especially in the PAG. Together with these developments, the infant shows the possibility of establishing visual expectations. This stage coincides with a great increase in the growth velocity of the mossy cells of the dentate gyrus of the hippocampus.[10]

Hypothalamus

The hypothalamus is almost fully developed at birth, and controls emotions in the newborn infant. It is the central core through which all emotions derive their motive force.[11] Endocrine, hormonal, visceral, and autonomic functions controlled by the hypothalamus are of utmost importance for the survival of the human infant. Paralleling these biological functions, and crucially important for the emotional survival, development, and attachment to the caregiver, are the emotional functions of the hypothalamus. Through this structure the newborn infant is capable of expressing aversion versus pleasure and rage versus quiescence. Vocalizations initially produced by the hypothalamus elicit maternal behaviors that attend to the basic needs of the infant, provide comfort, and are alerts to the need to be fed and cared for.

The hypothalamus consists of a complex number of nuclei, each with its subdivisions. However, in their extensive work on the neuroanatomy of the hypothalamus, Crosby and Woodbourne,[12] Crosby and Showers,[13] and Nauta and Haymaker[14] indicated that, for purposes of description, hypothalamic cell groups could be classified or subdivided into 3 longitudinal zones: periventricular, medial, and lateral.

The periventricular area is intrinsically associated with the neurohormonal control of the pituitary gland, and, as for stress, it plays a major role in the hypothalamic-pituitary-adrenal axis and is critically involved in the adaptation to stressful changes. From the point of view of the functional neuroanatomy of emotions, the medial and lateral nuclei play antagonistic but complementary functions. Electrical brain stimulation (EBS) with electrodes placed in the medial hypothalamic area in cats (and ventrolateral areas as well) resulted in what Flynn[15] called "attack with rage." Now called affective aggression, it is manifested by rage display (eg, hissing and growling), autonomic changes (eg, pupillary dilatation, piloerection), but at the same time with an aversion component, because trained cats try to stop the apparently unpleasant stimulation. A rat sharing the cage would not be hurt, as if the aggressive display was all for show.[9,15]

In contrast with EBS to the medial hypothalamic area, electrical stimulation of the lateral hypothalamic areas (specifically the dorsolateral area) elicited what Flynn[15] called "quiet biting attacks," which are now described in the scientific literature as predatory aggression. Cats stimulated with brain electrodes in this area move swiftly, with the nose close to the ground, stalking and going directly to the rat in the cage.

It may be useful clinically to conceptualize aggression under the subdivisions of predatory versus affective, because clinical assessment of the nature of aggression is often in one of these categories. Predatory aggression is goal oriented, planned, and controlled. The perpetrators hide their aggressive acts. The aggressors can control their aggressive acts. At the end, the predatory aggressors are proud of having been aggressive. This kind of aggression is seen in sociopathic behavior.

In contrast, affective aggression is reactive, unplanned, and uncontrolled. The aggressors may damage their own property with disregard to its value. They may be aggressive and lose control in front of other people, oblivious of shame in the heat of the moment. The aggressors expose themselves to physical harm. Children may fight with bigger, stronger children, disregarding the risk of being hurt. Aggression seems unplanned and to take place without an ultimate purpose. The aggressors may express remorse after the aggressive act.

EBS studies have the limitation that electrical stimulation may stimulate hundreds of thousands of emotions. A new, sophisticated technique developed by Karl Deisseroth and Ed Boyden at Stanford University can selectively stimulate a specially selected group of neurons (or their projection-specific dynamics) consisting of a promoter gene to an opsin (light-sensitive receptor) gene, which forms a construct that is expressed only on the specifically selected neuronal subpopulation (but not neighboring cells) when light is delivered to the brain through a fiberoptic cable (for a review see Tye and Deisseroth[16] and Fennol and colleagues[17]).

Using a variation of this technique, it has been shown that optogenetic stimulation of the ventromedial hypothalamus, ventrolateral part, causes mice to attack male and female mice and inanimate objects.[18] Optogenetic tools in the future will establish areas of dysfunction in psychiatric disease that are impossible to establish by any other means.[19]

According to Kagan and Baird's[10] ontogenetic model, the second transition occurs in most healthy infants between the ages of 7 and 12 months. During this period the infant is increasingly able to retrieve schemata (patterns of parents' physical features) and holds them along with current perceptions in a working memory circuit.[10] Separation fear occurs when the infant retrieves a schema of the mother's former presence held in a working memory circuit and tries to relate this to the discrepant perception of her current absence. Growth and development of the amygdala and prefrontal cortex are likely to be relevant to separation and stranger fear. Axonal projections from the amygdala to the anterior cingulate cortex through the capsula interna myelinize between postnatal months 7 and 10. This process coincides with the emergence of fears of strangers of separation from a caretaker.[10]

Amygdala

Experiments producing selective amygdala lesions in stressed infant monkeys, starting at 2 weeks of age, showed no difference in mother-infant interactions at 3 months of age. However, the one consistent and robust finding in both animal and human studies is that damage to the amygdala results in impairment in the danger-detection systems.[20–23]

The amygdala therefore plays a modulating role in social behaviors. The role of the amygdala as the detector of danger is to continuously evaluate the environment and surroundings for potential threats. These functions extend to social situations and generate appropriate physiologic/emotional responses.[23] Expanding on this concept, Buchanan and colleagues[24] postulated that what influences amygdala function is the unpredictable nature of social interactions. Damage to the amygdala results in inappropriate responses to ambiguous social cues.[24] Neonatal amygdala damage results in an inability to assess the degree of danger of a social situation and to modify behavior appropriately.[24]

Receiving sensory inputs from different parts of the brain, the amygdala monitors and abstracts the motivational significance from a wide array of multimodal sensory stimuli, from food to discrete social-emotional nuances.[11] It processes and funnels emotionally relevant sensory information from multiple neocortical and limbic areas and sends the processed data to the hypothalamus and brain stem, eliciting autonomic, endocrine, and emotional responses.[7] It responds mainly to danger/negative stimuli that evoke fear or defensive reactions but also responds to positive stimuli such as sexual attraction, positive emotional words, and appetizing foods.[7] It is responsive to somesthetic input and physical contact, both of which are necessary for maternal-infant bonding and the normal development of the amygdala.[8]

In general, there is a lateral-to-medial unidirectional flow and processing of information.[4,25] The lateral nucleus receives information from the neocortex and projects it to the basal and accessory basal nuclei, which in turn project it to the medial and central nuclei and form an output to visceral and autonomic regions. The centromedial amygdaloid complex forms a macrostructure with cell columns through the substantia innominata, including the bed nucleus of the stria terminalis portions of the nucleus accumbens, all of which makes up the extended amygdala.[26]

The amygdala analyzes information and transfers it back to the neocortex, with which it has extensive interconnections including the orbitofrontal and anterior cingulate gyrus. It projects to a much greater region of the neocortex than what it receives from the neocortex.[25] Hence, the normal amygdala is primarily wired to be able to adaptively sense, react, analyze, and respond to dangerous stimuli, rather than soothing and calming the individual. According to Amaral,[27] the amygdala is a protective device, designed to detect and avoid danger. It evaluates objects in the surroundings before interacting with them, and, based on this evaluation, coordinates species-typical responses.

The complexity of the small, almond-shaped amygdala cannot be overstated. It is heterogeneous in neurochemical organization, with rich intrinsic and extrinsic chemical neuroanatomy. The amygdala has the highest density of gamma-aminobutyric acid A receptors; a rich distribution of opiate receptors; and expresses as many neurotransmitters, peptides, and calcium-binding proteins as do the neurons in the neocortex.[25] Two major fiber systems, the stria terminalis and the ventral amygdalofugal pathway, connect the amygdala with the hypothalamus and other limbic structures involved in emotional expression.[28] In contrast with the hypothalamus, which can be immediately turned on and off, stimulation of the amygdala produces longer-lasting mood states after cessation of electrical stimulation.[11]

In the monkey, the amygdala receives input from area TE located in the anterior portion of the inferior temporal cortex. Area TE carries information from primary visual area V1, and comes at the end of the ventral stream of hierarchical visual processing. It is most responsive to complex visual objects like faces. It terminates in the lateral nucleus of the amygdala, which projects to the adjacent basal nucleus.[25] In the human brain, it is the fusiform gyrus that carries information of faces to the amygdala for processing. Social recognition requires the ability to recognize and remember other people before forming social relationships.[29] Lesions in the fusiform gyrus can abolish the ability to recognize faces. The right amygdala has a critical role in processing the emotional content of stimuli, including fearful facial expressions.[24,25,30]

The amygdala has a well-documented primary involvement in conditioned fear[4,31] and is prominently activated in response to fearful faces in subjects with PTSD compared with normal controls.[32]

Bilateral damage to the amygdala can result in an extreme lack of fear of dangerous stimuli and social situations. The case of S.M., a 44-year-old woman with bilateral amygdala damage as a result of lipoid proteinosis (Urbach-Wiethe disease), has been extensively studied.[33] She showed no fear of snakes and poisonous spiders when taken to an exotic pet shop. She was oblivious of danger when attacked with a knife in a park. She had an excessive degree of approach behavior and had a compulsive desire to touch and poke dangerous snakes, finding all of this interesting and amusing.[33]

Septal Nuclei

The septal nucleus attains greatest evolutionary development in humans. It is involved in emotional functioning and, like the amygdala and cingulate gyrus, it is capable of producing emotional vocalizations that may elicit care. It maintains a counterbalancing relationship with the amygdala, with antagonistic influence on the hypothalamus. The septal nucleus facilitates actions of the medial hypothalamus (whereas the amygdala mainly activates the lateral hypothalamus). It reduces extremes in emotionality and arousal and maintains a state of quiescence and readiness. It counters and inhibits aggressive behavior and suppresses expression of rage reactions following hypothalamic stimulations.[11] The septal nucleus exerts inhibitory influences on the amygdala, whereas the amygdala acts to facilitate or inhibit septal functions.[11] Development of the septal nuclei and anterior cingulate gyrus enable human infants to slowly develop a stable and selective loving attachment and, at around 6 months to 1 year of age, to show expressions of anger, joy, and fear. Normal, intact septal nuclei act to promote selective social attachments that are strengthened through positive reinforcement and caring parent-child interactions.

The septal nuclei undergo a more protracted rate of development than the cingulate gyrus. They do not reach adult levels of development until 3 years of age and continue developing into puberty.[8]

Anterior Cingulate Gyrus

The cingulum, formed by fibers from the cingulate gyrus, starts myelination in the second postnatal month, and completes its cycle of myelination about the end of the first postnatal year.[34] Through 7 to 8 months of age the septal nuclei and cingulate gyrus continue their development. The infant becomes more discriminating in interactions with others. Real and specific attachments are formed with the infant's caretaker.[8] Human attachment consequently becomes progressively more intense and stable as new synaptic connections are formed and reinforced.

From 9 to 12 months, the septal nuclei and cingulate gyrus development continues, together with that of the amygdala, which generates protective fear. About 90% of normal infants develop separation anxiety during these months. Indiscriminate social contact seeking is inhibited. Specific attachments are narrowed, strengthened, reinforced, and maintained.[8,11]

The anterior cingulate gyrus is thus of utmost importance in the formation of long-term attachments and maternal behavior. It participates with other limbic structures in the production of emotional sounds and the separation cry. Sounds generated by the infant promote intimate maternal behavior that responds, attends, and cares for the infant's needs, discomforts, or primitive emotions. A dyadic interplay seems to take place, because the sounds generated by the infant's anterior cingulate generate maternal instinctual feelings of tenderness, urgency, or care for the child. Destruction of the mother's anterior cingulate in nonhuman primates results in the loss of maternal responsiveness to the point that, if not rescued, infants may die from lack of care.[11] It is capable of processing and modulating expressions of emotional nuances, which is critical in the individual's response and adaptation in a social environment.[7]

During the first year of life, and before developing the capacity to express meaningful words, the infant develops what Joseph[8,11] calls the limbic language. Emotional sounds are initially produced by the hypothalamus, which, as mentioned previously, is fully functional at birth. The amygdala, septal nuclei, and cingulate gyrus are also capable of generating emotional sounds as they continue to mature during the first year of life. Socializations concomitantly become more complex and reflect specific mood states.[8,11]

The anterior cingulate gyrus, the largest limbic structure, functions in affective, autonomic, cognitive, social, and motor and motivational behavior.[7] It is a cortical suprastructure capable of initiating voluntary behavior and is able to produce emotional sounds that are not reflective of mood. As children grow older they develop more flexibility and increased voluntary control, and can mask a feeling state or deceptively pretend to have a different emotion.[8,11] Toddlers, aged 1 to 3 years, can whine, exaggerate feeling states, or simply imitate emotional sounds in order to manipulate a social situation, obtain a reward, or change the other person's behaviors; they can become experts at this.

Hippocampus

The hippocampus plays a major role in the storage and consolidation of information into long-term memory. It is of utmost importance in learning and memory encoding, providing long-term storage and retrieval of newly learned information.[7,11] The hippocampus has an intimate relationship with septal nuclei with which it is connected by fibers from the precommissural fornix. In concert with the medial hypothalamus and septal nuclei, it prevents extremes in arousal and maintains quiet alertness.[11] It is greatly influenced by the amygdala. It interacts with the amygdala in generating emotional imagery and is of paramount importance in learning and memory.[7,11] The amygdala and the hippocampus function in synchrony. Although the amygdala plays an important role in mediating emotional memory, the hippocampus has a major role in the organization of episodic memory.[35] Thus the hippocampus has an interdependent memory role with the amygdala. The amygdala is responsible for storing emotional aspects and personal reactions to events.[11] Functional imaging studies show that the amygdala becomes active when recalling personal and emotional memories. The hippocampus has a major role in contextual fear conditioning, contributing to the formation and retention of contextual fear associations.[4,31] There is a bidirectional neural communication between the hippocampus and the amygdala, which may provide the pathway of emotional reactions to contextual cues imparting emotional meaning to the context.[31] Projections from the amygdala to the hippocampal formation are stronger than vice versa, indicating that the amygdala provides an additional type of sensory information that is not reciprocated; perhaps the species-specific significance to an event.[25] The hippocampus interacts with the prefrontal cortex to recruit specific memories to guide planning and strategizing.[35]

In early infancy the greatest increase in the rate of growth of the hippocampus occurs between 2 and 3 months; the mossy cells of the hippocampus dentate gyrus undergo a spurt of differentiation. This differentiation probably contributes to the increased ability of a 2-month-old infant to recognize an event following a delay, and for a 3-month-old to establish expectations.[10]

EMOTIONAL ONTOGENY: FROM ZERO TO 3 YEARS

Emotions are almost fully developed by the age of 3 years, although further refinement and elaboration of emotions may take over after that time.[36] Thus, the first 3 years of life represent the major developmental leap in the emergence of human emotions.[36]

As previously discussed, the hypothalamus is almost fully developed at birth and is responsible for generating primitive emotions. At birth, children show what has been called a bipolar emotional life[36] (here, the term bipolar is not used to describe a mood disorder, but the manifestation of 2 distinct emotional poles). Although the newborn can show general distress manifested by crying and irritability (the negative pole), there is also pleasure reflected by satiation, attention, and responsivity to the environment, which represents the positive pole of this bipolar dichotomy.

The development of the social smile by the age of 3 months marks the emergence of joy in human infants. They show happiness and excitement (active and wiggling) when exposed to familiar or unfamiliar faces or even a cardboard Halloween mask when frontally presented.[37] During the same time, sadness emerges. Three-month-old infants react with sadness when their mothers stop interacting with them or on withdrawal of positive-stimulus events.[36] Infants react with joy and smiling when positioned in front of their mother's face. On the mother's presentation of a still face, 8-month-old babies first try to engage mothers by gesturing, making noises, and other maneuvers to attract the mother's attention. If the mother reengages in the interaction, the child's joy returns. However, if mothers are not available to reassume interactions with their infants, the results can severely impair the child's emotional development. Distaste, the precursor of disgust, also appears around this age and is manifested by spitting out and getting rid of unpleasant tastes in the mouth. Although some clinicians consider this to be evidence of disgust,[36] others have argued that true disgust does not appear as a separate emotion until the child is 4 to 8 years old.[38,39]

Anger emerges between 4 and 6 months of age. Anger is the adaptive action pattern that has evolved to enable humans to overcome a barrier to a goal. Anger thus results when the goal is blocked. Experiments with 4-month-old infants have shown that anger is manifested when children are frustrated (eg, when their hands are tied down and prevented from moving).[36] Anger expressions are targeted at other people by 7 months.[40]

Fearfulness emerges at around the age of 8 to 9 months. In order to develop fear, infants have to have the capacity to compare the event that frightens them with another event. For example, in the case of stranger anxiety, infants have to compare the face of the stranger with the mental representation of familiar faces. Fear results when there is a discrepancy between the new (stranger) face and the mental representations of familiar faces. Before developing this cognitive capacity, infants do not fear stranger faces, or even, as mentioned earlier, masks of human faces.

Surprise is another emotion that appears in the first 6 months. Children show a surprise response either when there is a violation of expected events or as a response to discovery. For example, when infants see a midget walking toward them, they show interest and surprise (rather than joy or fear), as a result of the discrepancy of seeing a small adult.[36]

The emergence of self-awareness during the second half of the second year of life gives rise to self-conscious emotions. These emotions include embarrassment, empathy, and envy. The emergence of embarrassment only takes place after children develop self-recognition. Embarrassment is measured by nervous touching, smiling, gaze aversion, and return behaviors.[36] Shame is closely related to embarrassment, but it is a more intense emotion accompanied by the wish to hide, disappear, or die and is a highly and painful emotional state that is difficult to dissipate.[41] Shame requires self-evaluation, which is a higher cognitive level than self-recognition or the consciousness that is required for the emotion of embarrassment. True empathy or veridical empathy develops at the end of the second year into the third year, when children become more aware that others can have their own thoughts, feelings, and desires.[42]

Self-conscious evaluative emotions require children to have the capacity to evaluate their behavior against a standard. This cognitive capacity emerges between 2 and 3 years of age. Besides shame, these complex social-evaluative emotions include pride and guilt. Evaluating self-conscious emotions of failure may result in shame, guilt, or regret, whereas self-perceived success gives rise to feelings of pride.

Therefore, by 3 years of age, normal children have formed the basis for an elaborate and complex emotional system that will expand in the years to come.[36] However, this normal development can be disrupted by excessive stress in infants or children as a result of neglect, physical or sexual abuse, or witnessing domestic violence. Individuals with poor attachment histories display empathy disorders: limited capacity to perceive the emotional state of others.[43]

PRINCIPLES OF NEURONAL DEVELOPMENT: IMPLICATIONS FOR CHILD ABUSE AND NEGLECT

The effect of child abuse and neglect on the limbic brain development at the cellular level can be conceptualized and organized under 4 closely interrelated developmental principles:

1. Hebbian synaptic modification
2. Experience-expectant learning
3. Sensitive periods of development
4. Self-organizing brain development

Influenced by the work of Spanish neurophysiologist Rafael Lorente de Nó, Canadian psychologist Donald Hebb[44] insightfully described a hypothetical mechanism of synaptic transmission that is still valid today. This hypothesis may be summarized as follows: synaptic knobs between communicating neurons develop with persistent neural activity and result in a lower synaptic resistance. The greater the contact area, the greater the chances that the action potential of the presynaptic cell will be decisive in firing another postsynaptic signal. The extent of the contact established is thus a function of joint cellular activity. As a result of the increased area of contact, firing of the efferent cell is more likely to follow the lead of the afferent cell.[44] Synaptic changes result in the consistent firing of 2 connecting neurons. Any 2-cell systems that are repeatedly active at the same time tend to become associated, forming what Hebb[44] called the cell assembly. These groups of reciprocally connected cells are simultaneously activated by the internal representation of an external event or object. If cell assemblies are repeatedly and persistently activated, consolidation occurs, making reciprocal connections more effective. Hence the observation that "neurons that fire together will wire together."[45]

The discovery of long-term potentiation (LTP) and its cellular and molecular mechanisms provided supporting scientific evidence for Hebb's[44] hypothesis. LTP results in long-lasting modifications in postsynaptic neurons, altering the synaptic structure permanently to facilitate future impulse transmission.[35] LTP has been demonstrated in the limbic system. Emotional states increase neurochemical excitation, which is essential for synaptic modification and learning. Amygdala-hippocampal synchrony mediates memory formation and consolidation.[35] LTP throughout the developing limbic system consolidates the infrastructure of intralimbic and corticolimbic circuits.

Hebbian modification of synapses resulting from the simultaneous activation of presynaptic and postsynaptic neurons enhances healthy, normal development in infants exposed to nurturing, caring environments that provide attention to basic needs, positive affections, maternal bonding, and positive sensory stimulations. However, in neglected or abused infants, this Hebbian modification can have the most detrimental and potentially long-lasting effects. These infants' brains establish, strengthen, and consolidate synaptic connections necessary for immediate survival, but, in the long run, are not adaptive or flexible enough to respond to normal environmental demands and proper learning. Moreover, development of emotions favors, strengthens, and consolidates connections that promote the expression of negative rather than positive emotions. In addition, those synapses that would provide healthy adaptation, learning, and positive emotions are not properly developed, retract, and are likely to be eliminated.

The second developmental principle is experience-expectant brain maturation. This principle is based on the theory that the neonatal brain is programmed to be stimulated by the environment in order to attain optimal development; it is experience expectant. Perinatal experiences, whether positive or adverse, play a crucial role in early brain development.[46] Experience-expectant learning implies that the developing brain expects and is primed to react to the exposure to environmental stimuli that will shape its development.[35] Rewiring and strengthening of connections and the maintenance of functional neuronal networks is achieved by epigenetic changes related to the interphase of genetic and environmental factors.[46] Experience-expectant learning takes place early in life. By contrast, experience-dependent learning refers to additional skills that the brain does not expect. It does not involve critical sensitive periods, but rather can be developed over a lifespan. Synapses are formed in response to, rather than in anticipation of, an experience.[35]

During early postnatal development, the brain expects to receive visual stimuli, including faces that are to become familiar, to develop language receptivity and the anxiety necessary for detecting danger, which will promote survival, and to establish the facial recognition necessary for bonding and so forth.

Limbic system circuit development requires extensive environmental stimulation. These circuits cannot achieve full functional potential under impoverished or adverse environmental conditions.[46] Experience-expectant emotional experiences during early infancy are crucial for interlimbic and prefrontolimbic pathway development during critical sensitive periods, and shape their function in adulthood. Neglected infants are particularly prone to this. Dysfunctional infant attachment may predispose the individuals to develop lasting, irreversibly impaired emotionality and social behavior later in life.[46]

The third developmental principle is that certain aspects of early brain development only take place during sensitive periods of development. Sensitive periods are developmental windows in which maturation and specific experiences interact to produce differential long-term effects on the brain and behavior.[47] During this time window a biological event develops more easily under the influence of an environmental stimulus. After this sensitive period has ended, learning is more difficult and less efficient. Examples of this are vision and language acquisition. Hubel and Weisel[48] performed experiments temporarily suturing the eyelids of kittens from birth to 3 months of age. These cats not only never fully developed vision through the blindfolded eye but also neurons in the occipital cortex receiving inputs from that eye greatly decreased their space compared with the increased cell growth of the cortex corresponding with the seeing eye. The deprived eye never develops normal vision later in life.

Some investigators distinguish between sensitive periods and critical periods. Sensitive periods start and end gradually and are particularly sensitive to certain types of stimuli. After the sensitive periods end, the individual can learn, but learning is more difficult, takes longer, and may require intensive interventions. An example of this is language acquisition. By contrast, critical periods are finite, compulsory, and are associated with a heightened sensitivity to a specific environmental stimulus that allows the development of a certain skill, after which acquisition is difficult or impossible. The example of vision fits this concept. Limbic and higher neocortical structures are open; that is, they change with experience during development. Lower structures like the hypothalamus and PAG are closed and change little or not at all.[9] However, limbic structures complete myelination in the second decade of life, much earlier than the neocortex.[34]

The principle of sensitive periods and critical periods has important implications for neglected or maltreated infants. Infants who do not regain adequate care after prolonged deprivation during the first year of life may be emotionally damaged for life.[37]

Finally, the fourth developmental principle conceptualizes brain development as a process of self-organization. Drawing from neurobiological research, Lewis[35] incorporated these data to formulate the principles and mechanisms of self-organization, with emphasis on the role of emotion in self-organizing neural systems.[35]

Brain development can be conceptualized as a process of self-organization, evolving in unpredictable and indeterminate ways through the repeated modification of synaptic systems.[35] Neural development organizes itself to achieve forms that were initially indeterminate. Self-organizing synaptic sculpting consists of 2 forces:

1. Synaptic elaboration (ie, proliferation and strengthening)
2. Synaptic pruning

Synaptic elaboration favors activity of some synapses rather than others. Pruning gets rid of underused synapses and consolidates synaptic stability. Neuronal substrates of emotion influence structural changes in all areas of development.[35] Emotional stress dysregulates neural activity in infancy by shutting down circuits for processing social information.[49] Self-organizing synaptic sculpting in infants exposed to neglect and abuse is expected to prune synapses promoting normal attachment and emotions, and proliferate and strengthen those maladaptive connections that express negative emotions and interpersonal difficulties.

THE PSYCHOANATOMICAL FORMULATION

Amy fulfills the Diagnostic and Statistical Manual of Mental Disorders, Fifth Edition (DSM-V) diagnostic criteria for disinhibited social engagement disorder[50] (this corresponds with the Diagnostic and Statistical Manual of Mental Disorders, Fourth Edition [DSM-IV] diagnosis of reactive attachment disorder of infancy and early childhood, disinhibited type). This disorder is characterized by a pattern of behavior in which a child actively approaches and interacts with unfamiliar adults, and in Amy's case this was manifested by reduced or absent reticence in approaching and interacting with unfamiliar adults. She also displayed overly friendly, familiar behavior. She showed willingness to go off with an unfamiliar adult with minimal or no hesitation, as when she tried to leave the house with strangers who came to the door. Amy also experienced a pattern of extremes of insufficient care, as shown by social neglect and deprivation in the form of a persistent lack of having emotional needs met for comfort, stimulation, and affection by caregiving adults. She also had repeated changes of primary caregivers (mother, relatives, and mother's friend), which limited opportunities to form stable attachments.

However, this diagnostic formulation does not provide insight into the underlying developmental/neuroanatomic mechanisms that are playing an important part in the manifestation of emotions and behavior in the patient. This author has developed the concept of psychoanatomical formulation, which is defined as the assessment/analysis of a clinical case based on the disturbed functional neuroanatomy underlying behavioral and emotional symptom expression. The earlier discussion of limbic nuclei development and function, development of emotions, and developmental principles as they relate to child neglect and abuse serves as a background for better understanding this formulation. This psychoanatomical formulation comes closer to National Institute of Mental Health (NIMH) Director Thomas Insel and colleagues'[51] efforts to develop research domain criteria that conceptualize mental disorders as disorders of brain circuits.

PSYCHOANATOMICAL FORMULATION OF CASE VIGNETTE

Amy is a 2.5-year-old girl with a history of severe early neglect during the first 20 months of life. During the first year of life, the amygdala, followed by the septal nuclei and anterior cingulate gyrus, are rapidly developing and forming synaptic connections. Physical contact and emotional parental involvement are crucial for the development and wiring of these limbic structures. The role of the amygdala is to detect danger and continuously evaluate the environment for surrounding threats. Amy's obliviousness of danger and her accident proneness seems to have resulted in an impairment in her danger-detection system. This amygdala deficiency extends to her social situations with strangers, and impairs her amygdala's ability to generate appropriate physiologic/emotional responses. Her poorly functioning amygdala is unable to respond appropriately to social cues and the unpredictable nature of interactions with strangers. As a result she is unable to assess the degree of danger when a stranger comes to her home door, and to modify her behavior accordingly. Because of extreme neglect, Amy did not receive the somesthetic stimulation and physical contact necessary for maternal-infant bonding and the normal development of the amygdala. Her lack of fear of dangerous stimuli and in social situations is also found in individuals with bilateral damage to the amygdala.

Amy's neglect continued through the second half of her first year of life, with the changing of caregivers. It can be inferred that neglect and lack of positive reinforcement from caring parent-child interactions during this time period interfered with the normal development of the septal nuclei and anterior cingulate gyrus, which are involved in the development of stable, selective, loving attachments. Because of the lack of normal development of the anterior cingulate gyrus and its synaptic connections, she did not develop the ability to be discriminating in interactions with others and to form real, specific attachments. Although not available by history, she probably never developed stranger and separation anxiety during the ages of 7 to 12 months. She was unable to form long-term attachment because of her exposure to neglect, the change of caregivers, and the resulting poorly developed anterior cingulate gyrus.

As the result of the stress caused by neglect and social impoverishment, Amy most likely established, strengthened, and consolidated the connections necessary for her immediate survival; however, now that she has been adopted into a caring and nurturing environment, these Hebbian modifications are maladaptive. She is not able to respond appropriately to her new environment and express positive emotions. Synapses that would provide healthy adaptation, learning, and positive emotions were not properly developed, ending up retracted and most likely eliminated.

Amy was not exposed to the normal environmental stimuli that a neonatal brain is programmed to receive in order to attain optimal development. She did not receive experience-expectant emotional experiences during the 20 months of life that are crucial for limbic and prefrontolimbic circuit development. Self-organizing brain development and synaptic sculpturing most likely proliferated and strengthened maladaptive connections, with synapses promoting positive emotions and secure attachments being eliminated. In addition, all of this neglect occurred very early in life, during the sensitive periods of emotional development. Recovery from the severe consequences of this neglect will be difficult, and most probably require intensive, long-term interventions. To her advantage is that she is still at a young age in which many limbic circuits have not finished myelinating. In addition, basic research has shown that afferents and new synaptic contacts from the amygdala to the medial prefrontal cortex increase significantly during the rat age equivalent to adolescence and early adulthood.[52] The implication here is that there is a second chance during adolescence for development of increased emotional control. It is thus possible that Amy may have another opportunity to improve emotional connections.

SUMMARY

Severe stress in the form of child abuse or neglect during early infancy may have serious, long-lasting effects on a person's brain development, affecting future manifestations of negative emotions, maladaptive behaviors, and conflictual attachments. As a result, individuals thus affected operate in a survival mode, rather than learning to flexibly adapt to environmental demands. More research is needed in order to understand the genetic and developmental protective factors that enable some persons to be less vulnerable and even more resilient to these extreme stressors, and for clinicians to learn to treat these patients more effectively.

The analysis and the correlation of external traumatic events with resulting structural brain changes provide a deeper, more detailed understanding of the classic nature-versus-nurture paradigm. This article is intended to stimulate psychiatrists and other mental health professionals to expand and incorporate their knowledge of neuroanatomy to conceptualize psychoanatomical formulations for patients with a variety of psychological disorders along the lifespan.

REFERENCES

1. US Department of Health and Human Services, Administration for Children and Families, Administration on children, youth and families, Children's Bureau.

Child maltreatment 2012. 2013. Available at: http://www.acf.hhs.gov/programs/cb/research-data-technology/statistics-research/child-maltreatment.

2. DeBellis MD. The psychobiology of neglect. Child Maltreat 2005;10(2):150–72.

3. Nemeroff CB, Binder E. The preeminent role of childhood abuse and neglect in vulnerability to major psychiatric disorders: elucidating the underlying neurobiological mechanisms. J Am Acad Child Adolesc Psychiatry 2014;53(4):395–7.

4. LeDoux J. The emotional brain: the mysterious underpinnings of emotional life. New York: Touchstone/Simon & Schuster; 1996.

5. Heimer L, Van Hoesen GW, Trimble M, et al. Anatomy of neuropsychiatry: the new anatomy of the basal forebrain and its implications for neuropsychiatric illness. Oxford (United Kingdom): Academic Press/Elsevier; 2008.

6. MacLean PD. The triune brain in evolution. New York: Plenum; 1990.

7. Devinsky O, D'Esposito M. Neurology of cognitive and behavioral disorders. Oxford (United Kingdom): Oxford University Press; 2004.

8. Joseph R. Environmental influences on neural plasticity, the limbic system, emotional development and attachment. Child Psychiatry Hum Dev 1999; 29(3):189–208.

9. Panksepp J. Affective neuroscience: the foundations of human and animal emotions. Oxford (United Kingdom): Oxford University Press; 1998.

10. Kagan J, Baird A. Brain and behavioral development during childhood. In: Gazzaniga MS, editor. The cognitive neurosciences III. 3rd edition. Cambridge (MA): MIT Press; 2004. p. 93–103.

11. Joseph R. Neuropsychiatry, neuropsychology and clinical neuroscience: emotion cognition, language, memory, brain damage, and abnormal behavior. 2nd edition. Baltimore (MD): Williams & Wilkins; 1996.

12. Crosby EC, Woodbourne RT. The comparative anatomy of the preoptic area and the hypothalamus. Association Research Nervous Mental Disorders Proc 1940; 20:52–169.

13. Crosby EC, Showers MJ. Comparative anatomy of the preoptic and hypothalamic areas. Hypothalamic nuclei and fiber connections. In: Haymaker W, Anderson E, Nauta WJ, editors. The hypothalamus. Springfield (IL): Charles C Thomas; 1969. p. 61–135.

14. Nauta WJ, Haymaker W. Hypothalamic nuclei and fiber connections. In: Haymaker W, Anderson E, Nauta WJ, editors. The hypothalamus. Springfield (IL): Charles C Thomas; 1969. p. 136–209.

15. Flynn JP. The neural basis of aggression in cats. In: Glass DC, editor. Neurophysiology and emotion. New York: Rockefeller University Press; 1967. p. 40–60.

16. Tye KM, Deisseroth K. Optogenetic investigation of neural circuits underlying brain disease in animal models. Nat Rev Neurosci 2012;13:251–66.

17. Fennol L, Yizhar O, Deisseroth K. The development and application of optogenetics. Annu Rev Neurosci 2011;34:389–412.

18. Lin D, Boyle MP, Dollar P, et al. Functional identification of an aggression locus in the mouse hypothalamus. Nature 2011;470:221–6.

19. Deisseroth K. Optogenetics and psychiatry: applications, challenges and opportunities. Biol Psychiatry 2012;71:1030–2.

20. Prather MD, Lavenex P, Maudlin-Jourdain ML, et al. Increased social fear and decreased fear of objects in monkeys with neonatal amygdala lesions. Neuroscience 2001;106:653–8.

21. Bauman MD, Lavenex P, Mason WA, et al. The development of mother-infant interactions after neonatal amygdala lesions in rhesus monkeys. J Neurosci 2004;24(3):711–21.

22. Bauman MD, Lavenex P, Mason WA, et al. The development of social behavior following amygdala lesions in rhesus monkeys. J Cogn Neurosci 2004;16(8): 1388–411.

23. Schumann CM, Amaral DG. The human amygdala in autism. In: Whalen PJ, Phelps EA, editors. The human amygdala. New York: Guilford; 2009. p. 362–81.

24. Buchanan TW, Tranel D, Adolphs R. The human amygdala in human function. In: Whalen PJ, Phelps EA, editors. The human amygdala. New York: Guilford; 2009. p. 289–318.

25. Emery NJ, Amaral DG. The role of the amygdala in primate social cognition. In: Lane RD, Nadel L, editors. Cognitive neuroscience of emotion. New York: Oxford University Press; 2000. p. 156–91.

26. Heimer L. A neuroanatomical framework for neuropsychiatric disorder and drug abuse. Am J Psychiatry 2003;160:1726–39.

27. Amaral DG. The primate amygdala and the neurobiology of social behavior: implications for understanding social anxiety. Biol Psychiatry 2002;51:11–7.

28. Nieuwenhuys R, Voogd J, van Huijzen C. The central nervous system. 4th edition. Berlin: Springer-Verlag; 2008. p. 917–46.

29. Lim MM, Young LJ. Neurobiology of the social brain. In: Beach SR, Wamboldt MZ, Kaslow NJ, et al, editors. Relational process and DSM-V: neuroscience, assessment, prevention and treatment. Arlington (VA): American Psychiatric Publishing; 2006. p. 21–37.

30. Clark DL, Boutrus NN, Mendez MF. The brain and behavior: an introduction to behavioral neuroanatomy. 3rd edition. Cambridge (United Kingdom): Cambridge University Press; 2010.

31. Le Doux J. Cognitive-emotional interactions: listen to the brain. In: Lane RD, Nadel L, editors. Cognitive neuroscience of emotion. New York: Oxford University Press; 2000. p. 129–55.

32. Shin LM, Wright CI, Cannistraro PA, et al. A functional magnetic resonance imaging study of amygdala and medial prefrontal cortex responses to overtly presented fearful faces in posttraumatic stress disorder. Arch Gen Psychiatry 2005;62:273–81.

33. Feinstein JS, Adolphs R, Damasio A, et al. The human amygdala and the induction and experience of fear. Curr Biol 2011;21:34–8.

34. Yakovlev PI, Lecours AR. The myologenetic cycles of regional maturation in the brain. In: Minkowski A, editor. Regional development of the brain in early life. Oxford (United Kingdom): Blackwell; 1967. p. 3–70.

35. Lewis MD. Self-organizing individual differences in brain development. Dev Rev 2005;25:252–77.

36. Lewis M. The emergence of human emotions. In: Lewis M, Haviland-Jones JM, Barett LF, editors. Handbook of emotions. 3rd edition. New York: Guilford; 2008. p. 304–19.

37. Spitz RA. The first year of life: a psychoanalytic study of normal and deviant development of object relations. New York: International Universities Press; 1965.

38. Ekman P. Emotions revealed: recognizing faces, and feelings to improve communication and emotional life. New York: Henry Holt; 2003. p. 174.

39. Rozin P, Haidt J, McCanley CR. Disgust. In: Lewis M, Haviland-Jones JM, Barret LF, editors. Handbook of emotions. 3rd edition. New York: Guilford; 2008. p. 757–76.

40. Lemerise EA, Dodge KA. The development of anger and hostile interactions. In: Lewis M, Haviland-Jones JM, Barett LF, editors. Handbook of emotions. 3rd edition. New York: Guilford; 2008. p. 730–41.

41. Lewis M. Self-conscious emotions: embarrassment, pride, shame and guilt. In: Lewis M, Haviland-Jones JM, Barett LF, editors. Handbook of emotions. 3rd edition. New York: Guilford; 2008. p. 742–56.

42. Hoffmann ML. Empathy and prosocial behavior. In: Lewis M, Haviland-Jones JM, Barett LF, editors. Handbook of emotions. 3rd edition. New York: Guilford; 2008. p. 440–55.

43. Schore AN. Affect regulation and the repair of the self. New York: Norton; 2003.

44. Hebb DO. The organization of behavior: a neuropsychological theory. New York: Wiley; 1949.

45. Bear MF, Connors BW, Paradiso MA, editors. Neuroscience: exploring the brain. Baltimore (MD): Williams & Wilkins; 1996.

46. Braun K. The prefrontal-limbic system: development, neuroanatomy, function, and implications for the socioemotional development. Clin Perinatol 2011; 38(4):685–702.

47. Penhune V, de Villers-Sidani E. Time for new thinking about sensitive periods. Front Syst Neurosci 2014;8:1–2.

48. Hubel DH, Weisel TN. Binocular interaction in striate cortex of kittens reared with artificial squint. J Neurophysiol 1995;26:994–1002.

49. Schore AN. Affect dysregulation and disorders of the self. New York: Norton; 2003.

50. American Psychiatric Association. Diagnostic and statistical manual of mental disorders. 5th edition. Washington, DC: American Psychiatric Association; 2013.

51. Insel T, Cuthbert B, Garvey M, et al. Research Domain Criteria (RDoC): toward a new classification framework for research on mental disorders. Am J Psychiatry 2010;167:748–51.

52. Cunningham MG, Bhattacharyya S, Benes FM. Amygdalo-cortical sprouting continues into early adulthood: implications for the development of normal and abnormal function during adolescence. J Comp Neurol 2000;453:116–30.

The Role of Stress and Fear in the Development of Mental Disorders

 CrossMark

Polaris Gonzalez, BA[a], Karen G. Martinez, MD, MSc[b],*

KEYWORDS

• Fear • PTSD • Stress • Extinction • Conditioning

KEY POINTS

• Stress and fear, in response to actual or possible threat, enhance the possibility of forming trauma-related memories leading to posttraumatic stress disorder (PTSD).

• Excessive fear responses in PTSD can be seen as physiologic reactions to trauma cues and alterations in arousal and reactivity increasing fear conditioning capacity.

• Predisposing factors such as childhood abuse increase the risk of fear conditioning, renewal, and reconsolidation.

• Studies on fear learning, extinction, and neuroimaging support the notion that increased fear is related to amygdala hyperresponsivity and dysfunctions in neural circuitry, specifically in the areas of the ventromedial prefrontal cortex that regulate fear.

• Severity of PTSD is associated with the inability to inhibit fear generalization, poor cognitive emotion regulation, and hippocampal damage affecting the memory processing of fear.

• Findings on fear have led to the identification of effective treatment modalities to reduce fear alterations in PTSD, such as effective pharmacotherapy including propranolol and selective norepinephrine reuptake inhibitors, cognitive behavior therapy, and exposure therapy.

Exposure to stress can lead to different psychiatric manifestations depending on the individual. One possible pathologic manifestation after a stressor is posttraumatic stress disorder (PTSD). Developing PTSD is closely related with predisposing factors such as genes and early traumatic experiences.[1] The Diagnostic and Statistical

This work was funded by National Center for Research Resources U54RR026139-01A1 and NIMHHD 8U54MD007587-03 (K.G. Martinez).
Disclosures: None.
[a] Ponce School of Medicine & Health Sciences, Clinical Psychology Program, PO Box 7004, Ponce, PR 00732-7004, USA; [b] University of Puerto Rico, Medical Sciences Campus, PO Box 365067, San Juan, PR 09936-5067, USA
* Corresponding author.
E-mail address: karen.martinez4@upr.edu

Psychiatr Clin N Am 37 (2014) 535–546
http://dx.doi.org/10.1016/j.psc.2014.08.010
0193-953X/14/$ – see front matter © 2014 Elsevier Inc. All rights reserved.

Abbreviations	
BDNF	Brain-derived neurotrophic factor
CBT	Cognitive behavior therapy
CR	Conditioned response
CS−	Safety signal
CS+	Threat signal
CS	Conditioned stimulus
Dl	Dorsolateral
DSM-IV-TR	Diagnostic and statistical manual of mental disorders, fourth edition, text revision
DSM-V	Diagnostic and statistical manual of mental disorders, fifth edition
fMRI	Functional MRI studies
HPA	Hypothalamic-pituitary-adrenal
NMDAR	N-Methyl-D-aspartic acid receptor
PTSD	Posttraumatic stress disorder
SCR	Skin conductance response
UR	Unconditioned response
US	Unconditioned stimulus
vmPFC	Ventromedial prefrontal cortex

Manual of Mental Disorders, Fifth Edition, (DSM-V) includes a category of trauma-related and stressor-related disorders that encompasses the variable clinical expressions of stress.[2] One of the most recognized expressions after a stressful stimulus is fear. Although fear is a natural response that protects against threats, when fear is excessive or expressed inappropriately it can become pathologic. Fear elicits natural autonomic responses such as increased heart rate, increased skin conductance, and activation of facial muscles that prepare the body to react to threat.[3] A possible pathologic manifestation of excessive fear after a stressor is PTSD.

The diagnosis of PTSD describes the cluster of symptoms that emerge after exposure to actual or threatened death, serious injury, or sexual violence. The person then develops intrusion symptoms associated with the trauma such as intrusive memories, distressing dreams, flashbacks or distress, or physiologic reactions on exposure to cues of the trauma. There is also the avoidance of the reminders of the trauma, alterations in memories or mood associated with the trauma, and marked alterations in physiologic arousal and reactivity. Projected lifetime risk for PTSD according to DSM-V is 8.7% in the United States, with lower prevalence in other countries. PTSD is a serious problem in certain samples such as war veterans, emergency medical personnel, and survivors of rape.[2]

FEAR EXPRESSION

In PTSD, a traumatic event causes a fear reaction that is excessively expressed. Based on DSM-V criteria, excessive fear can be seen as the physiologic reactions to trauma cues and the alterations in physiologic arousal and reactivity. Increased fear can be studied by evaluating the autonomic responses that are elicited, such as increased heart rate or skin conductance and activation of facial muscles, such as the startle response. Initial studies of fear responses in patients exposed to trauma showed increases in all of these autonomic responses to non–trauma-related stimuli.[4,5] Increased startle has even been reported in veterans with subthreshold PTSD symptoms.[6] These heightened responses seemed to be acquired as an effect of trauma exposure, as shown by twin studies in which the twin exposed to combat developed the increased physiologic responses, whereas the non–combat-exposed twin did not.[7] There is also evidence that pretrauma increased physiologic reactivity is a vulnerability factor in developing PTSD after exposure to trauma.[8] Findings from animal studies as well as functional MRI (fMRI) studies in humans describe activation of the amygdala during fear expression.[9,10] Neuroimaging studies support the notion of increased fear in PTSD because amygdala hyper-responsivity has been a consistent finding in such cases.[11]

FEAR LEARNING

Another characteristic that has been described in patients with PTSD is an increased capacity for conditioning fear responses. Patients with PTSD have an increased facility to associate fear responses with the trauma memory and trauma cues. Conditionability can be related to the DSM-V symptoms of intrusive memories/flashbacks as well as the distortions in the memories of the event.

Fear conditioning is the process by which a neutral or conditioned stimulus (CS) is paired with an aversive, unconditioned stimulus (US) that now produces a conditioned response (CR) to the CS. The unconditioned response (UR) is the natural response that would have been seen with the US alone, but when paired recurrently with the CS it results in the CR in the presence of the CS alone. In the laboratory, fear conditioning is usually measured by the skin conductance response (SCR) or startle responses. SCR is the changes in skin conductance that can be elicited when a US (usually an electrical shock to the fingers) is paired with neutral or unconditioned stimuli (UR; eg, images). Although many studies of SCRs in patients with PTSD have shown enhanced conditionability,[12–14] other studies have failed to find this enhanced conditioning.[15] Recent studies have even found that fear-potentiated startle responses discriminated better than SCR between healthy participants versus participants with PTSD.[16] Fear-potentiated startle response is another measure of conditioning in which the conditioned fear is measured by an increase in the amplitude of the acoustic startle reflex in the presence of a cue previously paired with a shock.[17]

There are various experimental factors that can affect the degree of conditioning. For example, when predictability is taken into account in patients with PTSD, heightened fear is seen during periods of unpredictable, but not predictable threat.[18] Fear conditioning also depends on the neutral stimulus that is chosen to be conditioned. Many laboratory fear conditioning studies use non–trauma-related CS, but recent studies using trauma-related CS also have shown increased conditionability.[12,19] Gender also plays a role in conditioning. In patients with PTSD, women show larger SCR than men.[20] In women, hormonal levels also affect conditioning, with studies showing that low estrogen levels are associated with greater fear-potentiated startle responses in patients with PTSD.[21] Another important finding seen in patients with PTSD during conditioning is that many such patients cannot verbally report the CS-US contingency,[22] pointing to a deficit in their declarative memory of the relationship between the trauma cues and the fear response.

Experimental studies of fear can also assess a safety signal (CS−). This assessment can be done by presenting another neutral stimulus similar to the CS but that is not paired with the US and thus creates an association between that stimulus and not receiving the US. For example, in a fear conditioning protocol in which a blue light is paired with an electric shock and a red light is not paired with an electric shock, the blue light is the CS+ (threat signal) and the red light is the CS−. In PTSD, some studies evaluating SCR have described increased reactions to the CS− that can be described as overgeneralization of the CS+ compared with the CS−.[13,14,22] Similar results have been found with fear-potentiated startle in that fear is potentiated to the safety cue in veterans with PTSD but not in healthy veterans.[23] Further exploring the processing of safety cues in PTSD has led to studies evaluating fear inhibition in the presence of safety cues; that is, the ability of the person to suppress fear with safety. The severity of the PTSD has been associated with the ability to generalize fear inhibition. For example, patients with more severe symptoms of PTSD have more difficulty with fear inhibition.[24] These studies have led to the proposal that CS− processing might require awareness of the CS-US contingency and if this process is affected, as often happens in patients with PTSD, then CS− will also be faulty.[24] Difficulties with fear inhibition have also been described in patients with acute stress disorder.[25]

The neural circuits involved in fear conditioning in humans have been described using fMRI and include activation of the amygdala, the dorsal anterior cingulate cortex, and the hippocampus.[10] These findings also relate to abnormal findings in fMRI of patients with PTSD during conditioning, which have found heightened amygdala activity,[26,27] especially the left side of the amygdala,[28] and diminished ventromedial prefrontal cortex (vmPFC) activity.[27] Dysfunctions in the connectivity between amygdala and vmPFC may mediate susceptibility to anxiety disorders.[29]

FEAR REGULATION

Once unwanted or excessive fear is present, it is important to have mechanisms to regulate this fear. Fear can be regulated by extinction, cognitive emotion regulation, active coping, reversal, or reconsolidation.[30,31] All these mechanism of change seem to be regulated by a common neural mechanism but evaluating each process can have important treatment implications.[31] Extinction is the process by which a new safety memory is created that can compete with the original conditioned memory. In other words, when a neutral stimulus produces a fear response because the person learned the contingency between CS and US, that fear response can decrease if the person then creates a new memory for which that CS is no longer paired to the US; this process is called extinction. Studies of patients with PTSD show slower extinction.[12,14,22] Patients with PTSD also show an overestimation of the probability of the US following CS+ during extinction.[22]

The neural circuits involved in extinction have been clearly delineated[10] and include interactions between the vmPFC, the amygdala, and the hippocampus. The amygdala activates in early extinction and this activation decreases across extinction training.[29] In fMRI of patients with PTSD during fear extinction there are reports of decreasing vmPFC activity[28] pointing to a possible neurofunctional deficit in the capacity to extinguish. Reduced extinction learning has also been related to risk of development of PTSD in firefighters[32] and Dutch soldiers.[33] The available evidence suggests a deficit in extinction that could be a risk factor for the development of PTSD.

In order for extinction to continue regulating fear, people need to be able to recall extinction memories when exposed to trauma cues. Studies of patients with PTSD have shown that, even if the subjects did not show increased conditioning or extinction, they still present difficulty using the extinction memory to control fear when exposed to the CS in the extinction context.[15,34] In fMRI studies, patients with PTSD show reduced activity in vmPFC and hippocampus but increased activity in dorsolateral PFC (dlPFC) during extinction recall.[34] Reduced vmPFC activity and increased dlPFC may mediate an inability to use contextual cues to predict safety.[29] Further studies have found that these impaired recall extinction findings are seen in participants with PTSD but not in their nontraumatized twins, which could mean this deficit is acquired and not a risk factor for PTSD.[15]

Fear can also be modulated in humans by cognitively regulating fear in which thoughts are used to diminish fear. In contrast with extinction, these techniques are thought to require active participation of the person. The available studies on how fear can be modulated cognitively could have important implications in the treatment of PTSD. For example, telling subjects that they will be shocked elicits a fear response and amygdala activation even if the shock is not given.[35] Instructions to regulate conditioned fear lead to reduced conditioned responses,[36] increased activation of the dlPFC, decreased activation of amygdala, and activation of the vmPFC.[37] Similar patterns of activation in amygdala and vmPFC are seen if fear is diminished by extinction or by cognitive regulation; only cognitive regulation activates dlPFC. One study has also found that the effect of cognitive reappraisal on fear is impaired by acute stress.[38] Data on cognitive regulation of fear in PTSD are limited, but, given that patients with PTSD show abnormalities in the same anatomic areas used for cognitive regulation, future studies could be used to better control fear.

Another way to modulate fear is through the disruption of reconsolidation. Every time a memory is retrieved the underlying memory trace is again labile and needs to reconsolidate; this reconsolidation period allows disruption of memory.[39] Because beta receptors regulate long-term memory storage, propranolol has been shown to decrease fear expression after activating a traumatic memory in patients with PTSD.[40] High levels of glucocorticosteroids can also interrupt the consolidation of the traumatic memory.[41] Reconsolidation manipulations might change the original conditioned memory and thus might be immune to the return of fear.[42]

FACTORS MODULATING FEAR

The process of extinction can be affected by several factors, such as how much time occurs between extinction trials, contextual cues, how related to the person's fear is the CS, the presence of other excitatory CS during extinction, or the introduction of inhibitory CS− during extinction.[43] In terms of inhibitory CS−, one study showed that the use of a button press to avoid shock prevented extinction in healthy subjects.[44] This finding is relevant for patients with PTSD because they tend to show avoidance of trauma cues to prevent physiologic arousal at the moment, but, given the studies with inhibitory CS−, this might worsen the fear responses in the long run.

There are several other factors that have been related to the return of fear even after adequate extinction, such as renewal, reinstatement, spontaneous recovery, or reacquisition.[45] Extinction is highly specific to the circumstances (context) in which the extinction occurs.[43] Presenting the CS in the context in which conditioning took place or in a new context can lead to renewal of fear. Renewal is greater when the conditioning context is encountered versus when exposed to a novel context.[46] Renewal is of particular relevance for PTSD because patients may learn to extinguish the conditioned fear responses to trauma cues in a safe environment but might have a return of symptoms if they encounter the same context but, in this case, where the trauma occurred.

Extinguished fear can also return if the US is presented again in the conditioning context; a process called reinstatement.[43] Extinction is also specific to time,[45] causing spontaneous recovery to occur with the passage of time.

INTERACTION OF STRESS AND FEAR IN THE DEVELOPMENT OF POSTTRAUMATIC STRESS DISORDER

The stress response of the hypothalamic-pituitary-adrenal (HPA) axis is closely related to fear expression and regulation. The amygdala has glucocorticoid receptors, which modulate fear memory consolidation.[47] One of the areas of convergence is the effect of early trauma on the circuits involved in fear. Early life trauma has been shown to sensitize the HPA axis producing an ineffective stress response system. For example, when exposed to stressful situations as adults, women with early life trauma have greater adrenal corticotropin hormone releases and increases in heart rates.[48] Stress in humans also may lead to hippocampal damage,[49–51] thus affecting the memory processing of fear. Childhood abuse is associated with increased startle reactivity in adults that cannot be accounted for by PTSD or depressive symptoms, suggesting that an increased startle may be a biomarker of stress responsiveness that is a persevering consequence of childhood trauma exposure.[1] The number of traumas a person has experienced also has implications for fear expression and PTSD symptoms. In a study of patients with PTSD who had multiple traumas, they did not present increased fear expression. These patients had lower skin conductance and startle responses than the patients who had only 1 traumatic event. Multiple traumas also had an effect on PTSD symptoms, because these patients also presented higher levels of avoidance and numbing than the patients with single traumas.[52]

TREATMENT IMPLICATIONS

The findings on fear processing in patients with PTSD can lead to better screening methods and treatments. In terms of using fear for screening, the genetic heritability of conditioning and extinction is 35% to 45%.[53] There is some evidence that genetic variation in the serotonin transporter gene affects conditionability, the catechol-O-methyltransferase gene affects fear memory consolidation, and the brain-derived neurotrophic factor (BDNF) val66met genotype has various effects on conditioning and extinction processes.[54] Thus the capacity for fear conditioning and/or extinction might be an inheritable risk factor for the development of PTSD and might be used as a way to identify people at risk before being exposed to trauma. The capacity to extinguish fear has been identified as a risk factor for the development of PTSD before trauma exposure in high-risk samples.[8,32,33] Longitudinal studies that measure fear conditioning or extinction capacity before trauma are needed in order to be able to classify these fear processes as biological risk factors (endophenotypes) for PTSD symptoms. There is also a need to evaluate how the factors affecting fear acquisition and extinction, such as consolidation and context, could also be used to prevent PTSD emergence when a person encounters the traumatic experience. For example, the production of the traumatic memory might be impaired if propranolol[55] or systemic glucocorticoids[41] are given before the initial consolidation of the fear memory.

Research on fear has also provided insight into the mechanisms of exposure therapy. Exposure therapy is thought to improve anxiety through emotional processing in which a fear network is activated and new incompatible information is added, which causes decreases in these fear responses within the therapy session (within-session habituation) and between therapy sessions (between-session habituation).[56] This theory could be described with fear terminology by stating that fear is elicited and then extinguished. Thus research on fear expression and extinction can lead to better understanding of exposure therapy and improvements for those patients who do not respond to therapy. Laboratory measures of extinction retention have been shown to predict degree of improvement with exposure therapy in social anxiety disorder but, to our knowledge, no studies of this kind have been done in PTSD.[57] Clinical measures of fear (self-report arousal symptoms) have also been related to cognitive behavior therapy (CBT) outcomes in general. For example, higher ratings of anxiety at the start of the first exposure were related to no improvement, whereas higher within-session habituation was related to improvement of anxiety symptoms.[58] Differential pretreatment conditioned responses were related to better responses of PTSD symptoms to the serotonin-norepinephrine reuptake inhibitor duloxetine.[59] Changes in symptom severity with trauma-focused CBT has also been associated with a decrease in physiologic reactivity.[60]

Studies on the factors that affect extinction learning can also improve exposure therapy. Studies with fMRIs have found that areas related to fear learning and extinction, such as greater activation of amygdala and ventral anterior cingulate region when viewing fearful faces before CBT, can predict who will have a better response to the therapy.[61] Also, one study has shown that the BDNF val66met polymorphism predicts response to exposure therapy in PTSD.[62]

Research on inhibitory CS during extinction has been done on the use of CS— in exposure therapy, which has been shown to impair positive outcomes in therapy.[43] Relapse or return of fear can affect as many as 33% to 50% of successfully treated individuals.[63] Return of fear has been seen when changing therapists or rooms in which exposure takes place.[64] Contextual stimuli might include external stimuli (room, place, background stimuli) or interoceptive stimuli (drug states, hormonal states, deprivation, expectation of events, time).[45] Drug states, as contextual cues, are particularly relevant in the treatment of PTSD because exposure therapy is frequently combined with pharmacotherapy. If the patient learns to extinguish fear under the effect of a medication, and after some time this medication is discontinued, that patient might be at higher risk of relapse because of a renewal effect,[65] possibly because the success was based on the neural pathways depending on the presence of medication; an example of state-dependent memory. To prevent relapses, these studies have provided information that using multiple context exposures or booster sessions (different contextual times) can improve outcomes of exposure therapy. It has also been recommended that, when using medications in combination with CBT, the medications should allow for the full activation of the fear structure with the least possible side effects to minimize this aforementioned state-dependent learning.[65]

Understanding the molecular mechanisms behind fear extinction can lead to novel treatments that enhance extinction learning or recall. One of the areas that have received the most attention is the N-methyl-D-aspartic acid receptor (NMDAR), because NMDAR antagonists block both fear and extinction learning, with the opposite being true of NMDAR agonists. This finding has led to the discovery that D-cycloserine, a partial agonist of NMDARs, facilitates fear extinction and has been tried with contradictory results during exposure therapy to enhance fear reduction.[65] Other areas of interest are the endocannabinoid system, with anandamide showing facilitation of fear extinction.[66] Although no adequate molecules have been found, the BDNF-tyrosine kinase B pathway and the pituitary adenylate cyclase–activating polypeptide are also areas of interest for the development of treatments because they have been shown to be implicated in fear extinction and in PTSD development.[67] Several other neurotransmitters, such as gamma-aminobutyric acid, dopamine, acetylcholine, norepinephrine, and opioids, are involved in the consolidation and extinction of fear but the clinical implications of these findings are still unclear.[68] Direct stimulation of the circuits involved in fear learning and extinction with devices and techniques such as deep brain stimulation, vagal nerve stimulators, and transcranial magnetic stimulation are also avenues of treatment that need further study.[69]

SUMMARY

The expression, conditioning, and regulation of fear have been implicated in the development of all of the symptoms of PTSD (**Fig. 1**). These fear processes have direct

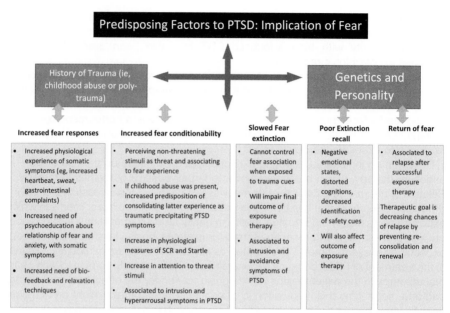

Fig. 1. Predisposing factors related to increased experience of fear in PTSD and their implications for treatment. Predisposing factors are a key to altering an individual's resiliency. Not only are genetic variances accountable for mental disorders but environmental experiences can either awaken or alter genetic behavior leading to mental disorders. In the development of PTSD, fear plays a crucial role.

relationships with stress responses because the traumatic experience starts a cascade in which fear circuits and the HPA axis are affected. Experimental and clinical measures of fear can be used to help in the understanding of how a stressful situation can lead to disorders and also serve in the development of better screening and treatment of patients with PTSD.

REFERENCES

1. Jovanovic T, Blanding NQ, Norrholm SD, et al. Childhood abuse is associated with increased startle reactivity in adulthood. Depress Anxiety 2009;26(11): 1018–26.
2. American Psychiatric Association. Diagnostic and statistical manual of mental disorders. 5th edition. Arlington (VA): American Psychiatric Association; 2013.
3. Lang PJ, McTeague LM. The anxiety disorder spectrum: fear imagery, physiological reactivity, and differential diagnosis. Anxiety Stress Coping 2009;22(1): 5–25.
4. Orr SP, Lasko NB, Shalev AY, et al. Physiological responses to loud tones in Vietnam veterans with posttraumatic stress disorder. J Abnorm Psychol 1995; 104(1):75–82.
5. Orr SP, Lasko NB, Metzger LJ, et al. Physiological responses to non-startling tones in Vietnam veterans with post-traumatic stress disorder. Psychiatry Res 1997;73(1–2):103–7.
6. Roy M, Costanzo M, Leaman S. Psychophysiological identification of subthreshold PTSD in combat veterans. Stud Health Technol Inform 2012;181:149–55.

7. Orr SP, Metzger LJ, Lasko NB, et al. Physiological responses to sudden loud tones in monozygotic twins discordant for combat exposure. Arch Gen Psychiatry 2003;60:283–8.

8. Guthrie RM, Bryant RA. Auditory startle response in firefighters before and after trauma exposure. Am J Psychiatry 2005;162(2):283–90.

9. Delgado MR, Olsson A, Phelps EA. Extending animal models of fear conditioning to humans. Biol Psychol 2006;73:39–48.

10. Sehlmeyer C, Schoning S, Zwitserlood P, et al. Human fear conditioning and extinction in neuroimaging: a systemic review. PLoS One 2009;4(6):e5865.

11. Etkin A, Wager TD. Functional neuroimaging of anxiety: a meta-analysis of emotional processing in PTSD, social anxiety disorder, and specific phobia. Am J Psychiatry 2007;164(10):1476–88.

12. Wessa M, Flor H. Failure of extinction of fear responses in posttraumatic stress disorder: evidence from second-order conditioning. Am J Psychiatry 2007; 164(11):1684–92.

13. Orr SP, Metzger LJ, Lasko NB, et al. De novo conditioning in trauma-exposed individuals with and without posttraumatic stress disorder. J Abnorm Psychol 2000;109(2):290–8.

14. Peri T, Ben-Shakhar G, Orr SP, et al. Psychophysiological assessment of aversive conditioning in posttraumatic stress disorder. Biol Psychiatry 2000;47: 512–9.

15. Milad MR, Orr SP, Lasko NB, et al. Presence and acquired origin of reduced recall for fear extinction in PTSD: results of a twin study. J Psychiatr Res 2008; 42(7):515–20.

16. Glover EM, Phifer JE, Crain DF, et al. Tools for translational neuroscience: PTSD is associated with heightened fear responses using acoustic startle but not skin conductance measures. Depress Anxiety 2011;28:1058–66.

17. Davis M, Falls WA, Campeau S, et al. Fear-potentiated startle: a neural and pharmacological analysis. Behav Brain Res 1993;58(1–2):175–98.

18. Grillon C, Pine DS, Lissek S, et al. Increased anxiety during anticipation of unpredictable aversive stimuli in posttraumatic stress disorder but not in generalized anxiety disorder. Biol Psychiatry 2009;66:47–53.

19. Wegener M, Blechert J, Kerschbaum H, et al. Relationship between fear conditionability and aversive memories: evidence from a novel conditioned-intrusion paradigm. PLoS One 2013;8(11):1–13.

20. Inslicht SS, Metzler TJ, Garcia NM, et al. Sex differences in fear conditioning in posttraumatic stress disorder. J Psychiatr Res 2013;47(1):64–71.

21. Glover EM, Jovanovic T, Mercer KB, et al. Estrogen levels are associated with extinction deficits in women with posttraumatic stress disorder. Biol Psychiatry 2012;72(1):19–24.

22. Blechert J, Michael T, Vriends N, et al. Fear conditioning in posttraumatic stress disorder: evidence for delayed extinction of autonomic, experiential and behavioural responses. Behav Res Ther 2007;45:2019–33.

23. Grillon C, Morgan CA. Fear-potentiated startle conditioning to explicit and contextual cues in Gulf War veterans with posttraumatic stress disorder. J Abnorm Psychol 1999;108:134–42.

24. Jovanovic T, Ressler KJ. How the neurocircuitry and genetics of fear inhibition may inform our understanding of PTSD. Am J Psychiatry 2010;167(6):648–62.

25. Jovanovic T, Sakoman AJ, Kozaric D, et al. Acute stress disorder versus chronic posttraumatic stress disorder: inhibition of fear as a function of time since trauma. Depress Anxiety 2013;30(3):217–24.

26. Rauch SL, Whalen PJ, Shin LM, et al. Exaggerated amygdala response to masked facial stimuli in posttraumatic stress disorder: a functional MRI study. Biol Psychiatry 2000;47(9):769–76.

27. Shin LM, Wright CI, Cannistrano PA, et al. A functional magnetic resonance imaging study of amygdala and medial prefrontal cortex responses to overtly presented fearful faces in posttraumatic stress disorder. Arch Gen Psychiatry 2005;62(3):273–81.

28. Bremner J, Vermetten E, Schmahl C, et al. Positron emission tomographic imaging of neural correlates of a fear acquisition and extinction paradigm in women with childhood sexual-abuse-related post-traumatic stress disorder. Psychol Med 2005;35(6):791–806.

29. Graham BM, Milad MR. The study of fear extinction: implications for anxiety disorders. Am J Psychiatry 2011;168:1255–65.

30. Hartley CA, Phelps EA. Changing fear: the neurocircuitry of emotion regulation. Neuropsychopharmacology 2010;35:136–46.

31. Schiller D, Delgado MR. Overlapping neural systems mediating extinction, reversal and regulation of fear. Trends Cogn Sci 2010;14:268–76.

32. Guthrie RM, Bryant RA. Extinction learning before trauma and subsequent posttraumatic stress. Psychosom Med 2006;68:307–11.

33. Lommen MJ, Engelhard IM, Sijbrandij M, et al. Pre-trauma individual differences in extinction learning predict posttraumatic stress. Behav Res Ther 2013;51:63–7.

34. Milad MR, Pitman RK, Ellis CB, et al. Neurobiological basis of failure to recall extinction memory in posttraumatic stress disorder. Biol Psychiatry 2009;66(12):1075–82.

35. Phelps EA, O'Connor KJ, Gatenby JC, et al. Activation of the left amygdala to a cognitive representation of fear. Nat Neurosci 2001;4(4):437–41.

36. Shurick AA, Hamilton JR, Harris LT, et al. Durable effects of cognitive restructuring on conditioned fear. Emotion 2012;12(6):1393–7.

37. Delgado MR, Nearing KI, LeDoux JE, et al. Neural circuitry underlying the regulation of conditioned fear and its relation to extinction. Neuron 2008;59:829–38.

38. Raio CM, Orederu TA, Palazzolo L, et al. Cognitive emotion regulation fails the stress test. Proc Natl Acad Sci U S A 2013;110(37):15139–44.

39. Ressler KJ, Mayberg HS. Targeting abnormal neural circuits in mood and anxiety disorders: from the laboratory to the clinic. Nat Neurosci 2007;10(9):1116–24.

40. Brunet A, Orr SP, Tremblay J, et al. Effect of post-retrieval propranolol on psychophysiologic responding during subsequent script-driven traumatic imagery in post-traumatic stress disorder. J Psychiatr Res 2008;42(6):503–6.

41. Schelling G. The effect of stress doses of hydrocortisone during septic shock on posttraumatic stress disorder in survivors. Biol Psychiatry 2001;50:978–85.

42. Monfils MH, Cowansage KK, Klann E, et al. Extinction-reconsolidation boundaries: key to persistent attenuation of fear memories. Science 2009;324(5929):951–5.

43. Hermans D, Craske MG, Mineka S, et al. Extinction in human fear conditioning. Biol Psychiatry 2006;60:361–8.

44. Lovibond PF, Mitchell CJ, Minard E, et al. Safety behaviours preserve threat beliefs: protection from extinction of human fear conditioning by an avoidance response. Behav Res Ther 2009;47:716–20.

45. Bouton ME. Context, ambiguity and unlearning: sources of relapse after behavioral extinction. Biol Psychiatry 2002;52:976–86.

46. Neuman DL, Kitlertsirivatana E. Exposure to a novel context after extinction causes a renewal of extinguished conditioned responses: implications for the treatment of fear. Behav Res Ther 2010;48(6):565–70.
47. Ursano RJ, Goldenberg M, Zhang L, et al. Posttraumatic stress disorder and traumatic stress: from bench to bedside, from war to disaster. Ann N Y Acad Sci 2010;1208:72–81.
48. Heim C, Newport JD, Heit S, et al. Pituitary-adrenal and autonomic responses to stress in women after sexual and physical abuse in childhood. JAMA 2000;284: 592–7.
49. Bremner JD, Narayan M. The effects of stress on memory and hippocampus throughout the life cycle: implications for childhood development and aging. Dev Psychopathol 1998;10(4):871–85.
50. Pitman RK, Shin LM, Rauch SL. Investigating the pathogenesis of posttraumatic stress disorder with neuroimaging. J Clin Psychiatry 2001;62(Suppl 17):47–54.
51. Bremner JD. Neuroimaging of childhood trauma. Semin Clin Neuropsychiatry 2002;7(2):104–12.
52. McTeague LM, Lang PJ. The anxiety spectrum and the reflex physiology of defense: from circumscribed fear to broad distress. Depress Anxiety 2012;29(4): 264–81.
53. Hettema JM, Annas P, Neale MC, et al. A twin study of the genetics of fear conditioning. Arch Gen Psychiatry 2003;60(7):702–8.
54. Londsorf TB, Kalisch R. A review on experimental and clinical genetic associations studies on fear conditioning, extinction and cognitive-behavioral treatment. Transl Psychiatry 2011;1:e41.
55. Pitman RK, Delahanty DL. Conceptually driven pharmacologic approaches to acute trauma. CNS Spectr 2005;10(2):99–106.
56. Foa EB, Kozak MJ. Emotional processing of fear: exposure to corrective information. Psychol Bull 1986;99:20–35.
57. Berry AC, Rosenfield D, Smits JA. Extinction retention predicts improvement in social anxiety symptoms following exposure therapy. Depress Anxiety 2009;26: 22–7.
58. van Minnen A, Hagenaars M. Fear activation and habituation patterns as early process predictors of response to prolonged exposure treatment in PTSD. J Trauma Stress 2002;15(5):359–67.
59. Aikins DE, Jackson ED, Christensen A, et al. Differential conditioned fear response predicts duloxetine treatment outcome in male veterans with PTSD: a pilot study. Psychiatry Res 2011;188:453–5.
60. Zantvoord JB, Diehle J, Lindauer RJ. Using neurobiological measures to predict and assess treatment outcome of psychotherapy in posttraumatic stress disorder: systematic review. Psychother Psychosom 2013;82(3):142–51.
61. Bryant RA, Felmingham K, Whitford TJ, et al. Rostral anterior cingulate volume predicts treatment response to cognitive-behavioural therapy for posttraumatic stress disorder. J Psychiatry Neurosci 2008;33(2):142–6.
62. Felmingham KL, Dobson-Stone C, Schofiel PR, et al. The brain-derived neurotrophic factor Val66Met polymorphism predicts response to exposure therapy in posttraumatic stress disorder. Biol Psychiatry 2012;73(11):1059–63.
63. Craske MG, Rachman SJ. Return of fear: perceived skill and heart-rate responsivity. Br J Clin Psychol 1987;26(Pt 3):187–99.
64. Rodriguez BI, Craske MG, Mineka S, et al. Context-specificity of relapse: effects of therapist and environmental context on return of fear. Behav Res Ther 1999; 37:845–62.

65. Hofmann SG. Enhancing exposure-based therapy from a translational research perspective. Behav Res Ther 2007;45(9):1987–2001.

66. Gunduz-Cinar O, MacPherson KP, Cinar R, et al. Convergent translational evidence of a role for anandamide in amygdala-mediated fear extinction, threat processing and stress-reactivity. Mol Psychiatry 2013;18:813–23.

67. Mahan AL, Ressler KJ. Fear conditioning, synaptic plasticity and the amygdala: implication for posttraumatic stress disorder. Trends Neurosci 2012;35(1):24–35.

68. Morrison FG, Ressler KJ. From the neurobiology of extinction to improved clinical treatments. Depress Anxiety 2014;31:279–90.

69. Marin MF, Camprodon JA, Dougherty DD, et al. Device-based brain stimulation to augment fear extinction: implications for PTSD treatment and beyond. Depress Anxiety 2014;31:269–78.

Stress in Service Members

R. Gregory Lande, DO[a,b,*]

KEYWORDS

- Military stress • Military culture • Deployment cycle • Alcohol use disorders
- Posttraumatic stress disorder • Early interventions • Nonpharmacologic treatment

KEY POINTS

- Understand the unique attributes of military life.
- Understand the common military stresses.
- Most service members adapt without difficulty.
- Stress is cumulative.
- Trauma exposure is common.
- Screen for posttraumatic stress.
- Screen for alcohol use disorders.
- Early intervention should emphasize nonpharmacologic management.

INTRODUCTION

Military service is a unique form of employment. It is one of the few occupations that modern societies can compel. Voluntary military service increases motivation but does not reduce the hazards or its stressors. Nations maintain militaries for many reasons, ranging from more offensive, aggressive purposes, such as the acquisition of territory, to more defensive reasons, such as protecting the citizenry from real or imagined threats. The purpose of any military is the projection of power, with the capability to initiate or repel an armed conflict. Whatever the inciting reason, Carl von Clausewitz, the erudite nineteenth-century German military strategist, summed it up best by declaring "that war is the continuation of politics by other means."[1]

Another distinctive aspect of military service is the ever present and persistent risk of death. This is not an existential threat. Even during periods of prolonged peace,

The views expressed in this article are those of the author and do not reflect the official policy of the Department of Army/Navy/Air Force, Department of Defense, or US Government.
[a] Medical Corps (RET), US Army, USA; [b] Psychiatry Continuity Service, Department of Psychiatry, Walter Reed National Military Medical Center, Building 8, 4th Floor, 8901 Wisconsin Avenue, Bethesda, MD 20889-5600, USA
* Psychiatry Continuity Service, Department of Psychiatry, Walter Reed National Military Medical Center, Building 8, 4th Floor, 8901 Wisconsin Avenue, Bethesda, MD 20889-5600.
E-mail address: Raymond.G.Lande.civ@health.mil

Psychiatr Clin N Am 37 (2014) 547–560
http://dx.doi.org/10.1016/j.psc.2014.08.007
0193-953X/14/$ – see front matter Published by Elsevier Inc.

Abbreviations	
AUD	Alcohol use disorders
GABA	γ-Aminobutyric acid
NMDA	N-Methyl-D-aspartate
PDHRA	Post-Deployment Health Reassessment
SBIRT	Screening, Brief Intervention and Referral to Treatment

military service members must confront the real potential for a sudden life-changing deployment. During war, the risk is naturally greater, both in terms of personal harm and collateral exposure from witnessing the morbidity, mortality, and destruction that conflicts create.

Aside from conscription and the risks of morbidity and mortality, military life introduces individuals to a subculture that requires adaptation for successful integration. As much as injury and death is a core facet of military life, so is a countervailing trend denying this possibility. The myth of invincibility or invulnerability is essential, honed through military training, and bolstering an unwavering confidence in the mission, weapons, and leadership.[2] Acceptance reduces anxiety but may also collaterally reduce group discussion about the horrors of war, almost as if talking about one's thoughts and feelings erodes the myth of invincibility. The service member's adoption of the myth seems to thrive, perhaps even intensify, after returning from combat, resulting in the further pursuit of risky activities.[3]

Other attributes of military life include obedience, regimentation, subordination of self to the group, integrity, and flexibility. Military training begins the conspicuous process of indoctrinating these values from the moment that a person first dons a uniform. The purpose is clear: to promote self-confidence and ensure faithful allegiance when it is most needed. The battlefield is not the place to argue. Each person has a purpose, guided through the leadership of more senior individuals. A predictable social structure, clearly visible on a military uniform, is a tangible reminder of authority, which offers the reassurance that comes from leadership.

One of the more important aspects of military life is unit cohesion. Unit cohesion, as the term implies, is an intangible glue the binds the individual members to the group. Each person draws both strength and comfort from the arrangement. Unit cohesion is particularly important on the battlefield, with mutual support affecting everything from the outcome of the conflict to the management of casualties. Various concepts promote unit cohesion, such as buddy support, but one of the defining values of military service is the expectation than no one is left behind.

In terms of assessing military stressors, it is important to understand the service member's environment. Those involved in combat operations experience periods of intense danger, which might alternate with periods of inactivity. Normal sleep is often one of the first casualties of combat. Communications with family and friends may be disrupted. The normal comforts of home are exchanged for the harsher, more spartan, battlefield. Privacy is often sacrificed. There is no real downtime; war demands a focused concentration, a watchful vigilance, and an energetic drive.

All service members in combat experience varying degrees of stress (**Box 1**). Military training is the tonic that reduces the stress sufficiently for service members to perform their job. Yet, training alone does not entirely determine the outcome. Each service member has their unique personality and coping styles. In some cases, the service member's constitutional makeup inhibits their integration. A clinical vignette helps show such a situation.

CLINICAL VIGNETTE: SERVICE MEMBER WITH A PERSONALITY DISORDER

The new recruit sailed through basic training, earning kudos for his hard work and serious demeanor. He benefitted from the highly structured nature of this entry-level military training, which directed every aspect of his life. Not being burdened by such common daily decisions as which clothes to wear, when to eat, and even who to socialize with left the new recruit free to concentrate on learning about military life. However, the highly regimented nature of basic training failed to expose the recruit's fundamentally aloof nature, pursuit of solitary activities, and interpersonal awkwardness. After completing basic training, he entered the next phase of his training, which would prepare him to be an infantry soldier. This training, although still highly organized, left the soldier with more leisure time. When the weekend rolled around, his buddies naturally expected him to join in their frivolous, often alcohol-laced, cavorting. Each time he was approached, the soldier dismissed the invitations with a haughty laugh. No one understood his refusal, but the soldier's preoccupation with video games, lack of friends, cold behavior, and indifference to criticism left him labeled as weird, odd, and crazy. Fellow soldiers soon avoided him, and during training no one trusted that this soldier "would have their back" in combat. He soon became an object of ridicule, which quietly angered the soldier. Toward the end of his infantry training, the soldier had an angry outburst, complaining bitterly that "everyone" was picking on him. His commander was alarmed by the outburst and referred the soldier to a mental health clinic, where a diagnosis of schizoid personality disorder was made. To the relief of all involved, the soldier was administratively separated from military service.

In this clinical vignette, the soldier's schizoid personality prevented him from binding with the other group members. His interpersonal deficits pushed people away, leaving him contentedly isolated. Teamwork is the epitome of military service, with reciprocal respect and trust being indispensable. The soldier was simply unable to function in this capacity, justifying his removal from active-duty military service.

The rigors of training and combat are unique military stressors, but service members are not immune from a panoply of other problems, ranging from the ordinary to the

Box 1
Summary of military stressors

Deployment to an area of combat operations

Trauma exposure

Frequent assignments, both stateside and overseas

Competitive career environment

Discipline and hierarchal structure

Termination from military service

Conflicts with supervisors and peers

Operational tempo

Housing problems

Financial problems

Medical fitness for duty

Marital conflicts

Deployment-related communication problems

Child care

extraordinary. Perhaps foremost among this list is notification of a pending deployment. Naturally, assignment to an area of combat operations is more stressful than a humanitarian deployment, but each may come with little advance notice. These sorts of deployments upend whatever stability the service member had achieved in their regular job. In short order, any number of actions might need to be accomplished, such as settling leases, selling a house, storing personal possessions (including automobiles), child care, and packing luggage.

Short of combat or humanitarian deployments, service members are subject to regular reassignments, often referred to as a permanent change of station. Some are more desirable locations than others, but all must be filled. Several factors aside from the imperative needs of the military determine who goes where, such as rank, experience, and history of previous assignments. In some cases, positions are competitive, such as senior leadership positions. Service members submit their wish lists and, based on various factors, may or may not realize their goals. The assignment process can be stressful, particularly if the final decision results in an undesirable choice. When assessing service members' stressors, clinicians can ask a series of questions probing this process.

Termination from military service is another potential stressor. Even when planned for, such as retirement after a rewarding 20-year career, the service member must manage the transition to civilian life. This transition again might involve relocation, but in most cases, might also involve decisions about future employment and education. A rough analysis predicting the degree of stress in this situation could, at least in part, rely on the service member's current job and its transferability to civilian life. For example, military health care providers might find the employment transition less stressful, given the similarity of duties.

In some cases, termination from the military is not planned. Certain medical conditions may leave the service member medically unfit for continued active duty. Service members who cannot adapt to military life, have substandard performance, or have recurrent disciplinary problems may be administratively separated. Serious misconduct might result in a court-martial, with subsequent punishment. Unplanned terminations raise a host of potential stressors, such as the type of military discharge, the impact on benefits, prospects for future employment, and the ignominious position of having to explain the outcome.

Career paths in the military require continuous learning. As a service member ascends the military hierarchy, education increasingly focuses on leadership. However, no amount of training can eliminate every disagreement or entirely inoculate the system from poor leaders or personality clashes. In this respect, military life may not seem dissimilar from civilian employment, with its inevitable workplace conflicts. However, there is 1 important distinction. Conflicts with a military supervisor can result in serious legal consequences, ranging from nonjudicial punishment to criminal charges. Service members may loathe confronting their supervisor, even when warranted. If the service member's particular coping style is less adaptive, this may leave few alternatives for conflict resolution, with a corresponding inability to effectively manage the relationship.

A panoply of other problems may plague the service member. The operational tempo of the environment may change dramatically at times, requiring longer work hours, with the accompanying infringement on personal time. Temporary duty assignments may require a geographic relocation, which may add further disruption. Military assignments may complicate housing and financial planning, and, depending on the location, may even expose the service member to a range of exotic infectious diseases.

Up this point, the stresses associated with the military have focused solely on the individual service member. Although the number fluctuates year over year, roughly half of all service members are married.[4] This dyad adds another source of potential stress as the couple adjusts to military life.

In the typical relationship, 1 partner is in the military, whereas the other is not. Perhaps the greatest adjustment the pair must overcome involves reassignments. If the relocation is within the Unites States, the couple must deal with the myriad of issues involved with a move. This relocation includes finding suitable housing, leaving friends and possibly family behind, addressing the spouse's employment, and making the necessary financial preparations. If children are involved, then, plans for day care and school are added to the list.

Assignments outside the Unites States place further potential strain on the family. Obviously, a service member's deployment to an area of combat operations or humanitarian need leaves the family behind. This factor leaves the civilian spouse in charge of the entire household, including children. Communication between the spouses may also be severely limited, given the military spouse's particular assignment.

Some overseas assignments permit the family to remain together. In these cases, the couple and any children face a new culture. The learning curve can be steep, as the family navigates such familiar obstacles as housing, employment, and education. The military provides a vast array of helpful services to smooth the transition, but the stress of moving overseas can be considerable.

Although the typical marriage is between a service member and a civilian, there are marriages between 2 service members. In most cases, the military tries to assign both persons together or in close proximity, but the overarching needs of the service may prohibit this. The daily struggles of managing joint military careers may be even more daunting when children are involved.

Despite the long list of military stressors, researchers have only recently focused on these issues. These studies provide confirmation and clarification and also identify service members' attitudes and behaviors that predispose to problems resolving these stressors. One service-wide behavior that seems to cut across all echelons of the military is a basic resistance to seeking help.[5] Barriers to seeking help include real and perceived threats to the service member's career.

An inability to manage the psychosocial stressors leads to impaired duty performance, absenteeism, and overall dissatisfaction with military service. This problem is most pronounced among younger service members, early in their military career.[6] Supervisors at all levels should be on the alert for changes in duty performance that might suggest a stress overload. Sometimes, the supervisor may be part of the problem. Not every leader develops the skills necessary to promote a good work environment, and should such an individual manage a large group of service members, the impact can be disproportionate and widespread. Even so, the most frequently cited dissatisfaction in 1 study singled out "too much work and too few people."[7]

Service members may come to the attention of health care providers through several different channels. Even although self-referral carries certain risks in the minds of many service members, it nonetheless is a means by which they access care. Service members have a variety of options when they decide to independently seek help, such as anonymous telephone help lines, chaplains, and an array of behavioral health care assets. Given the hierarchal nature of the military and training enforcing the importance and value of speaking with a supervisor, it is not unusual for a service member to request help from their chain of command. This individual may remedy this situation or refer the service member for additional help.

Military commanders and supervisors, based on their observations and judgment, can refer a service member for a behavioral assessment. The reasons are many and might simply be a reflection of the supervisor's concern for a service member's welfare. Disruptive behavior, absenteeism, moodiness, or even chronic sleepiness may justify a referral. After a discussion with the service member, the supervisor may conclude that psychosocial stressors are major contributors.

Another broad area leading to behavioral health referrals follows from some form of misconduct. This factor might include problems arising from substance misuse, mostly alcohol, or aggressive outbursts. Once again, an accumulation of military stressors, and an inability to effectively cope, might be the root cause of the behaviors.

CLINICAL VIGNETTE: THE IRRITABLE SERVICE MEMBER

The infantry sergeant had just returned from his third deployment to an area of combat operations. He had an exemplary career, was on the fast track for his next promotion, and was well respected. Roughly a month after returning home, he was assigned to a recruiting office in a large northern city. The hours were long and his supervisor's expectations high, leaving no doubt in the sergeant's mind that failure to meet a quota would be disastrous. Forsaking family life and enjoyable recreational activities, the sergeant attacked the assignment with vigor. Recruiting high-school students proved to be an uphill struggle, and despite his every effort, his numbers started slipping. Efforts to discuss the situation with his supervisor proved fruitless, leaving behind a bitter taste. Feeling isolated and under attack, yet determined to "suck it up," the sergeant was left with few options to relieve the mounting stress. Matters came to a head when the supervisor openly complained about the sergeant's poor work performance, prompting a violent outburst. After he struck a nearby table with his fists, the sergeant's agitation dramatically changed to uncontrolled crying. When the storm passed, the sergeant left the office and drove to a nearby military installation, seeking help in the hospital's emergency room. An astute physician listened to the sergeant's story and referred the reluctant soldier to behavioral health. From those visits, it soon became clear that unresolved traumatic experiences from multiple combat deployments had left the soldier anxious, dysphoric, and irritable. His limited repertoire of coping skills provided no means to resolve his traumatic experiences; a situation favorably fixed when he completed an exposure-based course of psychotherapy.

Certain coping styles seem to predict which service members become psychological casualties.[8] Service members, who are predominately passive, interpret their environment as highly stressful, and those who are more emotive than cognitive have more trouble adapting. Alternatively, those who actively use problem-solving techniques and avoid embellishment are less likely to suffer stress-related impairment.

The differences in adopting an active or passive response to stress were borne out in another study. Respondents were asked to pick from a list of behaviors they would pursue when "pressured, stressed, depressed, or anxious."[9] Choices were grouped among active and avoidant problem-solving behaviors. Active choices included such options as talking with a friend or planning a strategy, whereas avoidance choices included behaviors such as a reliance on alcohol or food. Gender differences emerged from the respondent's choices, with women more likely to seek help among friends and family and use food as a source of comfort, whereas men reached out less and turned to alcohol more.

A supportive home life helps service members weather the stresses of military life. The opposite is also true when a dysfunctional marriage or troubled children demand the service member's attention.[10] Long deployments, often coupled with an uncertain end date, can be particularly stressful for a spouse. Combine that situation with pregnancy, and both partners find themselves distracted and distraught by distance and impaired communication.

DEPLOYMENT-RELATED STRESS

For most service members, the greatest stressor involves assignment to an area of combat operations. Despite all the training received, nothing can fully prepare a service member for such a mission. Most service members clearly manage their anxiety, turning to their social support network, implementing problem-solving skills, and relying on their military experience. However, others develop varying degrees of incapacitating symptoms as they ineffectively cope with the stress. In most cases, the means by which the service members try to reduce their stress further aggravates their discomfort. Among this cohort, common outcomes include substance misuse, overeating, social withdrawal, depression, anxiety, and insomnia.

Assessing deployment-related stress benefits from an approach that recognizes 3 phases: predeployment activities, the deployment, and the postdeployment return home. Broadly understanding what typically accompanies each phase helps the clinician more accurately pinpoint problem-prone areas. This factor in turn may help the clinician more effectively design a therapeutic intervention.

Uncertainty is the theme uniting all 3 phases of deployment. Predeployment begins when the service member first receives news of the pending assignment. This news launches a combination of military training, relocation-related activities, and personal time with family and friends. Throughout it all, the service member experiences a swirl of emotions, in some cases proving overwhelming. Among this latter group, some may turn to alcohol or tobacco in an effort to quell their discomfort.

The deployment phase exposes the service member to varying degrees of privation and danger. A service member's specific job is another factor in the stress analysis. Direct combat duties clearly carry the greatest risks, but other occupations such as health care can also be stressful.[11] Constant exposure to battlefield injuries, whether physical or emotional, can erode the clinician's resilience. During unconventional warfare, in which enemy combatants blend into the civilian population and rely on tactics such as improvised explosive devices, there are no safe zones. Indiscriminate lobbing of mortars into supposedly more secure military facilities may not always do much physical damage, but it keeps service members perpetually on guard.

Even the daily hassles of battlefield life can slowly add up, drip by drip, sometimes unleashing a torrent of emotions. A catalog of daily hassles includes such minor irritants as the quality of food, the weather, lack of sleep, lack of recreational diversions, and limited communications with family and friends. The cumulative effect of nontraumatic deployment-experienced stressors may predispose the service member to more mental health problems than a specific traumatic event.[12] It could be that repetitive minor annoyances wear the service member down, albeit slowly, and contribute to a confidence-destroying pessimism. With this mind-set, depression has fertile ground to develop.

It is not uncommon for deployed service members to count down the days until departure. This anticipation allows many service members to ignore or at least minimize deployment-related stressors. Sometimes, the needs of the military delay the service member's departure. For some, this delay can be a particularly troubling development and, for the marginally compensated service member, may result in an incapacitating emotional disorder.

Postdeployment heralds the return home. For most, it is a joyous occasion, full of relief. The military takes this transition seriously and screens for any evidence of behavioral problems. All service members deployed to Iraq or Afghanistan completed the Post-Deployment Health Reassessment (PDHRA) screening instrument on return. The self-administered PDHRA screens for major depressive disorder, posttraumatic stress disorder (PTSD), and alcohol use disorders (AUD).[13]

The results of the PDHRA may lead to the service member's referral for an in-depth evaluation. As mentioned earlier, the PDHRA is just 1 channel leading to behavioral health care. Other pathways might include medical consultation, command referral, or self-referral. Regardless of the means by which the service member accesses behavioral health care, clinicians need to carefully analyze the symptoms in a military-oriented context. In many cases, the clinician identifies a significant mood or substance use disorder.

SUBSTANCE USE AND STRESS

Substance misuse and stress have a symbiotic relationship. A casual and widespread belief associating alcohol and drug misuse with stress is increasingly borne out by research. This factor is particularly true in the military, in which detailed epidemiologic studies track changes over time in the use of these substances.[14] Heavy drinking, defined as 5 or more drinks per occasion at least once a week during the preceding 30 days, increased from 15% to 20% from 1998 to 2008. During the same period, illegal drug use declined, with the notable exception of prescription drug misuse. Tobacco use declined up to 2008, with 31% of service members still smoking cigarettes.

Combat deployment may affect alcohol use. Results from a large survey[15] reported that service members deployed to an area of combat operations were significantly more likely to engage in binge drinking when compared with those not deployed. A closer examination showed that the highest-risk group of binge drinkers was not only combat veterans but also younger service members and those experiencing marital stress.

It seems intuitive that multiple combat assignments would, through an accumulation of traumatic and stressful events, increase the risks of problem drinking. In reality, most service members do not succumb to this conventional wisdom. Even so, a high-risk subgroup of service members do increase their drinking in proportion to the number and length of combat tours.[16] Clinicians uncovering such a pattern should explore this trend, looking for specific stressors that may be associated with the increased drinking.

Service members from the National Guard and Reserves deployed to an area of combat operations are more likely to develop new onset drinking than active-duty personnel.[17] The finding was particularly prominent among the younger service members. The higher rate of new onset drinking in National Guard and Reserve service members may relate to several factors. Perhaps foremost was the military's substantial mobilization of the National Guard and Reserve forces in Iraq and Afghanistan, no doubt an unexpected development for many of these part-time service members. The transition from a predominately civilian life to full-time military service was also a more abrupt and destabilizing experience for members of the National Guard and Reserve. Again, the clinically important point is assessing the context and avoiding a monolithic view of military service.

Much of the research exploring the relationship between alcohol use and stress comes through observations of the civilian workforce, with subsequent application to the military. Aside from the extraordinary stress associated with a deployment to an area of combat operations, the studies conducted in nonmilitary settings are still applicable to service members.

A national survey[18] collected data among a random sample of civilian employees in an effort to identify alcohol use during duty hours, within 2 hours of starting the work day, and reporting to work suffering a hangover. Based on the results obtained, the researchers extrapolated the findings to the American workforce and estimated that 15% of employees were alcohol impaired. A further breakdown of the data showed that 1.83% drank alcohol before reporting to work, 7.06% used alcohol during work, and 9.23% reported working with a hangover at least once during the preceding 12 months.

One of the more consistent associations with an AUD is a childhood history of abuse. Divorce and job loss are 2 other life stressors that also correlate with problem drinking.[19] Perhaps not surprisingly, a history of multiple traumas and other major life stressors seems to be cumulative and predispose younger individuals to an AUD.[20] Because this demographic is within the age range of many new recruits, such a history should be explored among service members. The relationship between major stressors and alcohol use may even follow a finer path. A large national epidemiologic survey[21] provided evidence of just such a relationship. The investigators of this study reported that heavy drinking, defined as 5 or more drinks for men and 4 for women consumed in 1 time, increased by 24% among men and 13% among women with each additional psychosocial stressor. This study suggests that in individuals already primed to misuse alcohol, there is a response to stress by consuming larger amounts of alcohol. A similar study once again confirmed that among individuals in remission from an AUD, the destabilizing stress associated with interpersonal conflicts such as divorce frequently led to a relapse.[22]

Stress plays an important role in a service member's choice to use alcohol. Of course, not every service member makes this choice, and even fewer develop an AUD. Despite the reported increase in heavy drinking, only 12% to 15% of service members deployed to Iraq indicated a concern about problem drinking when assessed 3 and 6 months after deployment.[23] The factors that mediate a normal response to a stressor that transitions to an AUD are the result of complex and not yet fully understood psychosocial and physiologic interactions.

An interesting psychosocial theory proposes that the workplace environment contributes to an employee's alcohol misuse.[24] In conceptualizing this approach, 3 different models are used to explain the deleterious interaction between the employee and their work, specifically social control, availability, and stress.

Social control is a measure of the person's integration into the work group.[24] An extension of this model to the military suggests that service members who are not integrated and remain detached are more likely to misuse alcohol. In some cases, this situation is aggravated by jobs with minimal supervision and low institutional visibility.

The availability model, as the names implies, suggests that workplaces in which alcohol is readily obtainable have a higher incidence of misuse. However, availability has 2 dimensions: physical and social. Physical availability is the ease of obtaining alcohol while at work, the prototype example being a bartender. Social availability is more of an expression of peer and leadership endorsement, with either implicit or explicit approval associated with higher rates of misuse. In the military, alcohol is not within arm's reach anywhere, and more austere assignments make it even more difficult.

In terms of social sanctions, the military has service-specific policies that deglamorize alcohol use and set strict standards for defining impairment. The Army policy for example states that "Commanders are encouraged to use drug or alcohol testing when there is a reasonable suspicion that a Soldier is using a controlled substance or has a blood alcohol level of .05 percent or above while on duty. This information will assist a commander in his or her determination of the need for counseling, rehabilitation, or medical treatment."[25] The Navy and Marine Corps have a more stringent policy involving random Breathalyzer tests.[26] Service members deployed to Iraq or Afghanistan were informed of General Order 1b, which prohibited the "introduction, possession, sale, transfer, manufacture or consumption of any alcoholic beverage within countries of Kuwait, Saudi Arabia, Pakistan, Afghanistan, and Iraq."[27]

The third psychosocial theory linking the workplace to increased alcohol use is the stress model.[24] From an organizational standpoint, employees are less likely to misuse alcohol if they have a meaningful job, have a voice in shaping their role, and are kept busy. The inverse, in which boredom reigns and a top-down management style limits employee participation, breeds stress and a higher likelihood of alcohol use.

Psychosocial factors interact with the person's physiology to complete the matrix that in some service members leads to an AUD. The biological contribution is complex and not fully understood but involves multiple neurotransmitters systems, the physiologic stress response of the body, and even genetic variations.

Alcohol is a potent chemical, which exerts its effects through multiple neurotransmitters. The 2 main systems affected include the excitatory neurotransmitter glutamate at the N-methyl-D-aspartate (NMDA) subtype of the glutamate receptor and the inhibitory neurotransmitter, γ-aminobutyric acid (GABA).[28] The major excitatory neurotransmitters in the human brain are glutamate and aspartate, which both exert their actions at the NMDA receptor. Alcohol consumption dampens the NMDA receptor activity, resulting in sedation. The opposite effect occurs at the brain's main inhibitory neurotransmitter GABA, with alcohol potentiating the activity of the receptor, producing a sedative and anxiolytic effect. The action of alcohol on these 2 neurotransmitters may also help to explain its well-known ability to impair memory.

The acute effects of moderate alcohol consumption stimulate the nucleus accumbens, an anatomic region located in the midbrain with neural links throughout the brain. The nucleus accumbens is an area rich with dopamine neurons and functions as a reward or pleasure center, motivating behaviors such as eating and sexual activity.[29] GABA neurons located in the ventral tegmental area of the brain project inhibitory impulses to the nucleus accumbens, completing a sort of reciprocal feedback circuit.[30]

Casual alcohol use activates the reward circuitry, producing the physiologically induced pleasurable experience that facilitates replication. A mild to moderate sedation is coupled with stress reduction. Even the memory impairment may, at least initially, be greeted as a positive development, an outcome favored for individuals trying to forget. The sedative effect of alcohol is also prized by some individuals suffering from a stress-induced hyperarousal that prevents sleep initiation. Recent animal research also suggests that alcohol use immediately after a stressor may improve cognition.[31]

Alcohol has a Janus-like quality, one face from casual use and the other emerging with chronic alcohol use. Most of the initial benefits of alcohol stemming from its anxiolytic and sedative qualities disappear with long-term use. The human brain adjusts to the chronic presence of alcohol through neuroadaptation.[32] This complex series of changes probably includes a reversal of acute effect of alcohol on neurotransmitters, resulting in hyperactivity at the NMDA receptor and hypoactivity at the GABA site. Chronic alcohol use also disrupts the brain's physiologic response to stress, as mediated through the corticotropin-releasing factor system.

Neuroadaptation contributes to the development of an AUD. The efforts of the brain to maintain homeostasis in the presence of long-term alcohol use results in cravings, negative emotional states, and the more severe alcohol withdrawal disorders.[33] Periods of abstinence result in a physiologic hypersensitivity to stress, along with irritability, dysphoria, and anxiety, all of which cause enough behavioral discomfort to motivate the individual to drink alcohol in an effort to quell these symptoms. This situation sets in motion a cycle of drinking, which perpetuates use and often culminates in addiction.

Increasingly, there also seems to be a moderate genetic risk associated with the development of an AUD.[34] Research suggests that service members with certain polymorphisms at the μ opioid receptor or the serotonin transporter may be at increased risk. From a clinical standpoint, this same research points toward linking identification of these polymorphisms with specific treatment interventions.

POSTTRAUMATIC STRESS DISORDER

PTSD is the signature military psychiatric disorder. In the decade that followed the start of the 2 wars in Iraq and Afghanistan, data collected from the Defense Medical Surveillance System[35] identified nearly 119,000 cases of PTSD. The numbers peaked in 2012, probably related to the removal of all US forces from Iraq, which occurred toward the end of 2011. The influx spotlighted the treatment of PTSD, which led to the publication of influential guidelines.

The Veterans Administration/Department of Defense practice guidelines provide a comprehensive approach for assessing and managing PTSD.[36] Of particular importance are early intervention strategies to help prevent the progression from an acute stress reaction to full-blown PTSD. The guidelines suggest that clinicians emphasize the use of extant social supports, offer psychoeducation, and attempt to normalize the service member's distress.

It is also important at this time to approach potential alcohol misuse through a systematic approach incorporating screenings, brief interventions, and possible referrals for treatment. The Screening, Brief Intervention and Referral to Treatment (SBIRT) is a public health initiative to identify hazardous drinking at an early stage and, through specific interventions, reduce the trajectory toward an AUD.[37] One of the key components of SBIRT is the definition of hazardous or risky drinking. The screening criteria differ by gender, with safe drinking for men occurring when no more than 4 drinks are consumed in a day and no more than 14 drinks in a week. For women, the limits are no more than 3 drinks in a day and no more than 7 drinks in a week.[38]

Aside from normalizing the stress and screening for alcohol misuse, the clinician should also determine the extent to which any of the military unique stressors may complicate the picture. Family problems, for example, may be an important complicating factor.

EARLY INTERVENTION CONSIDERATIONS

Clinicians should consult published treatment guidelines for current treatment recommendations for PTSD and other related psychiatric disorders. The principal focus of this section is to highlight various nonpharmacologic strategies that can be used in an effort to prevent the progression of a military stressor to a psychiatric disorder. The clinician's approach should be guided by thoroughly assessing military stressors in an attempt to normalize the stressful experience, mobilizing the service member's social supports, and where necessary, introducing nonpharmacologic interventions to reduce anxiety.

In the early stages of managing a stressor, nonpharmacologic interventions are a reasonable choice. Nonpharmacologic interventions avoid the systemic effects of medication and may reinforce healthy behaviors. Regular aerobic exercise is an example of this strategy, with studies finding that service members who maintain a regular physical exercise program are more resilient.[39,40] Closely allied with this health promotion concept is an effort to reduce hazardous drinking and any tobacco use.

Military clinicians might also consider other self-care options, such as progressive muscle relaxation, mindfulness-based stress reduction, and cognitive behavior treatments. A systematic review of randomized controlled studies examining the various approaches concluded by noting that "implementing these identified training programs into military settings appears highly feasible..."[41]

Other options are to consider taking advantage of newer technologies, which are generally well received among military service members. Perhaps foremost among this group is cranial electrotherapy stimulation.[42] This is a medical device that is approved by the US Food and Drug Administration for the treatment of depression, anxiety, and insomnia. This noninvasive treatment can be used in the early intervention treatment of anxiety and insomnia, 2 common symptoms of military stress. Simple biofeedback instruments and software programs that measure skin temperature, heart rate variability, or biorhythms can also help the service member make the connection between stress and the subsequent physiologic response.

SUMMARY

Military service is a rewarding occupation, but it differs from civilian jobs in terms of the unique stresses that service members experience. Among the differences are frequent deployments, which may involve an assignment to an area of combat operations. Other attributes of military life include obedience, regimentation, subordination of self to the group, integrity, and flexibility. The military culture emphasizes teamwork and peer support. In some cases, service members cannot adapt to military life, become overwhelmed by stress, or cannot overcome a traumatic experience. In these cases, clinicians should conduct a thorough evaluation, guided by an understanding of the military culture. Every effort should be made to identify the stress and the maladaptive response and, where possible, provide early nonpharmacologic clinical interventions to prevent progression.

REFERENCES

1. Paret P. Clausewitz and the state: the man, his theories, and his times. Princeton (NJ): Princeton University Press; 2007.
2. Hollingshead AB. Adjustment to military life. Am J Sociol 1946;51:439–47.
3. Kelley AM, Athy JR, Cho TH, et al. Risk propensity and health risk behaviors in US army soldiers with and without psychological disturbances across the deployment cycle. J Psychiatr Res 2012;46(5):582–9.
4. Wilmoth JM, London AS. Life course perspectives on military service. New York: Taylor & Francis; 2013.
5. Langston V, Gould M, Greenberg N. Culture: what is its effect on stress in the military? Mil Med 2007;172(9):931–5.
6. Hourani LL, Williams TV, Kress AM. Stress, mental health, and job performance among active duty military personnel: findings from the 2002 Department of Defense Health-Related Behaviors Survey. Mil Med 2006;171(9):849–56.
7. Pflanz SE, Ogle AD. Job stress, depression, work performance, and perceptions of supervisors in military personnel. Mil Med 2006;171(9):861–5.
8. Taylor MK, Mujica-Parodi LR, Padilla GA, et al. Behavioral predictors of acute stress symptoms during intense military training. J Trauma Stress 2009;22(3):212–7.
9. Bray RM, Fairbank JA, Marsden ME. Stress and substance use among military women and men. Am J Drug Alcohol Abuse 1999;25(2):239–56.

10. de Burgh HT, White CJ, Fear NT, et al. The impact of deployment to Iraq or Afghanistan on partners and wives of military personnel. Int Rev Psychiatry 2011;23(2):192–200.

11. Gibbons SW, Barnett SD, Hickling EJ, et al. Stress, coping, and mental health-seeking behaviors: gender differences in OEF/OIF health care providers. J Trauma Stress 2012;25(1):115–9.

12. Heron EA, Bryan CJ, Dougherty CA, et al. Military mental health: the role of daily hassles while deployed. J Nerv Ment Dis 2013;201(12):1035–9.

13. Skopp NA, Swanson R, Luxton DD, et al. An examination of the diagnostic efficiency of post-deployment mental health screens. J Clin Psychol 2012; 68(12):1253–65.

14. Bray RM, Pemberton MR, Lane ME, et al. Substance use and mental health trends among US military active duty personnel: key findings from the 2008 DoD Health Behavior Survey. Mil Med 2010;175(6):390–9.

15. Lande RG, Marin BA, Chang AS, et al. Survey of alcohol use in the US Army. J Addict Dis 2008;27(3):115–21.

16. Spera C, Thomas RK, Barlas F, et al. Relationship of military deployment recency, frequency, duration, and combat exposure to alcohol use in the Air Force. J Stud Alcohol Drugs 2011;72(1):5–14.

17. Jacobson IG, Ryan MA, Hooper TI, et al. Alcohol use and alcohol-related problems before and after military combat deployment. JAMA 2008;300(6):663–75.

18. Frone MR. Prevalence and distribution of alcohol use and impairment in the workplace: a US national survey. J Stud Alcohol 2006;67(1):147–56.

19. Keyes KM, Hatzenbuehler ML, Hasin DS. Stressful life experiences, alcohol consumption, and alcohol use disorders: the epidemiologic evidence for four main types of stressors. Psychopharmacology 2011;218(1):1–17.

20. Lloyd DA, Turner RJ. Cumulative lifetime adversities and alcohol dependence in adolescence and young adulthood. Drug Alcohol Depend 2008;93(3):217–26.

21. Dawson DA, Grant BF, Ruan WJ. The association between stress and drinking: modifying effects of gender and vulnerability. Alcohol Alcohol 2005;40(5):453–60.

22. Pilowsky DJ, Keyes KM, Geier TJ, et al. Stressful life events and relapse among formerly alcohol dependent adults. Soc Work Ment Health 2013;11(2):184–97.

23. Milliken CS, Auchterlonie JL, Hoge CW. Longitudinal assessment of mental health problems among active and reserve component soldiers returning from the Iraq war. JAMA 2007;298(18):2141–8.

24. Barling J, Cooper CL. The SAGE handbook of organizational behavior. Micro approaches, vol. 1. London: Sage; 2008.

25. The Army substance abuse program. Department of the Army. Army Regulation 600–85. Washington, DC; 2012. Available at: http://www.apd.army.mil/pdffiles/r600_85.pdf. Accessed September 11, 2014.

26. Secretary of the Navy Announces 21st Century Sailor and Marine Initiative. 2012. Available at: http://www.navy.mil/submit/display.asp?story_id=65698. Accessed April 8, 2014.

27. CENTCOM General Order 1B. Alcohol and drug abuse. 2009. Available at: http://www.arcent.army.mil/docs/2009-ig-bulletins/2009-03-mar-alcohol-and-drug-abuse.pdf?sfvrsn=2. Accessed April 8, 2014.

28. Valenzuela CF. Alcohol and neurotransmitter interactions. Alcohol Health Res World 1997;21(2):144–8.

29. Ikemoto S, Panksepp J. The role of nucleus accumbens dopamine in motivated behavior: a unifying interpretation with special reference to reward-seeking. Brain Res Brain Res Rev 1999;31(1):6–41.

30. Marty VN, Spigelman I. Effects of alcohol on the membrane excitability and synaptic transmission of medium spiny neurons in the nucleus accumbens. Alcohol 2012;46(4):317–27.

31. Gomez JL, Lewis MJ, Sebastian V, et al. Alcohol administration blocks stress-induced impairments in memory and anxiety, and alters hippocampal neurotransmitter receptor expression in male rats. Horm Behav 2013;63(4):659–66.

32. Cui C, Noronha A, Morikawa H, et al. New insights on neurobiological mechanisms underlying alcohol addiction. Neuropharmacology 2013;67:223–32.

33. Breese GR, Sinha R, Heilig M. Chronic alcohol neuroadaptation and stress contribute to susceptibility for alcohol craving and relapse. Pharmacol Ther 2011; 129(2):149–71.

34. Enoch MA. Genetic influences on response to alcohol and response to pharmacotherapies for alcoholism. Pharmacol Biochem Behav 2014;123:17–24.

35. Fischer H. A guide to US military casualty statistics: Operation New Dawn, Operation Iraqi Freedom, and Operation Enduring Freedom. Washington, DC: Congressional Research Service; 2014. Available at: http://fas.org/sgp/crs/natsec/RS22452.pdf. Accessed September 11, 2014.

36. The Management of Post-Traumatic Stress Working Group. VA/DoD Clinical practice guideline for management of post-traumatic stress. Washington, DC: Department of Veterans Affairs; 2010. Available at: http://www.healthquality.va.gov/guidelines/MH/ptsd/cpg_PTSD-FULL-201011612.pdf. Accessed September 11, 2014.

37. McCance-Katz EF, Satterfield J. SBIRT: a key to integrate prevention and treatment of substance abuse in primary care. Am J Addict 2012;21(2):176–7.

38. Lande RG, Marin BA, Chang AS, et al. Gender differences and alcohol use in the US Army. J Am Osteopath Assoc 2007;107(9):401–7.

39. Taylor MK, Markham AE, Reis JP, et al. Physical fitness influences stress reactions to extreme military training. Mil Med 2008;173(8):738–42.

40. Martins LC, Lopes CS. Rank, job stress, psychological distress and physical activity among military personnel. BMC Public Health 2013;13:716.

41. Crawford C, Wallerstedt DB, Khorsan R, et al. A systematic review of biopsychosocial training programs for the self-management of emotional stress: potential applications for the military. Evid Based Complement Alternat Med 2013;2013: 747694.

42. Lande RG, Gragnani C. Efficacy of cranial electric stimulation for the treatment of insomnia: a randomized pilot study. Complement Ther Med 2013;21(1):8–13.

Humor

Michel A. Woodbury-Fariña, MD, DFAPA, FAIS*,
Joalex L. Antongiorgi, MD

KEYWORDS

- Humor • Oxytocin • Freud • Albert Ellis • Melanie Klein • Playful therapy
- Laughter yoga • Locus of control

KEY POINTS

- Humor is related to changes in 5-hydroxytryptamine 1A and oxytocin.
- Humor can be adaptive or maladaptive.
- Humor can be expressed as protohumor, non-Duchenne smiles, Duchenne smiles, and laughter.
- According to the Humor Styles Questionnaire, 4 styles of humor have been identified: affiliative, self-enhancing, aggressive, and self-defeating.
- Other frequently used humor questionnaires are the State and Trait Cheerfulness Inventory, Coping Humor Scale, and 3-Witz-Dimensionen scale.
- Male and women tend to view humor differently and this difference is seen in the way they socialize with each other, as in dating.
- Men making women laugh is the usual social interaction.
- Freud is possibly one of the influences that have resulted in making clinicians believe that humor is inappropriate to use with patients.
- Albert Ellis embraced humor in his therapy.
- A Kleinian view of humor tries to solve splitting by fusing the serious with the humorous.
- Examples of playful therapy are giving a thumbs-up sign with good news.
- Everyone can develop a sense of humor.
- Laughter yoga is a type of yoga that is based on 20 minutes of nonstop laughter and can be extremely therapeutic.
- Humor helps to change to an internal locus of control.

INTRODUCTION

Humor is an amusing social interaction that occurs best between 2 or more persons.[1] Types of humor include sarcasm, slapstick, wit or punning, dry humor, and gallows humor. A sense of humor, and the ability and willingness to use the types

Disclosures: Speaker for Pfizer (M.A. Woodbury-Farina); none (J.L. Antongiorgi).
Department of Psychiatry, University of Puerto Rico School of Medicine, PO Box 365067, San Juan, PR 00936-5067, USA
* Corresponding author. Department of Psychiatry, University of Puerto Rico School of Medicine, 307 Calle Eleanor Roosevelt, San Juan, PR 00918-2720.
E-mail address: michel.woodbury@upr.edu

Psychiatr Clin N Am 37 (2014) 561–578
http://dx.doi.org/10.1016/j.psc.2014.08.006
psych.theclinics.com

Abbreviations	
CHS	Coping Humor Scale
LOC	Locus of control
STCI	State and Trait Cheerfulness Inventory
3WD	3-Witz-Dimensionen

of humor effectively, is considered a positive, desired social skill that attracts friendships[2] and is what most people want to have.[3] Humor can be associated with entertaining events that happen in daily life. In a therapeutic situation, humor can be enriched with personal experiences from other clinicians, to help establish new openings, restart conversations effectively, and bringing out a myriad of emotional issues.[4] In our personal experiences we have found it to be a link between patient and doctor, because most patients have thought that we have shown a more humane side to their treatment. This bond between speaker and listener has been documented as a meaningful role for humor.[5] This developing bond has led to a more personal and intimate connection with our patients, who echo this kind of treatment with some humor of their own as therapy progresses. From having seen famous clinicians like Patch Adams (see www.patchadams.org) portrayed in movies to personal experiences in clinical settings, we have seen that medicine can benefit from this bond seen in using humor. A sense of humor should be so important that an assessment of how much a patient laughs should be part of the clinical work-up. This can be as simple as asking how many times a patient laughs in a typical day. For more information on how to take the laugh history and how to organize the recommendations on who should increase humor according to illness see article by Hasan H and colleagues.[6] Humor should be a part of clinicians' treatment repertoire because the use of humor has been shown to mitigate the effects of negative life stresses, with those who do not use humor responding with depression to the same kind of stress.[7] It can also help all ages, because both Erikson[8] and recent studies about laughter in dementia[9] have proved humor to be a successful complement to traditional medicine. The global aspect of humor and the response of laughter that is evoked aids in the treatment of patients. The results of our interventions can be seen from the smile and innocent laughter in children to a grin or chuckle obtained in elderly patients. Theses results are validation and motivation for clinicians to continue to pursue different ways to use humor in their practices.

OXYTOCIN AND HUMOR

There is evidence from the effects of the drug 3,4-methylenedioxy-N-methylamphetamine (MDMA), also known as "ecstacy" causes users to be very giddy, that laughter stimulates the 5-hydroxytryptamine1A receptor that in turn stimulates oxytocin, the bonding or cuddling hormone.[10] Some clinicians think that the immunologic benefits of humor[11] are caused by an increase in oxytocin[12] because of the associated benefits in wound healing seen with such increases in oxytocin. With oxytocin, both cortisol[13] and the amygdala[14] are inhibited, thus decreasing the sense of danger. Thus, people who experience increases in oxytocin are not experiencing fear, which contributes to the desired relaxing effect. Since oxytocin increases the capacity to notice social cues one can surmise that one is especially attuned to the positive social signals that one sees when one laughs.[15] The question that will continue to be explored is how to take advantage of humor and in what setting. The approach to humor in medicine seems to be changing. Even in primary care, humor is being given more importance.[16,17] Hospitals are now using clowns to help with humor.[18] There might be other incentives to use humor because, in primary care, physicians who used humor, along with spending more time educating and facilitating understanding, were sued less.[19]

NEUROANATOMY OF HUMOR

Another interesting dimension of laughter is the neuroanatomic description of the process. Social laughter can involve auditory association cortices, the right dorsolateral inferior frontal gyrus, and brain areas linked to mentalizing and visual imagery.[20] Actually, laughter involves a voluntary and involuntary pathway that are controlled by a center in the dorsal upper pons.[21] The voluntary pathway goes from the premotor operular areas to the ventral brain stem. The involuntary or emotional pathway involves the amygdala, thalamus, hypothalamus, subthalamus and the dorsal brainstem. The Society for Neurosciences has divided up laughter into three areas: cognitive, which consists of the frontal cortex where we will understand the humorous situation, motor, which consists of the supplemental motor cortex that will coordinate the muscles needed for laughter and the emotional, which is centered in the nucleus accumbens where happiness originates.[22] Further on we will see more information on the actual gender differences in how the brain deals with humor.

EXPRESSION OF HUMOR

The responses to humor can go from playful verbal reactions to the smile and then to laughter. Laughter is divided into protohumor and the Duchenne smile/laughter. Humans inherited playful verbal interactions from our primate ancestors.[23] A smile forms when the muscles at both ends of the mouth (zygomatic major muscle) are flexed as well as the rest of the muscles of the mouth;[24] this is called a non-Duchenne smile. If the corners of the eyes also squint (orbicularis oculi muscle), giving what is known as crow's feet, then this is known as the Duchenne smile[25] and is thought to reflect positive emotions being sent to the receiver.[26] This kind of smile is effaced with Botox treatments because usually the crow's feet are eliminated, making the smile look fake.

Although smiles can also reflect contempt or embarrassment,[24] smiles usually make people seem friendly, are received well by the receivers, and are usually an open invitation to make social contact,[27] sometimes by simply returning the smile. Men find it appealing when women smile at them and rate happy, smiling women as being more attractive and sexy. The reverse is not always true because one study showed that women did not rate happy men as being attractive, preferring displays of pride and shame. Men were impressed with women who expressed shame but not with those women who expressed pride.[28]

Smiles do not always precede laughter but are associated with it. A milder form of laughter is called protohumor. It is a step above playful verbal social interactions that is also expressed in the context of a safe surrounding.[23] This form of laughter is the giggling that children express without laughing out loud. One famous comedian ensured a great response to his jokes by preselecting his audience to be those that expressed protohumor with him; that is, they giggled in his presence even without his telling a joke. True laughter, which means that a strong emotional feeling is being expressed,[29] is known as Duchenne laughter, involves Duchenne smiles,[23] and is the only laughter associated with emotional benefits.[30] The actual study of laughter is known as "gelatology".

STYLES OF HUMOR

Humor can be adaptive or maladaptive.[31] Using the Humor Styles Questionnaire (HSQ), four styles of humor have been identified: affiliative, self-enhancing, aggressive, and self-defeating.[32] Adaptive humor, which is associated with the benefits that result in better mental health, can be affiliative. In this case amusement is used to enhance interpersonal bonds by decreasing tension, as well as self-enhancing humor, which is when amusement is derived from pointing out the incongruities in life. Maladaptive humor, which has negative effects on mental health, can be aggressive (putting others down) or self-defeating (making fun of oneself).[32] Both affiliative and self-enhancing humor are thought to be advanced coping techniques because they are associated with psychological and emotional stability to the point of being protective against depression,[33] are part of extroversion, and are seen in those open to new experiences.[32] Because affiliative humor is the kind of humor used to decrease tension and enhance social bonding, this style has been associated with making friends.[34] Self-enhancing humor is seen in those with a positive attitude and who frequently find something humorous in almost any situation in such a nice way as to not be offensive.[35] Aggressive humor is used by those who do not really care how a joke will be interpreted by the receiver. Thus they do not mind if they hurt others when they jokingly put people down and can tease, laugh at, and ridicule another without much concern. Men use this humor more than women and seem less friendly[32] because of seeming to be too aggressive. Self-defeating humor is characterized by putting oneself down and is usually not appreciated by others.[32] Those who use this humor frequently are at risk for depression[32] because this style is considered to be a defense against truly negative feelings with the humor covering up the true feelings. Men also use this style more than women.[33] Other questionnaires on humor include one that separates state and trait humor, the State and Trait Cheerfulness Inventory (STCI),[36,37] another that identifies humor as a coping strategy (Coping Humor Scale [CHS][38]), as well as one that measures what types of humor are preferred (3-Witz-Dimensionen [3WD][39]). The STCI assesses humorous style by measuring factors that come under cheerfulness, seriousness, and bad mood.[36,37] Because it is a state-trait questionnaire, current humor (state) and how humorous the person usually is (trait) are evaluated. This scale was used to show that at 40 and 60 years of age there are significant increases in a person's ability to take adversities lightly.[40] The 3WD includes whether the person prefers incongruity resolution, silly jokes, or sexual jokes. For an extensive review of humor scales, see Köhler and Ruch.[41] In that review the conclusion was that a sense of humor is on a continuum between cheerfulness and seriousness. Extraverts are usually high on cheerfulness and low on seriousness, with psychoticism showing the opposite trend. Although cheerfulness was thought to be associated with emotional stability, the accuracy of the humor measurement is not thought to be satisfactory enough.[41]

Humor is thought to be the way that people deal with the imperfections of life so as to avoid having to deal with the ensuing negative emotions.[42] Humor improves emotional and physical health by attenuating the natural stress response by decreasing cortisol, dihydrophenylacetic acid (the major serum neuronal catabolite of dopamine), epinephrine, and growth hormone,[43] the result being that people are happier and smarter.[30,44–47] Men express humor through jokes and women express humor through pleasant experiences,[48] with women usually refraining from telling jokes.[49–51] Men use maladaptive humor, which includes not only aggressive and self-depreciating humor but also sexual humor,[52] much more than women.[32] Humor is associated with social bonding among groups.[53,54]

HUMOR AND SOCIALIZING

There are many studies that have shown that humor is associated with successful dating. One sign that the date is going well is that the man is making the woman laugh,[55] which can be done using affiliative and self-enhancing humor. Humor is so important that advice on how the man should go about seducing the woman frequently centers on how to make her laugh. Studies have shown that women evaluate the way men use humor to assess warmth and intelligence in them as well as whether men will be acceptable mates.[55] The way humor is handled behaviorally and neuroanatomically is different in adult men and women.[56,57] The different ways male and female children handle humor continues the same as they grow up into adults with no change in the neuroanatomical sites.[58] Differences in the importance that each sex gives to appreciating humor are seen as early as age 6 years of age. One study has shown that in children 6 to 13 years of age, there is a gender-related difference in their brain responses to humor.[59] In the study, 22 children of both sexes from 6 to 13 years of age were shown films that were humorous, neutral, or positive while they were being scanned with functional MRIs. The girls were amused with the humorous films and the boys had a stronger preference for the positive ones. The girls had bilateral temporo-occipital cortex, midbrain, and amygdala involvement with the humorous films and the boys had bilateral inferior parietal lobule, fusiform gyrus, inferior frontal gyrus, amygdala, and ventromedial prefrontal cortex activation with the positive clips. The differences between what was activated in the two situations are strong indicators that humor is a separate emotion from regular enjoyment.

What is not clear in the minds of many clinicians is at what time the encounter becomes romantic, because most people think that making the woman laugh is enough to make the encounter romantic. It is not. These moments of laughter establish friendship and not romance. For romance to occur there must be at least subtle statements reflecting the man's desire to have her sexually. Because the effects of humor are rarely studied in the field,[31] we consulted various blogs that in some way shared thoughts on what happens in dating. For instance, one blog, *How to Date a Girl by Making Her Laugh*, points out that even if the man can make the woman laugh, if the man does not let the woman know that there is lust, the man will be relegated to a nonromantic status. Unless otherwise stated, this article will now refer to the interactions of a male therapist with an adult female patient, following this social convention that dictates that men are almost programmed to make women laugh.

HUMOR IN THERAPY

There is a sense that it is taboo to use humor in the psychotherapeutic session, especially between a male therapist and a female patient. Some think that this probably started with Freud, who was actually a great joke teller according to Earnest Jones.[60] In fact Freud[61,62] published a book and an article specifically on humor. In his writings on humor, Freud has been seen as cautiously avoiding letting his unconscious intervene inappropriately (for a good review of this subject see Billig[63]) possibly because he was never analyzed. For a more complete review of his thinking as well as of humor in general readers are referred to Martin's[44] book. A summary of what Freud had to say is as follows. He was interested in what he called joke work and the reasons why jokes are made. He saw laughter as a way to release the libidinal drives that come from the id. Using his view of repression in his drive-defense theory, he thought that the unconscious expression of unacceptable desires (sexual and aggressive) that have to pass through the super ego[62] are defended against being expressed directly by the ego's use of jokes. Because the goal of the id is to derive pleasure either autoerotically or by getting more attention, laughter satisfies both these needs. The manner in which the drive will be expressed depends on the superego. Thus, humor is expressed as comforting if the superego is nurturing, upsetting if the superego is critical, and totally repressed if the superego is too critical. Thus, joke work can be obviously libidinal or aggressive (tendentious) or the opposite, not having any such themes (nontendentious). He and other psychologists rank defenses as being mature or immature, with humor having the potential to be one of the most mature.[64] This last fact is one of the few aspects that have been corroborated in his theory. Since he was more interested in understanding intrapsychic processes,[31] an increase in tension was seen as facilitating the access to the unconscious; humor was probably avoided because it would decrease tension.[65] Because he did not use humor with his patients, he does not give any hints on how to use it in therapy. At that time he was analyzing very sick, neurotic, hysterical women who probably were responding to men with such severe flashbacks of their imagined (or real) memories of having intimacy with their fathers that he had to use the couch to direct their visions away from him so as to avoid as much as possible any semblance of an erotic transference. He probably had to avoid any sort humor because these patients would misinterpret the roles of joke work in a normal social situation, which is that the man makes the woman laugh as an act of friendship and, misread the encounter as being romantic. Thus, Freud was taking his usual therapeutic approach, which was to avoid tainting the transference with anything that could be misinterpreted, here with humor, so as to avoid any semblance of having romantic desires because of these particular patients interpreting being friendly as being romantic. Freud was implying that making a patient laugh might be distorted and interpreted as a seduction of the patient with jokes to the point of stirring unresolved unconscious conflicts that result in transgressions of imaginary boundaries. However, the taboo was generalized to include all patients in psychotherapy, even those not in psychoanalysis.[65]

The difference between Freud's patients and ours is that hysterics are not frequently encountered in a regular practice. While they have been replaced with borderlines and posttraumatic stress disordered women who we usually accept were abused by someone in their past, these patients usually benefit from a myriad of therapies including pharmacotherapy. If strict psychoanalytic practices are to be used with them, or any patient in analysis, jokes have to be avoided. Even if not in psychoanalysis, we agree with Freud that jokes with patients with these severe disorders, and who are unmedicated, should be avoided or used cautiously. However, protohumor, affiliative, and self-enhancing humor styles have been well tolerated by them as well as by the rest of our patient population because none are in psychoanalysis. Aggressive humor in the form of teasing should only be done if the tease is not a demeaning insult and that there is a high level of familiarity with the patient. For instance, one stable schizophrenic patient told us that she was the daughter of the catholic Pope and the local cardinal. When I had a therapeutic relationship with her, I wanted to confront her delusion with humor so I smilingly said half-seriously that she was such a show-off, and I always greeted her as the show-off. Every time she chuckled happily with this, it was a sign that my intervention was appropriate. My confrontation was a way to acknowledge that fact she was indeed trying to be important and that I was going to reward her with a gentle reminder that I knew that she had chosen some very prominent fathers so it was not seen as a put-down. The stress here is on the tone of voice that is soft and affiliative. However, every time I said so, she kept on insisting that she had two famous fathers. I thus confirmed the continued presence of this delusion in a nonthreatening manner.

USE OF HUMOR IN MENTAL ILLNESS

Humor has been studied in schizophrenia. While the consensus is that the patients might not have all the neurocognitive hardware to understand humor[66] they not only appreciate it but respond to humor therapy with sustained gains in humor appreciation.[67] In one study of schizophrenics given the STCI, the schizophrenics did not seem to be very humorous as they had higher levels of seriousness and bad mood with lower scores on cheerfulness. Although there were no correlations between their scores and the ratings of positive and negative symptoms, bad mood was associated with higher depression scores. However, there were no differences in CHS scores or in humor preference as measured by the 3WD between the schizophrenics and controls. Laughter may also be associated with psychopathological states, including bipolar patients in manic phase, psychotic schizophrenics, and uninhibited patients with frontal lesions. Clinicians should be able to identify the degree of dysfunction that the patient has and develop a differential diagnosis based on the whole clinical picture. Responding to an extremely psychotic patient with humor may be seen as a challenge to their beliefs and may increase aggressive behavior, so the recognition and timing of the use of humor needs to be carefully evaluated.

With most of the patient population, Freud has hindered the use of humor because it is thought that humor is the factor that promotes a sexual relationship. As mentioned earlier, what transpires when clinicians are humorous with their patients is that the clinicians develop the nonsexual friendship relationship that is called the therapeutic alliance. At the other end of the spectrum there is Albert Ellis, a Freudian psychoanalyst who broke off from psychoanalysis in 1953,[68] who thought that the main problem in mental illness was that patients could not make light of their disorders.[69] He represented a major shift in how psychotherapy was done because he was very active in trying to deal with irrational thinking to the point of being confrontational and brusque. One author saw him once in action as he had people from the audience come up to the stage. He liked to use swear words to make his point and would use humor successfully as a method to try to deal with irrational distortions. Even in his descriptions of irrational thoughts he was playful. For example, he felt that depressed people feel that the only way to have any sort of worth was by being 100% effective in doing anything. They have such a drive to prove themselves that they MUST be able to do anything demanded of them, for instance at work or at home. In order to make light of this torment, he uses his wit to make this action humorous as he describes these people are "musterbating."[70] The pun, which is a classic element in the humor technique of wit, is with the word masturbating, which was part of the shock humor he liked to use. This way he could confront this maladaptive defense with humor. Although his theories have been extensively accepted, he had a particular confrontational style that has not been imitated by many. I think that people had a problem with how funny he was, because this is the problem with using humor in general: humor is not considered a serious subject.[31]

If we extrapolate from what has been presented, then when male clinicians smile too much, female patients will think that they are nice but not very smart. So, what is attractive to women? Remember, it is when men show pride or shame. Because clinicians rarely show shame, how do they show pride? We think that male clinicians show pride by being competent and showing off their ability to successfully treat their patients. This is one possibly important way that male clinicians "seduce" female patients, not when they joke around.

HOW TO USE HUMOR

There are some general rules to follow that can minimize the potential pitfalls of joke telling. As well-honed amateur joke tellers (as an adolescent, the senior author once got out of a fight by using a pun. He told the aggressor twice to cross the line that he had made in the dirt and after the other had crossed the 2 lines that the author had made, the author said "I do not fight double crossers." The other laughed so hard that the fight was off), we insist that in order to be able to tell jokes, especially in group therapy, you must be acutely aware of the nonverbal communications of the people to whom you are telling the jokes. If one is too distracted or impulsive to notice when the joke bombs then, jokes should be avoided because one is not going to know whether the others are appreciative of the jokes. As an indicator, laughter (or a chuckle) is the best sign that the clinician has been successful. If clinicians believe in the unconscious, can they avoid letting their unconscious belief express itself inappropriately in joke telling? Although the existence of the unconscious is controversial to some, we avoid any possibility of misinterpretations by not using jokes and instead using protohumor, affiliative humor, and self-enhancing humor with both sexes, which results in all the smiles, and at times laughter, that we need to promote the therapeutic alliance. When a joke is used, we usually use wit, Freud's favorite, as a means to increase insight such as when a patient is told that they are Egyptians because they live in "the Nile" (play on words with "DENIAL"). No offense is intended to the Egyptians as we are only refer-ring to the river. Usually the humor we use is conservative and our favorite tactic is coin-cidentally the one recommended in the previously mentioned blog, *How to Date a Girl by Making Her Laugh*, which is that men can be successful in making women laugh by not only seeing the positive in everything but also by making it funny. One perfect example was during an initial interview of a preadolescent who spontaneously cry whenever she was asked to talk about a recent time she had been corrected, because she had been very hurt by this. As an immediate intervention, she was told her that crying on demand was a great skill for her if she wanted to be an actress. She responded by laughing heart-ily. She kept on crying whenever the episode was recalled, but the alliance was made. There is actually a new psychology that Barbara Fredrickson has started that is based on positive emotions and is called the broaden-and-build theory of positive emotions.[71] Her group studies how positive emotions help the thinking process.[72,73] We encourage any attempt to operationalize positive emotions and laud Barbara Fredrickson's attempt to use mathematical models to understand changes in affect.[74] While she has been criticized,[75] she has accepted the errors saying that may be the mathematical models were not used appropriately.[76] However she does feel that there is ample evi-dence that positive emotions are better up to a point. We hope that these and any other attempts to make humor look more scientific will only help to make humor more respected.

HUMOR AND KLEIN

We are Kleinian in that we are aware of the splitting that can occur in our patients.[77,78] In a simplistic sense, by pointing out the positive, we are solving the splitting behavior and encouraging a move to a healthier manner of seeing the world. Klein[77,78] said that as the split of the all bad/all good paranoid position is resolved there is an integration of the good/bad that causes anxiety because the bad is so much stronger/scarier than the good that the bad can destroy the good, thus resulting in the sadness of the depressive position. Then, once good is stronger than bad, there is the resolution of the depressive position and the start of the relative calmness of object constancy. We are aware that cognitive behavior therapy explains the solving of the split as the correction of a cognitive distortion, a split being close to the all-or-nothing distortion. Here, we agree with Albert Ellis,[79] who thought that psychiatric patients do not notice the positive, dwell on the negative, and generalize that all is bad. Whichever the theory, humor that stresses the positive helps to foment the therapeutic alliance.

PLAYFUL THERAPY

There are many who have made directive and non-directive play therapy an acceptable treatment modality for children from 4-12 years of age, including, just to name a few, Ana Freud, Hermine Hug-Hellmuth, Melanie Kline.[80–82] A discussion of when to use directive versus non-directive play therapy is beyond the scope of this chapter. What we will be discussing is the use of directive play therapy techniques. There are a myriad of excellect resource books on the subject of directive playful therapy techniques,[83–85] some full of what many 50 therapists have found useful.[86–88] In our case, we have found that we can use directive playful therapy techniques effectively because of what we have learned from the book *Playful Parenting* by Cohen.[89] We recommend this book to parents/guardians who want to help their children grow up to love/respect and not fear authority by encouraging connection, security, and attachment through silliness and laughter. In *Playful Parenting*, the author points out that children know that supervising adults/parents are in charge and will always be in charge. Just because the supervising adult/parent playfully lets the child win does not mean that the balance of power will be upset. Instead, confidence is engendered. With children, Freud might say that successfully meeting the demands of an age appropriate competitive, phallic stage decreases the chance of a fixation at that stage. Cohen's[89] book is even appropriate for therapists as it teaches how to set up informal therapeutic interventions in therapy sessions that result in laughter. Our favorite is how he deals with guns, which he calls "love guns." If a child (usually a latency age or preteen) points a gun at him and shoots him, he calls the gun a "love gun" and goes after the child to give a kiss because they are shooting him with love. Once in therapy one of the authors taught a father to do this with his 11-year-old daughter. She squealed with laughter as he ran after her to kiss her each time she shot him. She enjoyed it so much that she 'shot' him various times. This interaction strengthened the bond between the two, a goal of therapy. We reiterate that chuckling/laughter is a sign that the clinician has been successful in communicating the desire for a positive bond.

In therapy with preadolescents, one of the authors uses the Thinking, Feeling, Doing game.[90] which is a simple board game that is well known to help clinicians retrieve fantasy material from young children (4–12 years of age) in a short time. For more information on how to use this game refer to Gelkopf M[91] and Gardner[92] To very briefly summarize the game, it consists of a trail that has colored squares that correspond to the matching colored cards that ask the child questions that make them think, feel, or do. Before starting, what one of the authors does is to tell the child not to worry because the therapist is very good at the game and that the therapist will almost surely win. As the game transpires, the chips are controlled by the therapist and the child receives many more chips for the answers than are given for the therapist's answers. At the end of the game, the therapist counts his measly 3 or 4 chips and claims to have won. Then, as the child's chips are counted, the therapist shows shock and wonderment that there are so many and the therapist says that surely the child has played the game before because the therapist has never been beaten so badly. These children always chuckle and go proudly to their mothers to tell of the defeat of the therapist. One mother even sheepishly asked whether it were true. With this approach, we have no problems with the therapeutic alliance because the children come back asking to play again.

We also try to relieve tension with humor. One common tactic that is used typically by one of the authors is used while doing an intake with the family and the child. If the parents have to tell of the child's bad grades and behavior, before they begin to give this information the therapist always starts with a smile and thumbs-up sign as he asks about grades. As they tell of the bad news, the therapist looks sad, says "Oh no-o!" and makes a thumbs-down sign. This response always gets a chuckle out of the child and avoids giving the impression that the therapist is only allied with the negative. With thumbs-up, thumbs-down, and happy and sad faces, the split is solved/undistorted, visually. Again it is an example of self-enhancing humor because this is the view that everything has a positive aspect, even if it is for a moment. By showing a thumbs-up there is the implication that the clinician knows that the child has potential even if the news is bad. We are always successful in solidifying the therapeutic alliance with the child with this approach. The parents have found this approach nonthreatening and appreciate the support of their concerns when there is a thumbs-down. At any time during therapy, whenever we hear good news we give a thumbs-up and even a high-five, which is appreciated by those of all ages, including the parents if we are doing family therapy. What we also do is to try to greet all the preadolescents and adolescents with a high-five and a big smile. We practice in Puerto Rico where the ritual of men greeting women is to kiss on the cheek, do nothing, or rarely give a handshake, depending on the familiarity. The high-five is a great solution especially for greeting the young female patients. With really young children, instead of giving a neutral handshake or nothing, we think it makes more sense to offer the raised hand so that they can happily "slap five". The high-five preceding the start of the therapy with preadolescents or adolescents of either sex is a way of starting the session on a positive note. At the end, the high-five starts the separation ritual.

In individual therapy with adults, we kid them a lot about skipping medications. When asked about taking a certain medication when it seems that they are not taking it, they are first asked whether a long time has lapsed since the last time the medication was taken, 6 to 8 months, for example. Before they answer, the therapist lets out a soft whistle sound and a wave of the hand upward, as if to say that someone forgot. They always chuckle. No confrontation, no reprimand. Just the hope that maybe they will take the medication. We of course follow up using standard approaches to try to analyze and solve their resistances, but do so with a positive start.

Playful therapy can help with teaching preadolescents and adolescents with learning disabilities, very short attention, impulsivity problems, and immature personalities (narcissistic) why they must behave. In one residential placement facility for female adolescents who cannot be with their families due to many dysfunctional situations such as sexual abuse, the staff tries to teach that oppositional behavior is not in their interest by telling these girls that they have to stop having an "attitude" when they have to complete a task. We know what that means, the staff knows, but the girls are clueless. Any attempt to define it usually ends up sounding like a personal grudge against the adolescent and the message goes over their heads. The definition has been simplified by saying that anything that will result in an imaginary boss firing them is considered an attitude. Here the boss is the bad guy and no one is blamed for unfairness. Even in more stable families it is pointed out that the family is a benign dictatorship that, along with school, is a training ground for how to keep a job. The money sign with the fingers (rubbing thumb against the first 2 fingers) is used as the patient is told that all the lessons learned will result in being able to keep a well remunerated job. Otherwise, if they do not shape up and follow the imaginary work rules, they will be fired. All the preadolescents and adolescents, even those with low intelligence quotients, understand and chuckle when they realize that they will be fired. This helps them to accept the behavior as being unacceptable; they can work to gain insight on how it is to their advantage that they know how their behavior affects future functioning in work, which is of interest to them because they all want to be gainfully employed.

Humor comes in when it is pointed out how swearing at the staff or at a foster mother will result in getting fired from an imaginary job. As they are told that they are going to be fired for their actions, staff can point to the door to show where they would go. They know this means that they would have been fired and they chuckle. Sometimes a flying figure with the hands can be added to operationalize how they will be fired, with the hand-figure crashing to the ground, while saying "O-oh no!", which always gets a laugh. Patients are never threatened as long as one makes a supportive gesture such as making a sad face as they are being fired. As has been stressed, a successful intervention is when one makes them laugh.

We want to point out again that a laugh is a sign that one person has successfully connected with the other person. This approach to the definition of attitude has been used by the staff and they have found it to drastically improve the ability to convey what is expected of the adolescents without causing undue stress. The confrontation is not seen as negative criticism as they accept that they have to learn the rules that will result in their being able to keep a job. Humor helps them to be able to accept that they have erred in what they were doing and need to work on improvement. This shows that humor can be used as complementary medicine to facilitate coping with symptoms, improving rehabilitation through its emotional, cognitive, social, and physiologic impact.[91]

HOW TO DEVELOP A SENSE OF HUMOR

Although humor is thought to be a stable personality trait,[93] we believe that humor is a skill that can be learned. To help do so, the Mayo Clinic doctors on their blog *Stress Relief from Laughter? It's No Joke* state that one should have funny clips within sight, watch funny movies and TV shows,[94] learn to laugh at yourself and the stresses around you ("it is hopeless but not serious"), hang around those that make you laugh, read up on jokes that make you laugh and then share them with friends, all the time avoiding laughing at the expense of others. They also agree with us that it is important to notice how the jokes are being received. Humor is not to be confused with lack of professionalism.[94] For other humor resources see Wooten[47] and read the old issues of the *Journal of Nursing Jocularity* or go to their blog under the journal's name.

There are also laughter clubs that practice laughter yoga (hasyayoga), a practice developed by Kataria.[95] With everyone looking playfully at each other, laughter is at first forced as if were an exercise, and, when it is a Duchenne laugh, the effort becomes spontaneous because this laughter is known to be contagious.[30] This routine usually lasts 20 minutes. In an elderly population of depressed women, the benefits of laughter yoga in mood equaled those seen in an exercise group,[96] both being more effective than controls. One doctor found this helpful with one severely bipolar patient who reached remission when she became an instructor.[5] See also www.laughteryoga. org for more information. Social laughter has been associated with decreased pain thresholds[97] caused by the rhythm of Duchenne laughter increasing endorphins, which in turn make people feel better emotionally.[98]

HUMOR AND LOCUS OF CONTROL

One researcher has been able to set up a 6-hour course that successfully trains participants to be humorous.[99] In one study of the effects of the course on humor, here on nurses, the test results were based on the concept of locus of control (LOC).[100] External LOC is associated with people thinking that they have no control over their fate and is considered unhealthy, with internal LOC meaning that people have control and is associated with healthy coping skills. After the humor course, the graduates had an increase in internal LOC and decrease in external LOC. Helping to make people have an internal LOC increases a sense of mastery known as cognitive control.[101] One last note: one study assessed whether humor was expressed by doctors as perceived by the patients and compared this with what the doctors thought they expressed. Patients saw doctors as having been funnier (60.4%) than the doctors thought themselves to have been (37.6%).[102] The implication is that because patients are smiling and laughing to calm down their nervousness, they pick up spontaneous humor or laughter more than intentional humor.[102]

SUMMARY

People smile at 3 months of age, start to laugh at around 4 months, with the laughter increasing to 400 times a day in children. Then adults decrease to about 4 times a day.[103] Thus, this article considers how clinicians might approach laughter, comedy, and humor in mental health and use such humorous approaches more than the usual 4 to 5 times a day to approximate the playfulness of our children. To help convince of the need to do so, the article begins with an understanding of humor as an entity in complementary medicine and then goes on to discuss how it may provide specific therapeutic and developmental insights while always monitoring the use of words. It is known that laughter via protohumor, affiliative, and self-enhancing humor styles may be a healthy expression of feelings, used as a defense mechanism or as part of a medical condition. Clinicians must take into consideration the cultural context (individualistic vs collectivist societies),[6] clinical picture, and differential diagnosis of their patients. As mentioned a laugh history should be taken.[6] Many bipolar patients in manic phases use laughter and humor in inappropriate ways, so it is the duty of clinicians to evaluate and regulate the setting in which that conduct takes place. As previously mentioned, if clinicians want to confront some of those delusions they must first establish a therapeutic alliance and make good choices with their words so that they are not perceived as a threat to the patient. This choice of words helps to establish a therapeutic alliance with the patient. By increasing the use of humor, clinicians can maintain a healthy relationship with their peers and patients. We do not suggest that doctors should become comic reliefs, but instead encourage them to take notice and see whether everyday humor is used at least the 5 times a day. As mentioned earlier, many physicians use humor unknowingly in their interactions with their patients. By using humor as a means of communication, clinicians can even improve interactions among their interdisciplinary team, because they feel more related to them.

Almost everyone has faced a situation in which they feel rejected when they think someone does not like them. This happens mostly when the other person presents with a serious attitude which can prevent further interactions. While most people cannot know the whole truth about how they affect others until they can explore it, most people can relate to the doctor who takes input and converts that into a thoughtful, positive message that uses humor when appropriate. An important factor to consider before using humor in therapy is that clinicians should know themselves in order to recognize their ability to adequately incorporate humor into therapy. Some people naturally have humor in their speech and actions and for them it is a process that seems fluid and natural. Others have limited skills, resulting in humor that seems to be forced and that may strain the therapeutic alliance. That is why we think that humor is a skill to be developed as a person would develop any psychotherapeutic skill: with practice and supervision anyone who is motivated can hone their skills. Psychiatrists in general are good communicators, but this does not mean they are good in every field of therapy. We suggest that clinicians seek out those who do use humor and ask for advice. In this way, humor, as a technique of complementary medicine to use with many future patients, increases clinicians' repertoire of possible interactions that will result in making the therapeutic alliance stronger not only in individual psychotherapy but also as an important part of group therapy.[91]

CONCLUSION

In our individual psychotherapy sessions, we have found humor to help in establishing a secure and strong therapeutic alliance, helping with issues regarding transference or countertransference and normalizing feelings that the patient may be having. An example of this is a patient who is currently depressed because of work conditions and is seeking help adjusting to new roles. If done correctly, the use of humor can help this patient understand the situation from a different perspective and establish a new way of dealing with this problem. As part of our group therapies, we have seen that humor helps with group cohesion, facilitates communication among patients and with staff, establishes empathy, and serves as a vehicle for communication. Humor in group therapy is especially helpful because it is used as a defense mechanism that facilitates communication. A patient may feel less judged about a personal image problem if a subtle thumbs-up is given for just about any reason. Significant progress is made in those groups in which there is cohesion between the patients, with humor being an effective way to help them to relate their own problems and feel less judged. Most patients in group therapy have social skills deficits so humor may be as beneficial as individual psychotherapy but with distinctive features.[91] It is our hope that all of this information can inspire clinicians to use humor in day-to-day interactions and progress to the use of humor in psychiatric interviewing/therapy when comfortable enough. Again, if in doubt, seek advice from your humorous peers!

REFERENCES

1. Chapman AJ, Chapman WA. Responsiveness to humor: its dependency upon a companion's humorous smiling and laughter. J Psychol 1974;88:245–52.
2. Sprecher S, Regan P. Liking some things (in some people) more than others: partner preferences in romantic relationships and friendships. J Soc Pers Relat 2002;19:463–81.
3. Apte M. Ethnic humor versus "sense of humor": an American sociocultural dilemma. Am Behav Sci 1987;30:27–41.
4. Prasad Rao G. Use of humour in psychiatric practice: can we do it properly? Indian J Psychiatry 2006;48(4):267–8.
5. Nasr SJ. No laughing matter: laughter is good psychiatric medicine. A case report. Current Psychiatry 2013;12(8):20–5.
6. Hasan H, Hasan TF. Laugh Yourself into a Healthier Person: A Cross Cultural Analysis of the Effects of Varying Levels of Laughter on Health. Int J Med Sci 2009;6(4):200–11.
7. Martin RA, Lefcourt HM. The sense of humor as a moderator of the relation between stressors and moods. J Pers Soc Psychol 1983;45:1313–24.
8. Capps D. Mother, melancholia, and humor in Erik H. Erikson's earliest writings. J Relig Health 2008;47:415–32.

9. Takeda M, Hashimoto R, Kudo T, et al. Laughter and humor as complementary and alternative medicines for dementia patients. BMC Complement Altern Med 2010;10:28.

10. Thompson MR, Callaghan PD, Hunt GE, et al. A role for oxytocin and 5-HT(1A) receptors in the prosocial effects of 3,4 methylenedioxymethamphetamine ("ecstasy"). Neuroscience 2007;146(2):509–14.

11. Berk LS, Felten DL, Tan SA, et al. Modulation of neuroimmune parameters during the eustress of humor-associated mirthful laughter. Altern Ther Health Med 2001;7(2):62–76.

12. Gouin JP, Carter S, Pournajafi-Nazarloo H, et al. Marital behavior, oxytocin, vasopressin, and wound healing. Psychoneuroendocrinology 2010;35(7): 1082–90.

13. Spitzer P. The clown doctors. Aust Fam Physician 2001;30:12–6.

14. Kirsch P, Esslinger C, Chen Q, et al. Oxytocin modulates neural circuitry for social cognition and fear in humans. J Neurosci 2005;25(49):11489–93.

15. Theodoridou A, Penton-Voak IS, Rowe AC. A direct examination of the effect of intranasal administration of oxytocin on approach-avoidance motor responses to emotional stimuli. PLoS One 2013;8(2):e58113.

16. Black DW. Laughter. JAMA 1984;252:2995–8.

17. Wender RC. Humor in medicine. Prim Care 1996;23:141–54.

18. Spitzer P. The clown doctors. Aust Fam Physician 2001;30:12–6.

19. Levinson W, Roter DL, Mullooly JP, et al. Physician-patient communication. The relationship with malpractice among primary care physicians and surgeons. JAMA 1997;277:553–9.

20. Wildgruber D, Szameitat DP, Ethofer T, et al. Different types of laughter modulate connectivity within distinct parts of the laughter perception network. PLoS One 2013;8(5):e63441.

21. Wild B, Rodden FA, Grodd W, et al. Neural correlates of laughter and humour. Brain 2003;126:2121–38.

22. Ariniello L. Brain Briefings, . Humor, Laughter and the Brain. Washington: Society for Neuroscience; 2001.

23. Gervais M, Wilson DS. The evolution and functions of laughter and humor: a synthetic approach. Q Rev Biol 2005;80(4):395–430.

24. Freitas-Magalhães A, Castro E. The neuropsychophysogical construction of the human smile. In: Freitas-Magalhães A, editor. Emotional expression: the brain and the face. Porto, Portugal: University Fernando Pessoa Press; 2009. p. 1–18.

25. Duchenne G. The mechanism of human facial expression. New York: Cambridge University Press; 1990.

26. Messinger DS, Fogel A, Dickson K. All smiles are positive, but some smiles are more positive than others. Dev Psychol 2001;37(5):642–53.

27. Gladstone G. When you're smiling, does the whole world smile for you? Australas Psychiatry 2002;10:144–6.

28. Beall AT. Happy guys finish last: the impact of emotion expressions on sexual attraction. Emotion 2011;11(6):1379–87.

29. Panksepp J. Affective neuroscience: the foundations of human and animal emotions. New York: Oxford University Press; 1998.

30. Keltner D, Bonanno GA. A study of laughter and dissociation: distinct correlates of laughter and smiling during bereavement. J Pers Soc Psychol 1997;73: 687–702.

31. Martin RA, Lefcourt HM. The psychology of humor: an integrative approach. Burlington (MA): EA Press; 2007.

32. Martin RA, Puhlik-Doris P, Larsen G, et al. Individual differences in uses of humor and their relation to psychological well-being: development of the Humor Styles Questionnaire. J Res Pers 2003;37:48–75.
33. Frewen P, Jaylene B, Rod M, et al. Humor styles and personality-vulnerability to depression. Humor 2008;2(21):179–95.
34. Yip J, Rod M. Sense of humor, emotional intelligence, and social competence. J Res Pers 2006;40(6):1202–8.
35. Martin R. Humor, laughter, and physical health: methodological issues and research findings. Psychol Bull 2001;127(4):504–19.
36. Ruch W, Köhler G, van Thriel H. Assessing the "humorous temperament": construction of the facet and standard trait forms of the State-Trait-Cheerfulness-Inventory—STCI. Humor 1996;9:303–39.
37. Ruch W, Köhler G, van Thriel H. To be in good or bad humor: construction of the state form of the State-Trait-Cheerfulness-Inventory—STCI. Pers Individ Dif 1997;22:477–91.
38. Martin RA. The Situational Humor Response Questionnaire (SHRQ) and Coping Humor Scale (CHS): a decade of research findings. Humor 1996;9:251–72.
39. Ruch W. Assessment of appreciation of humour: studies with the 3WD humor test. In: Spielberger CD, Butcher JN, editors. Advances in personality assessment, vol. 9. Hillsdale (NJ): Erlbaum; 1992. p. 27–32.
40. Sommer K, Ruch W. Cheerfulness. In: Lopez SJ, editor. The Encyclopedia of Positive Psychology. West Sussex, UK: Wiley-Blackwell; 2009. p. 144–7.
41. Köhler G, Ruch W. Sources of variance in current sense of humor inventories: how much substance, how much method variance? Humor 2009;9(3–4):363–98.
42. Hurley MM, Dennett DC, Adams RB. Inside jokes: using humor to reverse-engineer the mind. Cambridge, MA: MIT Press; 2011.
43. Berk LS, Tan SA, Fry WF, et al. Neuroendocrine and stress hormone changes during mirthful laughter. Am J Med Sci 1989;298:390–6.
44. Martin RA. The psychology of humor. An integrative approach. Burlington (VT): Elsevier Academic Press; 2007.
45. Neuhoff CC, Schaefer C. Effects of laughing, smiling, and howling on mood. Psychol Rep 2002;91(3):1079–80.
46. Rosner F. Therapeutic efficacy of laughter in medicine. Cancer Invest 2002;20(3):434–6.
47. Wooten P. Humor: an antidote for stress. Holist Nurs Pract 1996;10(2):49–56.
48. Crawford M, Gressly D. Creativity, caring, and context: women's and men's accounts of humor preferences and practices. Psychol Women Q 1991;15:217–31.
49. Three essays on the theory of sexuality. In: Freud S, editor. The standard edition of the complete psychological works of Sigmund Freud, vol. 7. London: The Hogarth Press and the Institute of Psychoanalysis; 1905. p. 123–246.
50. McGhee PE. Humor: its origin and development. San Francisco (CA): WH Freeman; 1979.
51. Grotjahn M. Beyond laughter: humor and the subconscious. New York: McGraw-Hill; 1966.
52. Spiegel D, Keith-Spiegel P, Abrahams J, et al. Humor and suicide: favorite jokes of suicidal patients. J Consult Clin Psychol 1969;33(4):504–5.
53. Dunbar RI. Mind the gap: or why humans aren't just great apes. Proc Br Acad 2008;154:403–23.

54. Dunbar RI. Mind the bonding gap: constraints on the evolution of hominid societies. In: Shennan SJ, editor. Pattern and process in cultural evolution. San Francisco (CA): University of California Press; 2009. p. 223–34.

55. Wilbur CJ, Campbell L. Humor in romantic contexts: do men participate and women evaluate? Pers Soc Psychol Bull 2011;37(7):918–29.

56. Azim E, Mobbs D, Jo B, et al. Sex differences in brain activation elicited by humor. Proc Natl Acad Sci U S A 2005;102(45):16496–501.

57. Kohn N, Kellermann T, Gur RC, et al. Gender differences in the neural correlates of humor processing: implications for different processing modes. Neuropsychologia 2011;49(5):888–97.

58. Neely MN, Walter E, Black JM, et al. Neural correlates of humor detection and appreciation in children. J Neurosci 2012;32(5):1784–90.

59. Vrticka P, Neely M, Walter Shelly E, et al. Sex differences during humor appreciation in child-sibling pairs. Soc Neurosci 2013;8(4):291–304.

60. Jones E. The life and work of Sigmund Freud. London: Penguin; 1964.

61. Freud S. Wit (jokes) and its (their) relation to the unconscious. New York: WW Norton; 1960/1905.

62. Freud S. Humor. Int J Psychoanal 1928;9:1–6.

63. Billig M. Freudian repression. Cambridge (United Kingdom): Cambridge University Press; 1999.

64. Vaillant GE. Adaptation to life. Boston: Little, Brown; 1977.

65. Gordon RM. To wit or not to wit: the use of humor in psychotherapy. Pennsylvania Psychologist 2007;67(3):22–4.

66. Bozikas VP, Kosmidis MH, Giannakou M, et al. Humor appreciation deficit in schizophrenia: the relevance of basic neurocognitive functioning. J Nerv Ment Dis 2007;195(4):325–31.

67. Witztum E, Briskin S, Lerner V. The use of humor with chronic schizophrenic patients. J Contemp Psychother 1999;29(3):223–34.

68. Abrams M, Abrams L. A brief biography of Dr Albert Ellis 1913–2007. 2012. Available at: www.rebt.ws/albertellisbibliography.html. Accessed August 21, 2014.

69. Ellis A. Fun as psychotherapy. Rational Living 1977;12(1):6.

70. Nemade R, Reiss NS, Dombeck M. Cognitive Theories of Major Depression - Ellis and Bandura. Depression: Major Depression & Unipolar Varieties. Available at: http://www.mentalhelp.net/poc/view_doc.php?type=doc&id=13006&cn=5. Accessed October 21, 2014.

71. Fredrickson BL. The Role of Positive Emotions in Positive Psychology Am Psychol 2001;56(3):218–26.

72. Fredrickson BL. What good are positive emotions? Review of General Psychology 1998;2:300–19.

73. Fredrickson BL. Positive emotions broaden and build. In: Devine P, Plant A, editors. Advances in experimental social psychology. San Diego, CA: Academic Press; 2013. p. 1–54.

74. Fredrickson BL, Losada MF. Positive affect and the complex dynamics of human flourishing. American Psychologist 2005;60:678–86.

75. Brown NJL, Sokal AD, Friedman HL. The complex dynamics of wishful thinking: The critical positivity ratio. American Psychologist 2013;68:1–13.

76. Fredrickson BL. Updated Thinking on Positivity Ratios. American Psychologist 2013;1–9.

77. Klein M. Notes on some schizoid mechanisms. In: Mitchell J, editor. The selected Melanie Klein. London: Penguin; 1986/1946. p. 19–46.

78. Klein M. A contribution to the psychogenesis of manic depressive states. Int J Psycho Anal 1986;16:145–74.

79. Ellis A. The essence of RET—1984. Journal of Rational Emotive Therapy 1984; 2(1):19–25.

80. Ciottone RA, Madonna JM. Play therapy with sexually abused children. A Synergistic Clinical-developmental Approach. Northvale, NJ: Jason Aronson Inc; 1996.

81. Axline VM. Play Therapy. Westminster, MD: Ballantine Books; 1981.

82. Axline V. Entering the child's world via play experiences. Progressive Education 1950;27:68–75.

83. Kenney-Noziska S. Techniques-Techniques-Techniques: Play-Based Activities for Children, Adolescents & Families. West Conshohocken, PA: Infinity Pub; 2008.

84. Drewes AA. Edit Blending Play Therapy with Cognitive Behavioral Therapy: Evidence-Based and Other Effective Treatments and Techniques. Hoboken, NJ: Wiley and Sons, Inc; 2009.

85. Gil E. The Healing Power of Play: Working with Abused Children. New York: The Guilford Press; 1991.

86. Lowenstein L. Creative Interventions for Troubled Children & Youth Paperback. Toronto, ON: Champion Press; 1999.

87. Lowenstein L. Assessment and Treatment Activities for Children, Adolescents, and Families: Vol 2. Practitioners Share Their Most Effective Techniques. Toronto, ON: Champion Press; 2010.

88. Lowenstein L. Assessment and Treatment Activities for Children, Adolescents and Families Vol 3. Practitioners Share Their Most Effective Techniques. Toronto, ON: Champion Press; 2011.

89. Cohen LJ. Playful parenting. New York: Ballantine Books; 2001.

90. Gardner RA. The talking, feeling, and doing game. In: Schaefer C, Reid SE, editors. Game play: Therapeutic Use of Childhood Games; Second Edition. New York: Wiley and Sons, Inc; 2001. p. 78–108.

91. Gelkopf M. The use of humor in serious mental illness: a review. Evid Based Complement Alternat Med 2011;2011:342837.

92. Gardner RA. The psychotherapeutic techniques of Richard Gardner. Chapter II-The Thinking, Feeling, Doing game. Cresskill, NJ: Creative Therpeutics; 1986. p. 609–84.

93. Willibald R. Explorations of a personality characteristic. New York: De Gruyter Mouton; 1998. p. 159–78.

94. Yates S. Finding your funny bone. Incorporating humour into medical practice. Aust Fam Physician 2001;30(1):22–4.

95. Kataria M. Laugh for no reason. 2nd edition. Mumbai (India): Madhuri International; 2002.

96. Shahidi M, Mojtahed A, Modabbernia A, et al. Laughter yoga versus group exercise program in elderly depressed women: a randomized controlled trial. Int J Geriatr Psychiatry 2011;26(3):322–7.

97. Dunbar RI, Baron R, Frangou A, et al. Social laughter is correlated with an elevated pain threshold. Proc Biol Sci 2012;279(1731):1161–7.

98. Zubieta JK, Smith YR, Buelle JA, et al. Regional μ-opioid receptor regulation of sensory and affective dimensions of pain. Science 2001;293:311–5.

99. Wooten P. Does a humor workshop affect nurse burnout? J Nurs Jocularity 1992; 2:42–3.

100. Lefcourt HM. Locus of control: current trends in theory and research. Hillsdale (NJ): Lawrence Erlbaum Associates, Inc; 1982.

101. Kabasa SC. Personality and social resources in stress resistance. J Pers Soc Psychol 1983;45:839–50.
102. Granek-Catarivas M, Goldstein-Ferber S, Azuri Y, et al. Use of humour in primary care: different perceptions among patients and physicians. Postgrad Med J 2005;81:126–30.
103. Freedman LW. Mosby's complementary and alternative medicine. A research-based approach. St Louis (MO): Mosby; 2004.

Diet and Stress

Michael J. Gonzalez, DSc, NMD, PhD[a],*,
Jorge R. Miranda-Massari, BS, BSPharm, RPh, PharmD[b]

KEYWORDS

• Diet • Stress • Nutrition • Supplementation • Vitamins • Minerals

KEY POINTS

• Nutrition, diet and stress.
• Stress and nutritional insufficiency.
• Nutrition for stress.

"Let food be your medicine and let medicine be your food."

—*Hippocrates*

INTRODUCTION

Stress in biological terms refers to the reaction of the body to the disturbance of the equilibrium given particular stimuli. A stressor can vary in intensity, and people have different levels of coping ability to respond well or fail to respond properly to an event that has occurred in their life, whether physical or emotional. Physiologic systems work in a complex and integrated manner. There are many factors of one's daily lifestyle that bring stress upon the body. Stress is a common problem in most modern societies, in which there are economic pressures; political, religious, and other social conflicts; overpopulation; contamination; and a food industry that provides main staple foods that are additional stressors (refined carbohydrates, excessive animal fats, artificial colors, preservatives, and sweeteners). Unhealthy eating patterns will only result in an increased level in stress, followed by further health problems in the near future if the issues are not resolved. With a healthy eating plan accompanied with scientific supplementation and a proper stress management program, one can overcome stress, prolong one's life span, and reduce the likelihood of stress-related illnesses.

The authors have nothing to disclose.
[a] Nutrition Program, Department of Human Development, School of Public Health, University of Puerto Rico, Medical Sciences Campus, GPO Box 365067, San Juan, PR 00936-5067, USA;
[b] Department of Pharmacy Practice, School of Pharmacy, University of Puerto Rico, Medical Sciences Campus, GPO Box 365067, San Juan, PR 00936-5067, USA
* Corresponding author.
E-mail address: michael.gonzalez5@upr.edu

Psychiatr Clin N Am 37 (2014) 579–589
http://dx.doi.org/10.1016/j.psc.2014.08.004
psych.theclinics.com
0193-953X/14/$ – see front matter © 2014 Elsevier Inc. All rights reserved.

Abbreviations	
ANS	Autonomic nervous system
DHA	Docosahexaenoic acid
EPA	Eicosapentaenoic acid
PMS	Premenstrual syndrome

The US population in general as a whole is overstressed. It is well understood that stress and perceived stress in adults contribute to a wide range of disorders including hypertension and elevated plasma cortisol,[1] cardiac and cardiovascular disease,[2] inflammatory bowel syndrome,[3] type 2 diabetes mellitus,[4] and a reduced quality of life among those suffering with cancer.[5–7]

Stress happens in 3 stages. The first is an initial state of alarm (fight or flight response), which produces an increase of adrenaline. Living organisms can withstand occasional extreme stress and still survive. The second stage is a short-term resistance mechanism that the body sets up to cope with the problem. The final stage is a state of exhaustion. The exhaustion stage occurs when the body has used up all its available resources. If the situation is not taken care of, stress can produce long-term damage to the body, including heart problems, high blood pressure, the immune system problems (susceptibility to infections and allergies), skin problems (acne, itchy rashes, psoriasis, and eczema), pain (neck, shoulder and back), diabetes, and infertility.[8]

Stress affects the whole body is the following sections provide a brief description of how stress affects different body systems.

Musculoskeletal System

When muscles are tense for prolonged periods of time, other reactions of the body promote stress-related disorders. Tension headache and migraine headache have been associated with chronic muscle tension in the area of the shoulders, neck, and head.

Respiratory System

Stress can make breathing more difficult. For those with asthma or a chronic obstructive disease, getting enough oxygen can become difficult.

Cardiovascular

Repeated acute stress and persistent chronic stress can induce inflammation in the vasculature, especially of the coronary arteries. This is one of the proposed mechanisms associating stress to myocardial infarcts. It addition, it has been shown that the way a person responds to stress can alter cholesterol levels.

Endocrine

Stress affects how the hypothalamus signals the pituitary gland and the autonomic nervous system to secrete the stress hormones epinephrine and cortisol. The hypothalamus stimulates the adrenal glands cortex to produce cortisol and the adrenal medulla to produce epinephrine. This gives the body the energy to run from danger.

The Nervous System

Chronic stress can result in a long-term drain on the body. As the sympathetic nervous system continues to trigger physical reactions, it causes a wear and tear on the body.

Excessive activation depletes the system of neurotransmitters, peptides, cofactors, and other mediators and also alters receptor response.[9]

NUTRITION, DIET AND STRESS: THE LINK BETWEEN STRESS AND NUTRITIONAL INSUFFICIENCY

Stress creates greater physiologic demands. More energy, oxygen, circulation, and therefore more metabolic cofactors are needed (eg, vitamins and minerals). The irony of stress is that people suffering stress need a more nutritionally dense diet but often opt for comfort foods lacking in the necessary nutrients, consequently inducing a situation of nutrient depletion that further compromises the metabolic systems. This situation can be further complicated by the use of medications that often contribute to nutrient depletion.

Stress can cause unhealthy eating habits. People who often endure stress have no time to fit a balanced nutrition around their busy schedule. Moreover, stress makes the body crave foods that are high in fats and sugars. This eating problem in time will inflict a greater stress on the body, plus a nutritional insufficiency state that poses a threat to one's physical and mental health. Stress can have the effect of making people skip or forget to eat their meals. Also people under stress use coffee or other stimulants to assist them and help them cope. The problem with coffee is that it contains caffeine, which, if taken in large quantities, can have negative adverse effects on the body. One problem is that the person is using coffee to stay awake when rest is obviously needed. Caffeine also has an impact on the hormones in the body. Adrenaline and cortisol are increased under the influence of caffeine. The neurotransmitter dopamine is also increased, all with possible negative adverse effects. The increased amount of cortisol produced by stress gives the person a strong urge to eat foods that are high in carbohydrates, sugars, and fats. This eating pattern will result in excess fat being stored. When someone is stressed and does not eat the right amount of food or the correct amount of nutrients, he or she will start to encounter inconsistencies in their blood sugar and other metabolic reactions. These inconsistencies lead to problems such as tiredness, lapses of concentration, and mood swings. If stress is not dealt with properly, the body will suffer in the long run problems that are much more serious, such as diabetes.

DIET AND STRESS
The High-Fat Diet and the Stress Response

Kitraki and colleagues[10] published a study in 2004 using Wister rats, investigating the effects of a diet high in polyunsaturated fat (corn oil) corresponding with a deceased consumption of carbohydrates and reduced intake of protein over 7 days on both energy consumption and a subsequent stress reaction to a short stressor (swimming). Comparing levels of stress hormones in the high-fat/low-protein/low-carbohydrate diet rats and normally fed rats, they found that the levels of corticosterone in both sets of rats were not different during the application of the stressor. Additionally, corticosterone concentrations appeared to not be affected by the different diets. However, further analysis of the blood showed elevated levels of glucocorticoid receptors within the hypothalamic area of the rats fed a normal diet, while lower glucocorticoid receptors levels were found in the rats fed the high-fat/low protein/low-carbohydrate diet. The results highlight how quickly an improper diet with high fat intake and lacking in other nutrients can adversely impact the balance of stress hormones as evidenced by lower glucocorticoid receptors in the hypothalamus known to mediate the effects of cortisol.[11]

Omega-3 and Perceived Stress

Bradbury, Myers, and Oliver (2004) did a study to determine if perceived levels of stress can be lowered through consumption of the omega-3 fatty acid docosahexaenoic acid (DHA).[12] Participants scoring high on a scale of perceived stress were randomly assigned to either a group taking fish oil supplements containing DHA or a group (placebo group) taking supplements of olive oil for 6-weeks. For the analysis, both the fish oil group and the olive oil placebo group were compared with each other as well as against a larger control population. Following the 6-week trial, results showed that perceived stress levels were significantly lower among both the fish oil and olive oil groups. When comparing perceived stress levels between the fish oil group and the larger population, the fish oil group had significantly lower perceived stress. Further analysis showed that there were no significant differences in perceived stress levels between the fish oil and olive oil groups, and no significant difference in perceived stress levels between the olive oil and the control groups. At the end, only the fish oil group showed significant reductions in perceived stress compared with the control sample, consistent with the conclusion that omega-3 attenuates perceived stress.

Diet, Stress, and Inflammation

Inflammation is a biomarker of stress. Hänsel, Hong, Cámara, and von Känel[13] demonstrated that situations such as work-related stress, stress associated with living in poor socioeconomic conditions, stressful events suffered in childhood, and stress associated with caring for another all contribute to chronic stress and influence the function of the immune system. Furthermore, Hänsel and colleagues[13] described how chronic stress impacts the HPA axis and the autonomic nervous system (ANS), resulting in increased levels of inflammation. Galland[14] did research exploring the impact of nutrition and patterns of food consumption on immunologic indicators of inflammation (eg, interleukin-6, tumor necrosis factor alpha, and C-reactive protein). Galland[14] showed healthier, anti-inflammatory influences with food consumption patterns that result in a greater monounsaturated fat to saturated fat ratio, a greater omega-3 to omega-6 ratio, and greater levels of vegetable, fruit, whole grain, and legume consumption.

Bakker and colleagues[15] did research to see if dietary changes could reduce moderate levels of chronic inflammation in individuals identified as being overweight. They provided men who were overweight with a mix of nutrients known to deliver anti-inflammatory effects (vitamin C, omega-3, and extracts derived from green tea and tomatoes) for 5 weeks. Measures were taken of blood plasma, fat tissue, and metabolic enzymes. At the end of the 5 weeks, there were no changes in measures of inflammation (C-reactive protein). Yet, there were small changes indicating some attenuation of inflammation in fatty tissues as indicated by improved performance of endothelial tissue and oxidation of fatty acids in the liver. The outcome indicates that adopting a diet high in anti-inflammatory and antioxidant properties may have beneficial impacts on inflammation and oxidative stress. It is possible that the nutrients provided were not given in enough quantities to have a more profound effect on inflammatory parameters.

Vitamins and Stress

As mentioned earlier, supplementation with vitamins may reduce stress and improve overall mood. The benefit of vitamin supplementation in reducing stress and improving mood and mental performance was shown by Kennedy and colleagues[16] in a sample of working men between the ages of 30 and 55. These men were required to fill out questionnaires measuring their mood state and perceived stress, and assessing their overall health. Cognitive functioning, mood change, and fatigue were also assessed during a battery of cognitive tests. The men where then randomly assigned to an experimental or control group. For 30 days, the men in the experimental group received dietary supplements of vitamins and minerals. During the last day of the trial, all men were asked to walk on a treadmill as they were engaged in a test of cognitive function. Analysis showed that the men who received supplements of vitamins and minerals exhibited improved cognitive performance, lower rated stress, and improved mental functioning.

Another study conducted by Mishra and colleagues[17] further demonstrates how insufficient amounts of vitamins, specifically B vitamins, can contribute to distressed mood. They assessed the impact of vitamin levels (vitamins B6, B12, niacin, and folate) taken as a child and taken as an adult on women's psychological state during adulthood. Using a standardized questionnaire to assess levels of psychological distress and a memory recall session to assess patterns of food consumption and vitamin intake during childhood, they collected food intake information from a sample of women. They found that only deficient levels of vitamin B12 taken at their current adult age had an association with higher reporting of psychological distress. With respect to diet, improper nutritional balance, insufficient vitamin intake, and excess consumption of fat have been shown to exacerbate the stress response and create unhealthy balances of stress hormones. The dietary patterns shown to create positive protective effects against stress and inflammation are consistent with the Mediterranean diet, consisting of increased levels of vegetables, fruit, whole grain, nuts, seeds, beans, eggs, and higher levels of fiber along with lower levels of red meats. Stress reduction is also aided by supplementation with vitamins and minerals including magnesium, calcium, manganese, B vitamins, and vitamins C and E. Additional stress protection was shown with the intake of omega-3 fatty acids, particularly DHA from fish oil, and increasing the ratio of monounsaturated fats (omega-9) to saturated fats.

NUTRITION FOR STRESS

"Don't be foolish enough to dig your own grave with a fork and spoon."
—Anonymous

It cannot be overstated that emotional stress affects all aspects of nutrition. A wide variety of foods needs to be consumed in order to remain healthy. This is because there is not 1 food available that contains all the necessary nutrients that are required for optimal health. Therefore a selection of healthy foods is needed. Nutrients needed include minerals, vitamins, proteins, and fatty acids. Consuming the required nutrients (typically between 40 and 60 nutrients) per day is essential to a healthy, well-protected body. Sadly, most physicians have no background in nutrition. Sugar is one of the foods we should eliminate. Sugar itself contains no required vital nutrients. Sugar may produce a burst of energy for a short period of time only. When this high runs out, the person will suffer a crash.

One of the main problems with on-going stress is the depletion of nutrients. The stress response is fight or flight; either action requires lots of energy. Stress utilizes many nutrients for energy production, even if one sits in front of a computer screen all day.

B vitamins are essential for coping with stress, as they are used in most metabolic enzymes. Substances like sugar, alcohol, and caffeine will drain these resources and affect the functionality of the body and the brain. When under stress, the body uses reserve B vitamins.

Foods can help relieve stress in several ways. Comfort foods, like a bowl of warm oatmeal can boost levels of serotonin, a calming brain chemical. Other foods can cut levels of cortisol and adrenaline, stress hormones that take a toll on the body over time. And a healthy diet can counter the impact of stress, by revving up the immune system and lowering blood pressure. One of the best ways to reduce high blood pressure is to get enough potassium, and half an avocado has more potassium than a medium-sized banana. Guacamole, made from avocado, just might be a healthy alternative when stress has one craving a high-fat food.

Carbohydrates prompt the brain to make more serotonin. For a steady supply of this feel-good chemical, it is best to eat complex carbohydrates, which are digested more slowly and have a lower glycemic index. Good choices include whole grain breakfast cereals, breads, and pastas, as well as old-fashioned oatmeal. Complex carbohydrates can also help one feel balanced by stabilizing blood sugar levels. Carbohydrates at bedtime can speed the release of serotonin and help one sleep better. Because heavy meals before bed can trigger heartburn, stick to something light, such as fruit and low-fat yogurt. Another bedtime stress buster is a glass of warm milk. Research shows that calcium eases anxiety and mood swings linked to premenstrual syndrome (PMS). The authors recommend organic, skim, or low-fat milk.

Oranges provide vitamin C. Studies have demonstrated that this vitamin can curb levels of stress hormones while strengthening the immune system. In a study of people with high blood pressure, high cortisol levels (a stress hormone) returned to normal quicker when people took vitamin C.

Crunchy raw vegetables can help ease stress in a purely mechanical way. Munching celery or carrot sticks helps release a clenched jaw and may ward off tension. Spinach and all green leafy vegetables are a good source of magnesium. Insufficient magnesium may trigger headaches and fatigue, compounding the effects of stress. Cooked organic soybeans or a filet of salmon can also provide magnesium.

Omega-3 fatty acids, found in fish such as salmon and tuna, can prevent increases in stress hormones and may help protect against heart disease, mood disorders like depression, and PMS. For a steady supply of feel-good omega-3s, aim to eat 3 ounces of fatty fish at least twice a week.

Pistachios, as well as other nuts and seeds, are good sources of healthy fats. Eating a handful of pistachios, walnuts, or almonds may help lower cholesterol, ease inflammation, reduce the risk of diabetes, and help protect against the effects of stress. Almonds are full of helpful vitamins: vitamin E to increase the immune system, plus B vitamins, which may make one more resilient during bouts of stress such as depression. Snack on a quarter of a cup every day.

Drinking black or green tea may help one recover from stressful events more quickly. One study compared people who drank 4 cups of tea daily for 6 weeks with people who drank another beverage. The tea drinkers reported feeling calmer and had lower levels of the stress hormone cortisol after stressful situations. When it comes to stress, the caffeine (in coffee) can boost stress hormones and raise blood pressure.

Caffeine can be responsible for inducing the first stage of stress (alarm stage). Caffeine is also responsible for making people hyperactive and nervous. Because of this, the person's sleeping pattern can be affected significantly by caffeine. If one has trouble controlling stress and always feels tired, one should look at his or her diet to see if there are any nutrient deficiencies or insufficiency. When the body is under stress, it has been proven that the body uses up its resources until they are finished. Following a diet plan will strengthen the body against stress and other illnesses.

The following are the main nutrients that the body will use up

1. B vitamins. These help the body cope with stress (build metabolism) and control the whole nervous system
2. Proteins. Assist in growth and tissue repair
3. Vitamin A. Essential for normal vision
4. Vitamin C. Protection of the immune system (eg, antioxidants and diabetes protection), lowers the amount of cortisol in the body
5. Magnesium. Needed for a variety of tasks such as muscle relaxation, fatty acid formation, making new cells, and heartbeat regulation

There are many herbal supplements that claim to fight stress. One of the best studied is St. John's Wort, which has shown benefits for people with mild-to-moderate depression. This herb also appears to reduce symptoms of anxiety and PMS. Valerian root is another herb that has a calming effect. Health care providers should be told about any supplements a patient is taking, especially herbs, so they can check on any possible interactions with any medication.

DIETARY TIPS TO IMPROVE DIET TO HELP COPE WITH STRESS
Tip # 1 Eat a Variety of Different Color Foods

The colors and their intensity are a guide to the variety of phytochemical (pigments) and their concentrations.

The color blue/purple on fruits and vegetables reveals the presence of natural plant phytochemicals called anthocyanins, which act as powerful antioxidants, protecting cells from damage. In general terms, the darker the color means the higher the phytochemical concentration. Anthocyanins have been shown to have a role in the support of healthy blood pressure, the prevention of blood clot formations, the improvement of memory function, and in lowering the risk of cancer.[18–20]

Blue/purple on fruits and vegetables also shows that they contain flavonoids that support blood vessels, help prevent short term memory loss, and even prevent urinary infections by precluding bacteria from sticking in the epithelium of the urinary tract.

Green fruits and vegetables reveal chlorophyll content. Another phytochemical found in green colored food is lutein, which is important for eye health.Lutein works with zeaxanthin (found in corn, red peppers, and grapes) to reduce the risk of cataracts and macular degeneration.[21]

Other nutrients present in green food include the indoles in broccoli, cabbage, and other cruciferous vegetables, which may help protect against some types of cancer.[22]

Many green plant foods are also rich in isothiocyanates, which stimulate enzymes in the liver that assist the body in removing potentially carcinogenic compounds. Greens (especially dark leaves) are also rich sources of folate, vitamin K, potassium, some carotenoids, and omega-3 fatty acids.

Red fruits and vegetables reveal lycopene and anthocyanins. Lycopene is a powerful antioxidant that is found in plants such as tomatoes, watermelon, and pink grapefruit. Anthocyanin is found in fruits such as strawberries, raspberries, and red grapes and has powerful antioxidant activity. Lycopene is believed to reduce risk of myocardial infarcts and certain types of cancer, especially prostate.[23,24]

Yellow/orange
Orange/yellow fruits and vegetables reveal carotenoids. Beta-cryptoxanthin, beta-carotene, and alpha-carotene are all orange-friendly carotenoids that can be converted in the body to vitamin A. Vitamin A is important for vision and immune function,

as well as skin health. There are scientific reports on carotenoid-rich foods helping to reduce the risk of cardiovascular disease and some cancer.[25,26]

In conclusion, many phytonutrients are essential in helping the body fight oxidation and degenerative diseases.

Tip #2 Eat Antioxidant-Containing Foods

Most phytochemicals are known to have antioxidant activity. Free radicals are oxygen molecules with an aberrant electron. Metabolically speaking, this unbalanced electron configuration causes damage to the following: cell membranes, DNA, RNA, and mitochondria. Free radicals are a hazard to the body's integrity at the cellular and tissue level. They have been associated with the development of cancer and heart disease, and other diseases as well. Antioxidants destroy free radicals. The 4 major antioxidants are: carotenes (precursors to vitamin A) vitamin C, vitamin E, and the mineral, selenium. Antioxidants are found mostly in fruits and vegetables.

Tip # 3 Choose Organic Foods (Whenever Possible)

In simplest terms, currently available foods are full of chemicals: synthetic fertilizers, pesticides, herbicides, and fungicides. Organic foods will largely reduce the burden of contaminants.

Tip #4 Drink Filtered Water

In general, people are usually dehydrated. People do not drink enough water! Many beverages (eg, coffee, tea, sodas) act as diuretics, meaning they increase the loss of water through urination, thus promoting dehydration. Various studies show that the water supply is not as clean as it should be. City drinking water may contain sizable traces of antibiotics, hormones, and chemicals.

It is in the best interest to install a high-end water filter system to be used for all drinking water (and cooking). Remember to replace the filter once a year (or as often as needed). One should also know that there is no federal regulation on bottled water. Most bottled water is ordinary tap water, sitting in plastic containers on pallets, stored in warehouses months before store delivery. It might be best to carry one's own filtered water in a suitable water bottle.

The importance of being hydrated cannot be overemphasized. Water helps flush out metabolites, waste products, and toxins for elimination. Dehydration will compromise this process. How much water is enough per day?

The authors suggest the best indication of being hydrated is producing near-clear urine (since dark urine may be a sign of dehydration).

Tip # 5 Eat Herbs and Spices

Use fresh spices and herbs to cook and in salads. Prepare a backyard garden with herb plants that may include rosemary, thyme, sage, cilantro, oregano, garlic, and many others. These spices and herbs are not only added for taste, they have health benefits (essential oils of herbs enhance the immune system and may have antimicrobial and other beneficial properties). The leaves, stems, and roots of these plants contain phytochemicals such as bio-flavonoids and antioxidants. There are several mushrooms (shitake, maitake and reishi) that are known to enhance the immune system as well.[27,28]

Tip # 6 Consume Free Range Meats and Poultry and Wild Caught Fish

Free range means that the cattle are allowed to eat as they roam around the pasture for their entire lives. Nonfree range refers to those animals that are raised on factory farms, live in overcrowded conditions and fed corn and other grains. Once again, corn is not a food source and is not found in their normal diet. The problem is that it may contain synthetic fertilizers, herbicides, fungicides, or pesticides. Also, living in such close quarters gives rise to infections; hence more antibiotics are used even prophylactically. Hormones and steroids are also given to increase yield. As for the consumption of beef, chicken, mutton, pork, and salmon, the best way to go is organic.

Tip # 7 Eat Fiber

Fiber (roughage) is found in fruits, vegetables, grains, and legumes (eg, peas, beans, and lentils). These are complex carbohydrates that are not digestible. Fiber sweeps out both the small and large intestine, carrying fat molecules (which is why fiber is said to lower cholesterol) and toxins. The World Health Organization suggests that each person consume 30 to 40 g of fiber a day. One should try to consume a good amount of fruits and vegetables each day.

Tip #8 Consume Omega 3s

Omega 3 and omega 6 oils are essential fatty acids. This means that one's body cannot produce them, and hence they must be obtained from the diet.

People have an imbalance of fatty acids in their diet; it is overloaded with omega 6s (vegetable oils) and severely lacking in omega 3. The standard American diet, which is high in omega 6 oils, tends to favor inflammation. Sources of omega 3s include cold-water fish (eg, salmon, cod, and tuna), flax seed oil, and walnuts. Omega 3 fats act as anti-inflammatory agents. They are also essential for brain cells and the retina. DHA comprises about 97% of all the omega-3 fatty acids in the human brain and 93% of those in the retina. Low concentrations of eicosapentaenoic acid (EPA) and DHA have been shown to result in an increased risk of death from all causes and accelerate cognitive decline.[29-32] There is evidence that omega 3 oils may also help to prevent and combat cancer. If one chooses salmon, the authors recommend buying wild Alaska salmon or Norwegian salmon, not farm-bred salmon. The latter is known to have a high polychlorinated biphenyl content (a known carcinogen).

Tip # 9 Take a Multivitamin and Mineral Formula with a High Content of B-Complex

B-complex vitamins are known to act as a stress fighter vitamin, because many of the B vitamins are used to assist metabolic processes for energy production (fight or flight).

SUMMARY

The impact that stress can have on one's health is serious and can cause problems to every major system of the body. With the right nutrition, one can reduce the impact that stress has on the body and effectively repair any damage that has been done. Proper nutrition prepares the body for any stress. When the body becomes stressed, it craves foods that are high in fats and sugars. These are the foods that need to be avoided, as they only provide someone with a small burst of energy, which will result in a long period of fatigue. On the other hand, a high-fiber diet rich in fresh fruits, vegetables, nuts, and whole grains provides greater appetite satisfaction over a longer period than processed, high-fat, and high-sugar snacks. But even more important, when one replaces junk foods with fresh, high-fiber plant foods, one is more likely to consume greater amounts of vitamins A, B6, and C, and the B vitamins niacin, thiamin, riboflavin, and folate. One will also have a higher intake of magnesium, iron, selenium, zinc, phosphorus, and calcium. These nutrients are all vital to a healthy metabolism and provide significant stress protection.

REFERENCES

1. Esler M, Eikelis N, Schlaich M, et al. Presence of biological markers of stress. Clin Exp Pharmacol Physiol 2008;35(4):498–502.
2. Stanley R, Burrows G. Psychogenic heart disease - stress and the heart: a historical perspective. Stress & Health: J of the Intern Soc for the Investigation of Stress 2008;24(3):181–7.
3. Jordan C. Stress and inflammatory bowel disease: encouraging adaptive coping in patients. Gastrointest Nurs 2010;8(10):28–33.
4. Heraclides A, Chandola T, Witte D, et al. Psychosocial stress at work doubles the risk of type 2 diabetes in middle-aged women: evidence from the Whitehall II study. Diabetes Care 2009;32(12):2230–5.
5. Hansen F, Sawatzky JV. Stress in patients with lung cancer: a human response to illness. Oncol Nurs Forum 2008;35(2):217–23. http://dx.doi.org/10.1188/08.ONF. 217-223.
6. Kreitler S, Peleg D, Ehrenfeld M. Stress, self-efficacy and quality of life in cancer patients. Psychooncology 2007;16(4):329–41.
7. van de Wiel H, Geerts E, Hoekstra-Weebers J. Explaining inconsistent results in cancer quality of life studies: the role of the stress–response system. Psychoon-cology 2008;17(2):174–81.
8. Carlson NR. Physiology of behavior. 8th edition. New York: Allyn & Bacon; 2004.
9. American Psychological Association. Psychology help center: stress effects on the body. Available at: http://www.apa.org/helpcenter/stress-body.aspx. Accessed May 27, 2014.
10. Kitraki E, Soulis G, Gerozissis K. Impaired neuroendocrine response to stress following a short-term fat-enriched diet. Neuroendocrinology 2004;79(6): 338–45.
11. Manary M, Muglia L, Vogt S, et al. Cortisol and its action on the glucocorticoid receptor in malnutrition and acute infection. Metabolism 2006;55(4):550–4.
12. Bradbury J, Myers SP, Oliver C. An adaptogenic role for omega-3 fatty acids in stress; a randomised placebo controlled double blind intervention study (pilot). Nutr J 2004;3:20.
13. Hänsel A, Hong S, Cámara RA, et al. Inflammation as a psychophysiological biomarker in chronic psychosocial stress. Neurosci Biobehav Rev 2010;35(1): 115–21.
14. Galland L. Invited review: diet and inflammation. Nutr Clin Pract 2010;25(6): 634–40.
15. Bakker GC, van Erk MJ, Pellis L, et al. An antiinflammatory dietary mix modulates inflammation and oxidative and metabolic stress in overweight men: a nutrigenomics approach. Am J Clin Nutr 2010;91(4):1044–59.
16. Kennedy DO, Veasey R, Watson A, et al. Effects of high-dose B vitamin complex with vitamin C and minerals on subjective mood and performance in healthy males. Psychopharmacology 2010;211(1):55–68.
17. Mishra G, McNaughton S, O'Connell M, et al. Intake of B vitamins in childhood and adult life in relation to psychological distress among women in a British birth cohort. Public Health Nutr 2009;12(2):166–74.
18. de Pascual-Teresa S, Moreno DA, García-Viguera C. Flavanols and anthocyanins in cardiovascular health: a review of current evidence. Int J Mol Sci 2010;11(4): 1679–703.
19. Lilamand M, Kelaiditi E, Guyonnet S, et al. Flavonoids and arterial stiffness: promising perspectives. Nutr Metab Cardiovasc Dis 2014;24(7):698–704.

20. Spencer JP. The impact of fruit flavonoids on memory and cognition. Br J Nutr 2010;104(Suppl 3):S40–7.
21. Zampatti S, Ricci F, Cusumano A, et al. Review of nutrient actions on age-related macular degeneration. Nutr Res 2014;34(2):95–105.
22. Ahmad A, Sakr WA, Rahman KM. Anticancer properties of indole compounds: mechanism of apoptosis induction and role in chemotherapy. Curr Drug Targets 2010;11(6):652–66.
23. Kelkel M, Schumacher M, Dicato M, et al. Antioxidant and anti-proliferative properties of lycopene. Free Radic Res 2011;45(8):925–40.
24. Holzapfel NP, Holzapfel BM, Champ S, et al. The potential role of lycopene for the prevention and therapy of prostate cancer: from molecular mechanisms to clinical evidence. Int J Mol Sci 2013;14(7):14620–46.
25. Ciccone MM, Cortese F, Gesualdo M, et al. Dietary intake of carotenoids and their antioxidant and anti-inflammatory effects in cardiovascular care. Mediators Inflamm 2013;2013:782137.
26. Tanaka T, Shnimizu M, Moriwaki H. Cancer chemoprevention by carotenoids. Molecules 2012;17:3202–42.
27. Johnson JJ. Carnosol: a promising anti-cancer and anti-inflammatory agent. Cancer Lett 2011;305(1):1–7.
28. Gebreyohannes G, Gebreyohannes M. Medicinal values of garlic: a review. Intern J of Med and Medical Sci 2013;5(9):401–8.
29. Wennberg M, Bergdahl IA, Hallmans G, et al. Fish consumption and myocardial infarction: a second prospective biomarker study from northern Sweden. Am J Clin Nutr 2011;93(1):27–36.
30. Montgomery P, Burton JR, Sewell RP, et al. Low blood long chain omega-3 fatty acids in UK children are associated with poor cognitive performance and behavior: a cross-sectional analysis from the DOLAB study. PLoS One 2013; 8(6):e66697.
31. Lee LK, Shahar S, Chin AV, et al. Docosahexaenoic acid-concentrated fish oil supplementation in subjects with mild cognitive impairment (MCI): a 12-month randomised, double-blind, placebo-controlled trial. Psychopharmacology (Berl) 2013;225(3):605–12.
32. Stonehouse W, Conlon CA, Podd J, et al. DHA supplementation improved both memory and reaction time in healthy young adults: a randomized controlled trial. Am J Clin Nutr 2013;97(5):1134–43.

The Role of Nutrient-Based Epigenetic Changes in Buffering Against Stress, Aging, and Alzheimer's Disease

Simon Chiu, MD, PhD, FRCP, ABPN[a],[*],[1],
Michel A. Woodbury-Fariña, MD, DFAPA, FAIS[b],[1],
Mujeeb U. Shad, MD, MSCS[c],[1], Mariwan Husni, MD, MRC (Psy), FRCP[d],[e],[1],
John Copen, MD, MSc, FRCP[f],[1], Yves Bureau, PhD[g],[1],
Zack Cernovsky, PhD, CPQ, ASPB[h],[1], J. Jurui Hou, PhD[i],[1],
Hana Raheb, BA Honors[i],[1], Kristen Terpstra, MSc (Neurosciences)[j],[1],
Veronica Sanchez, MSc[k],[1], Ana Hategan, MD, FRCP[l],[1],
Mike Kaushal, MD[i], Robbie Campbell, MD, FRCP[a],[1]

KEYWORDS

- Alzheimer dementia • Cognition • Stress • Epigenetics diet • Nutraceuticals

Potential conflict of interests: As lead investigator of the Epigenetics Research Group, Simon Chiu, MD, PhD, FRCP, ABPN, declares no potential conflict of interests. The authors acknowledge the financial support from Stanley Medical Research Institute for studies on Ginsana-115 in schizophrenia and from SignPath Pharm. Co. PA, USA for funding of the study of LipocurcR in a Parkinson disease model.
Conflict of interests: Michel A. Woodbury-Fariña, MD, DFAPA, FAIS is Speaker for Pfizer.

[a] Department of Psychiatry, Schulich School of Medicine & Dentistry, The University of Western Ontario, London, ON N6G 4X8, Canada; [b] Department of Psychiatry, University of Puerto Rico School of Medicine, 307 Calle Eleonor Roosevelt, San Juan, PR 00918-2720, USA; [c] Oregon Health & Science University, Department Psychiatry, 3181 South West Sam Jackson Park Road, Portland, OR 97239-3098, USA; [d] Northern Ontario Medical School/Lakehead University, 955 Oliver Road, Thunder Bay, ON P7B 5E1, Canada; [e] Faculty of Medicine, Imperial College London, London SW7 2AZ, UK; [f] Vancouver Island Health Authority, Department of Psychiatry, Victoria, BC, University of British Columbia-Victoria Medical Campus, Island Medical Program, University of Victoria, 3800 Finnerty Road, Victoria, BC V8N-1M5, Canada; [g] Department of Medical Biophysics, Schulich School of Medicine & Dentistry University of Western Ontario, London, ON N6G 4X8, Canada; [h] Certificate Professional Qualification (CPQ), Clinical Psychology, Association of State and Provincial Psychology Board (ASPB): USA and Canada; [i] Epigenetics Research Group, Lawson Health Research Institute, St Joseph Health Care, 268 Grosvenor Street, London, ON N6A 4V2, Canada; [j] Accelerated B.Sc.N. Nursing Program, Lawrence S. Bloomberg, Faculty of Nursing, University of Toronto, 155 College Street, Suite 130 Toronto, ON M5T 1P8, Canada; [k] McGill University, Meakins-Christie Labs, 3626 St., Urbain Street, Montreal, QC H2X 2P2, Canada; [l] Geriatric Psychiatry Division, St. Joseph's Healthcare Hamilton /McMaster University Health Sciences, West 5th Campus 100 West 5th Hamilton, ON L8N 3K7, Canada
[1] Contributed equally toward Epigenetics Research Group, Lawson Health Research Institute, St Joseph Health Care, 268 Grosvenor Street, London, Ontario N6A 4V2, Canada.
* Regional Mental Health Care London, 850 Highbury Avenue, London, Ontario N6A 4H1, Canada.
E-mail addresses: schiu3207@rogers.com; Simon.chiu@sjhc.london.on.ca

Psychiatr Clin N Am 37 (2014) 591–623
http://dx.doi.org/10.1016/j.psc.2014.09.001
0193-953X/14/$ – see front matter © 2014 Elsevier Inc. All rights reserved.

psych.theclinics.com

KEY POINTS

- The marked increase in the incidence of Alzheimer dementia (AD) has become a global health issue.
- Early detection and prevention of AD is feasible with imaging biomarkers.
- Stress-related disorders (metabolic, cardiovascular diseases, posttraumatic stress disorder, late-life depression) are recognized as risk factors for AD.
- Stress and the limbic-hypothalamic-pituitary-adrenal axis intersect with epigenetics in a reciprocal manner, with both positive and negative effects on brain health.
- Chronic stressors affecting hippocampal neurogenesis may set the stage for accelerated aging and cognitive impairment.
- Epigenetics regulation at DNA methylation near stress gene loci may be the missing link in stress responses and AD.
- There is good evidence in support of epigenetic shift regarding epigenetic processes such as DNA methylation, histone modification, and microRNA for aging-related cognitive impairment and AD.
- An epigenetics diet and nutraceuticals targeting epigenomics (omega 3-fatty acids, cocoa, caffeine, spices, red wine, vegetables, fruits, nuts, and dietary supplements) hold promise in epigenetic reprogramming of the aging brain and AD. Preventive trials are needed to examine efficacy in preventing cognitive decline in aging and AD.
- Epigenetics signatures and epigenomics targets represent a new frontier in AD research and geriatric care.
- An integrated service model may be the best approach for translating personalized epigenetics dietary intervention to an integratred care model of psychiatric practice.

INTRODUCTION

Recently, social media has heightened interest toward the public health issue of cognition changes in aging. The estimated global prevalence of Alzheimer disease or Alzheimer dementia (AD) of 24 million in 2005 is expected to increase by 4-fold by the year 2050.[1,2] Regarding the incidence and prevalence of AD, North America and Western Europe rank highest, followed by Latin America and China. The incidence rate of AD rises exponentially with advancing age, reaching the peak around the seventh and eighth decade. Each year, an estimated 4 to 6 million new cases are identified. Dementia has a projected worldwide incidence of more than 30 million by 2040. In the United States, an estimated 5.2 million Americans are diagnosed with AD: 5 million as late-onset AD (LOAD), and 0.2 million as early-onset dementia (EAD). If the onset of AD can be deferred by as little as 1 year, the prevalence can be reduced by 10%. Early-onset autosomal dominant AD is caused by mutations of genes encoding amyloid precursor protein (APP), presenilin 1 (PSEN1), and presenilin 2 (PSEN2). The ε4 allele of the apolipoprotein E (APOE) gene is now considered as a major genetic risk factor for AD.[3]

Health economics data conclude that AD has taken a heavy toll on health care costs across the world. A disturbing trend has recently been found in the United States. Between 2000 and 2010, AD-related mortality increased disproportionately in relation to a decrease in deaths from other medical diagnoses. Mortality from AD increased by 68%, compared with reduced mortality rates from cardiovascular disease (16%),

Abbreviations

5-hmC	5-Hydroxymethylcytosine
5-mC	5-Methylcytosine
AD	Alzheimer dementia
AGE	Advanced glycation end product
AMP	Adenosyl monophosphate
APOE	Apolipoprotein E
APP	Amyloid precursor protein
BBB	Blood-brain barrier
BDNF	Brain-derived neurotrophic factor
CBF	Cerebral blood flow
CHS	Cardiovascular Health Study
CNS	Central nervous system
CSF	Cerebrospinal fluid
CTE	Chronic traumatic encephalopathy
DHA	Docosahexaenoic acid
DNMT	DNA methyltransferase
EAD	Early-onset dementia
EGCG	Epigallocatechin gallate
ENCODE	Encyclopedia of DNA Elements
FTD	Frontotemporal dementia
GABA	γ-Aminobutyric acid
GR	Glucocorticoid
HAT	Histone acetyltransferase
Hcy/SAM	Homocysteine/S-adenosylmethionine
HDAC	Histone deacetylase
HOMA	Homeostasis Model Assessment
HPA	Hypothalamic-pituitary-adrenal
IRS	Insulin receptor substrate
LHPA	Limbic-hypothalamic-pituitary-adrenal
LOAD	Late-onset Alzheimer dementia
MCI	Mild cognitive impairment
MD	Mediterranean diet
miRNA	MicroRNA
MMSE	Mini-Mental State Examination
MRI	Magnetic resonance imaging
MUFA	Monounsaturated fatty acid
ncRNA	Noncoding RNA
NMDA	N-Methyl-D-aspartic acid
NST	Neural stem cells
NVC	Neurovascular coupling
PC-AD	Preclinical sporadic stage of AD
PET	Positron emission tomography
PSEN1	Presenilin 1
PSEN2	Presenilin 2
PTSD	Posttraumatic stress disorder
PUFA	Polyunsaturated fatty acid
SAM	S-Adenosylmethionine
Sir2	Sirtuin gene
SIRT	Sirtuins
SPECT	Single-photon emission computed tomography
T2DM	Type 2 diabetes mellitus
TBI	Traumatic brain injury

stroke (23%), and prostate cancer (8%), respectively.[2] The total aggregate payments for health care, long-term care, and hospice services for people aged 65 years and older with dementia are expected to reach $203 billion, far exceeding the budget for cancer and cardiovascular care. Caregiver burden adds yet another fiscal and human dimension to the health care landscape for AD care in the United States. Despite the alarming trend in health care costs, current AD therapeutics fail to prevent, delay, or modify the course of AD.[4]

The diagnostic scheme of AD has experienced a radical paradigm shift during the past few years. In 2012, the National Institute of Aging and the Alzheimer's Association for the first time proposed a new set of guidelines and criteria to categorize regional changes in the brain associated with AD and other dementias.[5] Using positron emission tomography (PET) and/or magnetic resonance imaging (MRI), levels of the putative biomarkers amyloid-β (Aβ) and tau proteins are to be combined with clinical assessment in the proposed diagnostic criteria. More significantly, the new criteria emphasize the evidence that changes in the brain begin before any symptoms develop. Infact, in the preclinical sporadic stage of AD (PC-AD), the individual may have Aβ deposits before the onset of symptoms. PET allows measurement of brain amyloidosis with specific imaging ligands such as ^{11}C-labeled Pittsburgh compound-B to identify Aβ.[6] Hypometabolism in the temporal-parietal brain regions can be visualized with ^{18}F-fluorodeoxyglucose PET. Furthermore, MRI can demonstrate medial temporal atrophy, and single-photon emission computed tomography (SPECT) can delineate brain hypoperfusion. The battery of AD biomarkers (PET imaging for Aβ, cerebrospinal fluid [CSF] Aβ, and tau protein), when combined with the APOE e4/4 carrier genotype, has been shown to be relatively robust in detecting early AD.[2]

The US National Institute of Aging has recently proposed to subdivide the preclinical stages of AD into Stage 0 and Stages 1, 2, and 3[7,8] as follows:

- Stage 0: Older individuals with no biomarker evidence of AD abnormality
- Stage 1: Asymptomatic cerebral amyloidosis with PET or CSF measures of Aβ accumulation
- Stage 2: Cerebral amyloidosis plus evidence of neurodegeneration or neuronal injury (elevated CSF tau levels or abnormalities on functional or structural neuroimaging)
- Stage 3: Amyloidosis plus neurodegeneration plus evidence of subtle cognitive impairment and decline

The transition from PC-AD to the stage of mild cognitive impairment (MCI) and from MCI to AD may be related to certain cascade events targeting neuronal apoptosis and neuroinflammation.[9] The stage of AD begins when the affected individual exhibits symptoms of AD consistently. On the other hand, 10% to 20% of patients older than 65 years may initially present with MCI symptoms. In one study, the annual rate of MCI converting to AD was estimated to be 23%. Taken together, the stages of AD span across a greater part of the adult life cycle.

From the pragmatic perspective, the 20-year period of occurrence of amyloid deposits without any clinical symptoms in the PC-AD and MCI stage offer a new exciting "therapeutic window" for prevention interventions. Converging evidence strongly suggests that stress derived from cardiometabolic, traumatic, and behavioral health domains is the final common pathway for cognitive decline and LOAD.[10] In this respect, research advances in epigenetics as mediator/moderator of stress pathways offer the best evidence-based approach to link stress to stress-related disorders targeting cognition.

The next section evaluates the strength of evidence in support of epigenetics in modulating stress-related disorders.

EPIGENETICS REGULATION OF STRESS RESPONSES AND RISKS OF ALZHEIMER DEMENTIA
Stress Vulnerability and Resilience in Aging

The stress paradigm consists of 3 components: a stimulus capable of challenging the homeostasis of the individual, the stressful response to the stimulus, and the consequences of the response.[11] The stressful response does not simply encompass the neural-behavioral domain, but hormonal, gender-specific, age-specific, and sociocultural arenas. Stressors are often coupled with stress responses, which can be adaptive or nonadaptive. The holistic term allostasis has been proposed to summarize the process by which variations in the internal milieu allow an organism to achieve stability despite changes in the environment.

Berger and colleagues[12] proposed 3 categories of molecular signals that culminate in the development and establishment of a stable heritable epigenetic state: "Epigenator," "Epigenetic initiator," and "Epigenetic maintainer" signals. The Epigenator originates from the environment and triggers an intracellular pathway. The Epigenetic initiator signal responds to the Epigenator and is essential in delineating the precise loci of the epigenetic-changes. The stability of the epigenetic system depends on the functioning of the Epigenetic maintainer signal for maintaining the chromatin environment in the initial state and for the future generations. Within the framework of molecular and cellular footprints, the Epigenator denotes differentiation of extracellular signals, presumably from the stem cells. The Epigenetic initiator role is fulfilled by DNA-binding protein and noncoding RNA, and the Epigenetic maintainer is mediated through histone variants and histone/DNA modifications within the nucleus.

The authors propose an integrated model of the epigenetic dysregulation modified from the Berger model of epigenetic state[12] and from the adaptive model of neuronal functioning, coined "neuro-hormesis" (**Fig. 1**).[13] The model attempts to explain the complex interplay of stress, stress response, and epigenetics dysregulation in aging. The biological system theory takes into account the internal milieu, adaptive

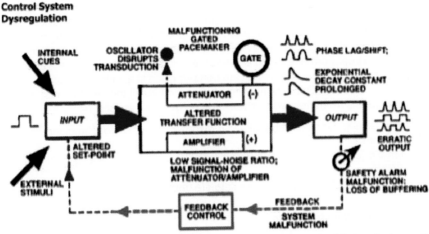

Fig. 1. Multi-level dysregulation of stress responses in aging and Alzheimer's dementia: buffering role of epigenetics diet.

physiological responses, and the regulation and control mechanisms within the organism to maintain homeostasis. The authors adopt the biological control system model to better conceptualize the distinction between adaptive and maladaptive stress responses. The "sensor" corresponds to the "Epigenator" in Berger's model.[12] The intrinsic stimuli can be defined as the sum of biological signals: metabolic, hormonal, cardiovascular, or respiratory stimuli, and affective and cognitive processes. The extrinsic stimuli refer to changes in the external social and physical environment. The sensor can be turned to high gain: the amplifier is turned on to maintain the constancy of the internal milieu. The dynamic processes of transfer function and feedback control are equivalent to the multiple roles of the Epigenator and Epigenetic maintainer. Malfunctioning of the attenuation and feedback control leads to dysregulation of the control system. The faculty memories, through earlier imprinting and learning paradigms,[14] become the substrates for the vicious cycle of age-related cognitive impairment. The instability and chaos reflect the loss of control of the Epigenator and Epigenetic maintainer. According to the integrated model, the feedback control is regulated by the fine balance between the "attenuator function" and "the amplifier function". Homeostasis depends upon the optimal functioning of the feedback control matching the output responses with the input signals.

Successful aging depends on the resilience of the so-called adaptive stress response, in contrast to stress vulnerability, which is the driver for accelerated aging and cognitive decline. The adaptive stress response always seeks to achieve a fine balance between signal/noise ratio and input/output as regulated by the feedback loop. Maladaptive stress responses result when the stressors become excessive and overwhelming to the extent that the system becomes destabilized, with erratic output and oscillations. In other words, stress vulnerability at risk is linked to maladaptive stress response. Stress resilience or stress protection results in an adaptive neuronal stress response. The threshold of adaptive versus maladaptive response will determine the likelihood of the crossover from health to disease domains. Maladaptive responses may self-multiply when the feedback in a physiological system changes from negative to positive. Under the biological system theory, the array of stressors (metabolic, cardiovascular, psychosocial, and traumatic) becomes excessive, or prolonged, and the repertoire of maladaptive responses may accelerate aging. A second seemingly innocuous "hit" suffices for successful cognitive aging to cross over to the "diseased domain "of cognitive impairment and AD. The feedback loop is transformed to a positive feedback loop characterized by waves of oscillations, high signal-to-noise ratio, hypersensitivity toward signals, and unpredictable amplifier/attenuation function. This process may reflect the prodromal stage of stress-mediated AD and accelerated aging. In this respect the buffering roles of stress hormones such as neurosteroids against the deleterious effects on neuronal survival and neuroprotection are compromised in accelerated aging.[15]

The risk factors for AD are categorized under the overall theme of central nervous system (CNS) disorders related to stress and epigenetics as follows:

1. Cardiovascular stress (cerebrovascular disorder, hypertension, smoking)[16]
2. Dyslipidemia[17]
3. Traumatic stress (traumatic brain injury [TBI], posttraumatic stress disorder [PTSD])[18]
4. Cumulative psychosocial stressors (late-life depressive disorder)[19]

Epigenetics and the Stress Response

Earlier studies on the stress response focus heavily on the importance of the hypothalamic-pituitary adrenal (HPA) axis. Recently the HPA axis has been refined and expanded to include the role of the limbic and paralimbic cortex to become the limbic-hypothalamic-pituitary-adrenal (LHPA) circuitry.[20] Because the limbic and paralimbic cortex encompass the hippocampus, prefrontal cortex, amygdala, and striatum, the LHPA circuitry network is strategically positioned to be an important niche where the multiple interactions of the various neurotransmitters N-methyl-D-aspartic acid (NMDA), glutamate, γ-aminobutyric acid (GABA), serotonin, dopamine, and acetylcholine will modulate aging. It is noteworthy that the hippocampus is the substrate for learning and memory, emotional regulation, sustaining neurogenesis, and synchronizing behavioral responses. Proinflammatory cytokines and hippocampal neurogenesis may be the missing links for the glucocorticoid (GR)-mediated stress response and age-related cognitive impairment. During the acute response phase, the GR complexes with the cortisol released from the adrenal glands. Once the GR-cortisol complex is activated, cross-talks between proinflammatory cytokines in astrocytes and microglia with the peripheral lymphocytes lead to dysregulation of immune responses. With chronic stresses, GR modulation of neurogenesis in the hippocampus is adversely affected.[21] GR resistance leads to erratic cytokine production.

There is converging evidence to suggest that stress produces enduring effects on gene expression through the traumatic memories: the biological effects are expressed within the LHPA network. Stress and the LHPA axis interact with epigenetics signatures in a reciprocal fashion. The epigenetics machinery plays a pivotal role in modulating both the intensity and direction of stress responses as risk factors for AD. Epigenetics (epi meaning "above" or "beyond" genetics) was first described by Conrad Waddington, the Scottish geneticist, to denote heritable changes in gene expression in the absence of any changes in the nucleus DNA sequences.[22–24] The epigenetic script is not encoded in the primary DNA sequence but creates a de novo cellular phenotype without any changes in genotype. Epigenetics creates novel cellular "phenotypes" without any intrinsic "genotype" change and brings into sharp focus the pivotal role of chromatin remodeling. In this respect, epigenetic machinery fulfills the transducer function in orchestrating the variety of adaptive stress responses (Figs. 2 and 3). The 3 basic elements of epigenetics consist of: (1) DNA methylation; (2) histone posttranslational modifications; and (3) noncoding RNA (ncRNA).

There is a growing body of evidence suggesting that epigenetic modifications are highly sensitive to early adverse stressful events. As a key partner of the LHPA network, GR receptor gene (Nc3c1) has drawn most of the attention in the field of stress research.[25] In a recent postmortem study, hypermethylation of Nr3C1 promoter gene was found in the hippocampus of suicide victims with a history of childhood abuse.[26] A recent study found that in examining the human genome locus of 281 differential methylated regions, 136 regions displayed a distinct methylation profile in suicide subjects with a history of early childhood abuse, compared with 126 regions in the control group.[27]

It is intriguing how closely rodent models parallel human epigenetic studies of maternal care regarding the impact on LHPA responses (reviewed in Refs.[28,29]). In the rodent model of maternal care, adult offspring of high-maternal-care mice showed reduced DNA methylation but enhanced acetylation of the Histone H-3 (H3k9) protein. The epigenetic changes were highly correlated with loss of fearfulness and dampened poststress corticosterone levels. Prenatal exposure to maternal depressive and anxious states was found to result in increased methylation of the Nr3c gene promoter in the CpG-rich region in the promoter and exon IF of the human GR gene. The epigenetics change correlated with activation of LHPA-mediated salivary cortisol response at 3 months postnatally.[30]

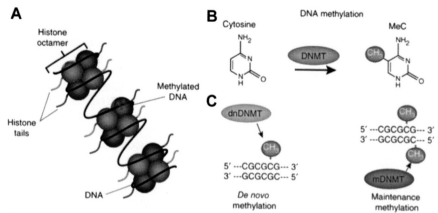

Fig. 2. DNA methylation. (*A*) Inside a cell nucleus, DNA is wrapped tightly around an octamer of highly basic histone proteins to form chromatin. Epigenetic modifications can occur at histone tails or directly at DNA methylation. (*B*) DNA methylation occurs at cytosine bases when a methyl group is added at the 5′ position on the pyrimidine ring by a DNA-methyltransferase (DNMT). (*C*) Two types of DNMTs initiate DNA methylation. De novo DNMTs methylate previously nonmethylated cytosines, whereas maintenance DNMTs methylate hemimethylated DNA at the complementary strand. (*From* Day JJ, Sweatt JD. DNA methylation and memory formation. Nat Neurosci 2010;13:1319–23; with permission.)

Taken together, the marked parallelism of human and rodent studies concludes that epigenetics-mediated stress responses can be transmitted in a transgeneration manner.[14] Suicide epitomizes how early adverse life events are consolidated in the "memory genes," which synergize with "depressive genes" in completed suicides.

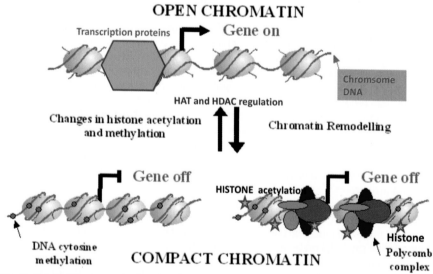

Fig. 3. Epigenetics control of gene expression: role of histone deacetylase (HDAC) and histone acetyltransferase (HAT). (*Adapted from* Dennis ES, Peacock WJ. Arabidopsis—what can crop breeders learn from a weed? In: New directions for a diverse planet. Proceedings of the 4th International Crop Science Congress. Brisbane (Australia): 2004. Available at: www.cropscience.org.au.)

Epigenetics can amplify the impact of environmental factors on the stress response through activation of the GR receptor. The release of GRs in response to stress enhances the memory and affective signaling pathways: MEK-ERK1/2, MSK1, and Elk-1 in the hippocampus. The signal cascade results in phospho-acetylation of histone H3 and modifications of gene expression, including upregulation of immediate early genes such as c-Fos.[14,23] These considerations provide further evidence for the roles of GR receptor and epigenetic signals in coordinating the gene transcription networks in the hippocampus. Both GR receptors and corticotropin-releasing hormone drive epigenetic modifications and chromatin conformation states, which in turn facilitate the expression of neuroplasticity genes specific for stress-related learning and memory paradigms.[31,32]

Epigenetics: Missing Links Connecting Stress to Risk of Alzheimer Dementia?

While cumulative stressors from early adverse events may contribute towards late-life depressive disorder, the paradigm of stress risks produce a well-defined constellation of psychiatric symptoms characterized as PTSD.[32] Both civilian-related and combat-related PTSD have captured much attention from worldwide social media. The prevalence of PTSD for US veterans returning from Iraq or Afghanistan is estimated to be as high as 17%.[33] It is evident that stress risks outweigh stress-protective factors in combat-related PTSD. In a recent study, the level of NR3C1-1$_F$ promoter methylation seems to be related to combat-related PTSD symptoms. In the lymphocyte model, combat veterans with PTSD had reduced Nr3c promoter methylation compared with non-PTSD combat-exposed veterans.[34] The change in Nr3C1-1$_F$ promoter methylation was inversely correlated with HPA measures and PTSD symptoms. A case-control study of predeployed and postdeployed US military personnel found preliminary evidence for DNA methylation pattern in Alu repetitive elements as a protective factor against PTSD.[35] Before exposure to the traumatic event, a stress-protective effect may be inferred from lower levels of Alu repetitive elements, in contrast to the higher levels of Alu element conferring stress vulnerability. Because long methylated domains reside primarily in tandem repetitive elements that comprise 50% of the human genome, the preliminary findings highlight the role of DNA methylation in PTSD in gene silencing and expression.[36]

The series of PTSD studies among military servicemen calls into question the missing links between traumatic stress and AD.[37] A stratified retrospective cohort study followed 181,093 veterans aged 55 years and older without any dementia at baseline, from 2000 to 2007. The veterans with PTSD were found to have a highly statistically significant 7-year cumulative incident dementia rate of 10.8%, compared with 6.6% in the control group.[17] The study adjusted for the high prevalence of comorbid medical conditions such as depressive disorders, diabetes mellitus, and TBI. However, the incidence in civilian-related PTSD population exposed to natural disasters, war trauma, and abuse, and the subsequent development of AD is unknown. A recent study found that both combat veterans and Holocaust survivors experienced substantial impairments in learning, free and cued recall, and recognition memory, without evidence for progressive memory loss or accelerated aging.[38] Given the substantial health care costs of AD and cognitive decline among combat veterans and military staff,[39] large-scale longitudinal studies are urgently needed to corroborate retrospective studies. Military risk factors for PTSD have been proposed, and await further longitudinal validation.[40]

Recently, the epidemiological relationship between TBI and AD has stimulated considerable controversy.[39,41] Earlier, the severity of TBI as measured using the degree of loss of consciousness was considered as the rare but robust environmental risk factor for AD. The syndrome of chronic traumatic encephalopathy (CTE) has recently been characterized as the neurological sequela following repetitive concussion injuries.[42] A recent meta-analysis reduplicated the findings of the first meta-analysis and concluded that there was a significant association between head injury and AD, but only in males.[43] World War II veterans who suffered severe to moderate head injury had a 2- to 4-fold risk of developing AD. CTE bears some of the clinical and neuropathological features of frontotemporal dementia (FTD) while overlapping with AD features.[44] Core PTSD symptoms have also been reported following TBI. Regarding Tau pathology, TDP-43, a neurofilament protein, is implicated in FTD and CTE.[45] Neuropathological findings in boxer-related CTE revealed loss of pyramidal neurons and Purkinje cells, and degeneration of substantia nigra melanin-containing cells. Neurofibrillary tangles with diffuse amyloid deposits or senile plaques were observed, implying an overlap with AD.[46] Functional MRI studies reveal similar imaging evidence of neuronal injury in the hippocampus: hippocampal atrophy was associated with a decrease in N-acetylaspartate levels in PTSD.[47]

The Innate immune system, once activated, can produce low-grade systemic and neuroinflammation, and will intersect with the LHPA axis in TBI and PTSD.[48] PTSD was shown to correlate with changes in circulating proinflammatory markers, increased reactivity to antigen skin tests, lower natural killer cell activity, and lower total T-lymphocyte counts.[49] It is likely that the epigenetics network modulates the interaction of the LHPA axis with the immune system. Although various biomarkers have correlated with PTSD and TBI, no specific putative biomarker has been validated to predict with high sensitivity and specificity AD progression from PTSD or TBI.[50] In in vitro and in vivo models of TBI, the putative histone deacetylase (HDAC) inhibitors, curcumin and sodium valproate, restored behavioral deficits and nerve growth factor-mediated cell survival in the TBI model.[51] Recruitment of brain-derived neurotrophic factor (BDNF) and enhancement of GABA neuronal tone reversed contextual fear conditioning, targeting the amygdala in a PTSD model.[52]

Cardiovascular signaling and metabolic stressors are increasingly recognized as modifiable risk factors for AD. Epidemiological evidence identifies hypertension at mid-life (40–60 years) as the most significant vascular risk for cognitive impairment in late life.[53] The vascular component of AD has increasingly been recognized as overlapping with vascular dementia.[54] The arterial spin label-MRI technique has consistently demonstrated reduction in cerebral blow flow (CBF) in AD.[55] The decrease in CBF and brain hypoperfusion most likely occurs secondarily to disruption of the blood-brain barrier (BBB), and may result in a mismatch of oxygen-dependent cerebral perfusion with the constant demands of neuronal activities. Reduction in CBF can even predict vascular stress risk in preclinical AD subjects.[56] In this respect, defects in neurovascular coupling (NVC) have been shown to correlate with cognitive decline in AD.[57] The model of dysregulation of NVC proposes that oxidative stress and inflammatory responses converge at the endothelium of the BBB to trigger the signal cascade of neurodegeneration.[58] Vascular endothelium is recognized as regulating the dynamics of the transport of neurotropic and vascular factors, and is highly sensitive to altered redox signaling, with a direct impact on neuronal survival. Microglial inflammatory responses at the BBB, along with faulty amyloid clearance, are among the negative spinoffs from endothelium dysfunction.[59] Neuroinflammation may likewise underscore late-life depression.[60] A meta-analysis of late-life depression studies further identified late-life depression as a significant risk factor,[18] echoing abnormalities of cerebral vascular signaling originating from changes in cerebral endothelium.[61]

Over the past decade, epidemiological evidence has pointed to T2DM as a putative risk factor for AD.[9,62] The shift in insulin uptake from the peripheral to the BBB is thought to desensitize brain insulin signaling mediated through the insulin receptor–mediated signal transduction pathway.[63] The construct of AD as "cerebral type 3 diabetes"[64] has been proposed, based on postmortem studies of brains from AD patients. T2DM brains showed substantially downregulated expression of the insulin receptor, the insulin-like growth factor 1 receptor, and the insulin receptor substrate (IRS).[65] On the other hand, the central theme of insulin resistance arising from oxidative stress in the mitochondria is likely the missing link in AD.[66] Evidence suggests the metabolic culprits as being progranulin[67] advanced glycation end products (AGEs), and an associated receptors named Receptor for advanced glycation end products,[68] in linking cognition decline in T2DM and AD. Abnormal accumulation of AGEs can accelerate aging.[68] Hence, targeting insulin resistance and brain energy metabolism can be therapeutic in AD. Controlled clinical trials on intranasal insulin and insulin sensitizers in AD have produced highly promising findings.[69,70] Intriguingly enough, phytopolyphenols from food sources are well known to sensitize IRs, and to restore insulin signaling and lower insulin resistance.[71]

The close link between metabolic syndrome and oxidative stress underscores the detrimental effects of metabolic stress on cognition.[72] Metabolic syndrome summarizing the cluster of cardiovascular and metabolic disturbances (hypertension, abdominal obesity, dyslipidemia, fasting hyperglycemia) has been demonstrated to link with cognitive deficits through changes in insulin resistance. Aberrant regulation of insulin signaling and endothelial dysfunction adversely affects cerebrovascular reactivity.[72–75] The vascular impairment often co-occurs with neuroinflammation, oxidative stress, and abnormal brain lipid metabolism. Imaging studies in T2DM have consistently shown reduced brain glucose metabolism, cortical and hippocampal atrophy, and a mismatch in neural network connectivity.[76]

EPIGENETICS AND ALZHEIMER DEMENTIA
Epigenetics Regulatory Network

As discussed earlier, epigenetics research is rapidly growing to address the classical issue in medicine: nature versus nurture. Interaction between genes and environment has finally been transformed to molecular epigenetics signatures, and more recently an epigenetics road map, in many diseases ranging from cardiovascular diseases, diabetes mellitus, and obesity to AD.[77,78] Epigenomics, defined as the pattern of epigenetics modification in the genome, extends above and beyond the 3 billion base pairs identified initially in the Human Genomes project. The ENCyclopedia Of DNA Elements (ENCODE) project is a public research consortium that aims to identify all functional elements of the human genome sequence, with far-reaching implications for advancing our understanding of CNS disorders.[79] The project consists of 1640 data sets from 147 different cell types, and the findings were released in a coordinated set of 34 peer-reviewed journals. Epigenomics has been applied to all of medicine.[80] For the past few years, there has been a sharp increase in the number of epigenetics studies in CNS disorders. This section highlights the more recent updates of epigenetics relevant to AD and aging.[81–88]

Epigenetics modifications consist of 3 major regulatory elements: (1) DNA methylation; (2) histone posttranslational modification and chromatin; and (3) ncRNA.[19] MicroRNAs (miRNA) are among the common kinds of ncRNA. Classical epigenetic mechanisms, including DNA methylation and histone modifications, refer to the process of transfer of activated methyl group from the donor, S-adenosylmethionine (SAM) to the 5′ position of cytosine residues as CpG dinucleotides. The so-called 1-carbon metabolism is highly regulated by vitamin B_{12} (cyanocobalamin) and folic acid. DNA methylation is regulated by the 3 members of the family of enzymes named DNA methyltransferase (DNMT) (see **Fig. 3**).

The chromatin is considered the functional architecture of the brain. Increased frequency of DNA methylation patterns often leads to restricted transcription from the promoter gene region (**Fig. 4**). Histone posttranslational modification is carried out through the activity of the nucleosome.[81,89] As the elementary unit of chromatin, the nucleosome consists of 146 bp of DNA coiled two-and-half times around the octamers of histone proteins H2A/H2B/H2/H4, as shown in **Fig. 2**. Acetylation and methylation are the commonly studied steps in histone modification. The degree of acetylation of the histone tails determines the relative intensity of transcription activity. Increased frequency of histone acetylation parallels enhanced transcript activity of the gene promoter regions.

The functional role of the ncRNA (or commonly named miRNA) has been vigorously redefined and expanded.[90] The miRNA consist of 21 to 23 single-stranded noncoding nucleotides capable of suppressing gene expression through altering the stability of gene transcripts, in addition to selecting gene transcripts for degradation. The ncRNAs can integrate sequence information from the DNA code, and unravel the epigenetic regulation and functions of multimeric protein complexes to provide the instant readout of the epigenetic status and transcriptional network in any given cell. Interestingly enough, miRNA play a major role in posttranscriptional regulation of gene expression and regulate more than 50% of all the protein-coding genes.

There is evidence for an epigenetic paradigm shift in aging and AD.[91] Remodeling of chromatin has direct consequences on transcriptional regulation. The epigenetics machinery can orchestrate the transcriptional responses to both internal and external

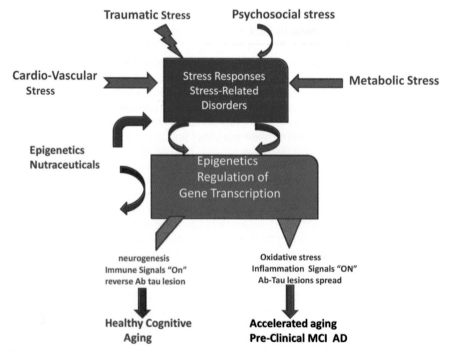

Fig. 4. Integrated model of epigenetics: stress cascade, cognitive aging, and AD. Ab, antibody; MCI, mild cognitive impairment.

signals and consolidate the long-lasting storage of regulatory data in the genome, after the signals are processed and dissipated. Over the past decade, it has become clear that the neuroepigenetics machinery encompasses both the neural development and neurodegenerative cycles of neurological and neuropsychiatric disorders. Epigenetics, through regulating the "on-off" switches of transcription, can orchestrate multiple signal pathways specific for cellular differential, survival, network connectivity, microglia integrity, and neuronal plasticity. The epigenetics regulatory network is functionally active across the entire life span of the organism from prenatal to aging. In this respect, epigenetics neural circuits derived from cross-talks among miRNA networks, histone modifications, and DNA methylations have been shown to be disrupted in neurons and glial cells in AD.[88] Disturbance in miRNA regulatory networks can affect Aβ production, which in turn can alter miRNA expression.

DNA Methylation, Histone Modification, and MicroRNA

In AD there is evidence from the genome-wide association study and postmortem brain studies for global hypomethylation of DNA.[92] Redox signaling is known to modify DNA methylation effects on gene regulation. 5-Methylcytosine (5-mC), the key epigenetic marker of AD, is oxidized to 5-hydroxymethylcytosine (5-hmC). Whereas 5-mC is associated with repression of gene expression, 5-hmC facilitates increased gene expression and is involved in diverse cellular processes of differentiation, development, and aging.[93] DNA methylation is also sensitive toward redox signaling in regulating gene transcription.[94] The balance between 5-mC and 5-hmC in DNA methylation may hold the key toward deciphering the epigenetic code.

Studies aimed at exploring role of DNA methylation in Aβ and tau phosphorylation have met with mixed findings. No direct correlation between APP methylation and AD was noted.[95] An in vitro study revealed that in the neuroblastoma cell line, the gene encoding glycogen synthetase kinase, the major kinase regulating phosphorylating tau, displayed hypermethylation at the promoter region.[96] Cognitive decline in aging is also reflected in the metabolic pathway of DNA methylation, targeting specifically the homocysteine/S-adenosylmethionine (Hcy/SAM) cycle.[97] Under normal circumstances, DNA cycling depends on the availability of the activated methyl donor, S-adenosylmethionine (SAM), which can donate the methyl group to the cytosine as the substrate that can drive the DNA methylation cycle. However, dietary deficiency of folate and vitamin B_{12} (cyanocobalamin) will prevent the recycling of homocysteine and SAM and excessive accumulation of homocysteine. Hyperhomocysteinemia is considered the vascular risk factor for cognitive impairment. Preliminary studies of folate and vitamin B12 supplementation showed positive results in MCI and early AD; although the long-term effects on modifying the course of AD are unknown.[98,99]

Histone Modification and MicroRNA

Studies in memory models imply that histone changes correlate with neuroplasticity. In rodent models, hippocampus-dependent memory formation and consolidation run parallel with posttranslational modifications of histone tails.[100–102] During associative learning tasks histone (H4K12Ac) levels increased on the gene bodies of learning-associated genes, showing posttranscriptional elongation in memory formation. It is likely that the genome-wide pattern of acetylated histone marks can be mapped fully in both human and rodent brains.

Converging evidence strongly suggests that the different members of the HDAC family interact differently to modulate cognition. Genetic reversal of the epigenetic blockade unlocks the repression of "memory genes," restores neuronal plasticity, and facilitates extinction of fear. HDAC-1 activation improves fear extinction, whereas HDAC-4 knockout worsens cognition.[103] Furthermore, loss of HDAC-5 impairs memory function without affecting amyloid pathology.[104] Aged SAMP8 mice showed global reduction in the histone H-3 acetylation level and corresponding changes in genes involved in histone acetylation homeostasis, silent mating type information regulation 2 homolog (sirtuin)s or (SIRT)-1 and HDAC-6.[105] Postmortem brain samples from AD confirmed differential changes in HDAC and SIRT in AD. Histone acetylation was reduced in temporal lobes of AD subjects.[106] Accordingly, the HDAC inhibitors curcumin and phenylbutyrate merit consideration of their therapeutic potential for the treatment of AD and have been tested for their efficacy in translational AD models.[107]

The search for longevity is a common theme cutting across geographical boundaries. The family of HDAC enzymes play a pivotal in regulating histone post-translational modifications and are divided into four classes, based uon their homology to the yeast specieis: Class-I, Class-II, Class-III and class-IV. While class I, class-II and class IV are zinc-dependent enzymes, Sirtuin belongs to nicotinamide-dependent class III HDAC. The discovery of Sirtuins as the central regulators of aging has recently created unprecedented wave of excitement in aging research.[108] SIRT-1 belongs to the class of NADPH+ dependent HDAC was significantly reduced in the parietal cortex of AD brains and correlated significantly with Aβ and tau hyperphosphorylation.[109] SIRTs are unique in that they require NAD(+) as an integral cofactor for enzyme activity in multiple energy-dependent metabolic processes; this determines the crucial link between SIRTs and the energy-dependent regulation of gene transcription. The multi-task roles of the SIRTs are further illustrated by the versatile target substrates functioning as modulators of the cell cycle, neuronal survival, and cellular oxidative stress, especially in the aging.[110] In yeast the SIRT gene, Sir2, extends their life span by 30%. Longevity effects have been extended to other invertebrate species such as nematodes. In mammals, SIRT-1 behaves similarly to Sir2 in the yeast species. Seven families of sirtuins (SIRT-1–SIRT-7) have been characterized with unique cellular distributions and exhibit pleiotropic actions: regulating cellular survival, protecting against inflammation, and maintaining metabolic balance through insulin signaling. SIRT-1 is the prime modulator of the p53-mediated posttranslational acetylation process in aging.[111] Overexpression of SIRT-1 blocks oxidative stress-induced apoptosis in a neuronal model. Conversely, gene knockout or downregulation of SIRT-1 produces a phenotype resembling AD: Aβ accumulation and tau hyperphosphorylation. Interestingly enough, SIRT-1 is regulated by miRNA.[112] Resveratrol isolated from grapes was first characterized as a SIRT-1 activator.[113] Since then, SIRT-1 modulators have been synthesized and have undergone clinical investigations to evaluate efficacy in boosting metabolic, cardiovascular, and brain health.[114]

Rapid advances have been made to fast-track miRNA as a diagnostic tool. A recent study found that in the hippocampus at postmortem, the expression profiles of miRNA-16, miRNA-34c, miRNA-107, miRNA-128a, and miRNA-146a were differentially regulated. Low CSF levels of miR-146a were associated with AD.[115] In peripheral lymphocytes, the upregulation of miR-128 identified in the monocytes correlated with impaired clearance in the Aβ clearance mechanism.[116]

Integrative Model of Stress-Coupled Epigenetics Dysregulation

In summary, the authors propose an integrative stress-induced metaplasticity model to account for the 3 stages of AD (see **Fig. 4**). Metaplasticity comprises changes that modify the properties of synaptic plasticity owing to a priming or preconditioning event or series of events. The operational framework of epigenetics already defined in molecular signatures and environmental stressors fits well into the scheme of priming stimulus or cues.[117] The authors consider the 4 pillars of stressors, namely metabolic, traumatic, cardiovascular, and psychosocial, as a priming cascade of events interacting with the epigenetics regulatory networks. Stress-induced metaplasticity at the synapse level spreads to the behavioral domain and comprises synapses, transsynapses, and changes in social behavior. The key elements of epigenomics are DNA methylation, histone modification, and miRNA, and the cross-talks among them. The outcomes depend heavily on whether AD protective genes or AD at-risk genes are turned on. Hence, dietary epigenetics interventions are strategically positioned to shape the crucial outcomes. With cardiometabolic, traumatic, and psychosocial stressors as priming events, epigenetics modifications intersect the vascular and metabolic signaling mechanisms in a bidirectional manner to bring about enduring changes in synaptic functions and behavioral and cognitive processes as outcome measures.[72–75,77] The model accounts for the efficacy of preventive and treatment trials of AD that target epigenetics regulatory networks from the microscopic to macroscopic levels.

EPIGENOMICS DIET AND NUTRACEUTICALS: ROLE IN ALZHEIMER DEMENTIA

Based on evidence in support of epigenomics in regulating gene expression in stress-mediated AD risk factors, and the pathophysiology of AD, there has been growing interest in examining whether diet and nutraceuticals targeting epigenomics may prevent, delay, or reverse the course of AD. It seems paradoxical that an epigenetics diet has been concurrently tested all across the world for efficacy in the treatment and prevention of cancer.[118] Despite divergent causes, the "odd couple" of cancer and AD as the prototypical neurodegenerative disorder, overlaps in the reprogramming of epigenetic networks in cancer cells and overstressed "traumatized" neurons. On the other hand, as the precursor to the epigenetics diet, the Mediterranean diet (MD) diet has undergone vigorous testing (**Fig. 5**). This section briefly reviews the updates on the bioactive food ingredients of the epigenetics diet and nutraceuticals (summarized in **Fig. 6**) in cognitive aging in the context of relevance to AD.

Mediterranean Diet and Omega-3 Fatty Acids

With recent increased media coverage of the cardiovascular risks of trans fatty acids, there is global action to regulate and even to ban the sale of trans-fats in food.[119] The accumulative epidemiological and biochemical evidence suggests that excessive trans fats in the diet are a significant risk factor for cardiovascular events. A 2% absolute increase in energy intake from trans fats has been associated with a 23% increase in cardiovascular risks. Trans fats have to be distinguished from monounsaturated fatty acids (MUFAs) or polyunsaturated fatty acids (PUFAs). The MD, originating from Southern Europe, places a heavy emphasis on a high intake of vegetables, fruits and nuts, legumes, cereals, fish, and olive oil, with relatively low intakes of meat and dairy products.[120] The MD accepts a moderate consumption of red wine as the source of alcohol. Olive oil, highly enriched in MUFAs, is considered the hallmark of this diet. The salient features of the MD are summarized in the MD food pyramid (see **Fig. 5**).

Regarding the specific components of the MD, controlled studies of total olive oil (MUFA) show a positive effect on cognition among the elderly. In the recent Three-City study recruiting 6947 subjects, olive oil consumption patterns were associated with reduced odds of cognitive decline in visual memory and verbal fluency.[121] During the 4-year follow-up, the association with intensive use was significant for visual memory but not for verbal fluency in multivariate analysis. In the United States and Canada,

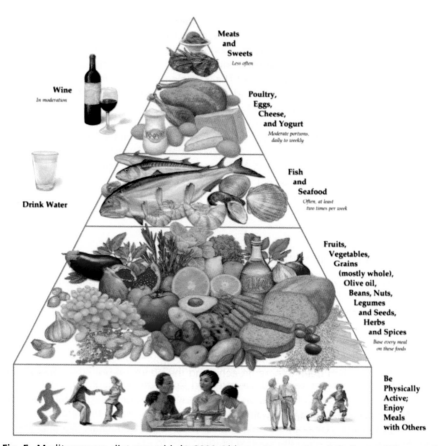

Fig. 5. Mediterranean diet pyramid. (© 2009 Oldways Preservation & Exchange Trust; used with permission. Available at: www.oldwayspt.org. Accessed September 5, 2014.)

canola oil is the most common source of MUFAs. A randomized controlled trial of supplementation of the MD with extra-virgin olive oil found additional benefits in improving cognitive performance.[122] The multi-faceted actions of MUFA are further illustrated by the protective actions against cardiovascular and metabolic events.[123] A recent meta-analysis of the MD reveals that it offers protection against T2DM. Greater adherence to an MD is associated with a significant reduction in the risk of diabetes (19%: moderate quality evidence).[124] Because both metabolic and vascular stress events are risk factors for AD, the MD offers additional therapeutic advantage in cognition and in AD-preventive trials.

The results of the longitudinal studies found the MD to be beneficial in preserving cognition and selectively enhancing cognition measures.[125] Two longitudinal studies from the United States by Samieri and colleagues[126] a Women's Health Study (n = 6174; 3–10 years) and a Nurses' Health Study (n = 16,058; 11–15 years),[127] reported female subjects who reported that MD adherence over the 12-year period led to better cognitive outcome. On the other hand, the French study by Kesse-Guyot and colleagues[128] (n = 3083, 11–15 years) found that lower adherence to the MD resulted in poorer cognitive outcome. Whether the findings can be generalized to the male gender remains to be examined in the future.

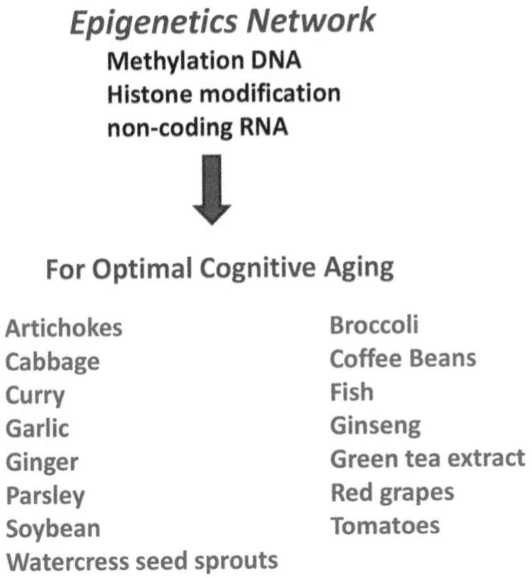

Epigenetics Network
Methylation DNA
Histone modification
non-coding RNA

For Optimal Cognitive Aging

Artichokes	Broccoli
Cabbage	Coffee Beans
Curry	Fish
Garlic	Ginseng
Ginger	Green tea extract
Parsley	Red grapes
Soybean	Tomatoes
Watercress seed sprouts	

Fig. 6. Epigenetics diet and nutraceuticals. (*Data from* Tollefsbol TO. Dietary epigenetics in cancer and aging. Cancer Treat Res 2014;159:257–67; and Hardy TM, Tollefsbol TO. Epigenetic diet: impact on the epigenome and cancer. Epigenomics 2011;3(4):503–18.)

Recently there has been interest in achieving the optimal ratio of n-3 versus n-6 PUFA because n-3 PUFA is anti-inflammatory, in contrast to n-6 PUFA which is proinflammatory.[129] Fish oil is a better source of n-6 than α-linolenic acid. The optimal ratio of n-3:n-6 PUFA in the healthy diet for AD prevention is tentatively set at less than 5:1, and the general recommendation from the Centers for Disease Control and Prevention for consuming 2 to 3 fish meals per week still commands the best evidence-based practice.

In the MD, moderate use of alcohol is recommended. Epidemiological data have suggested that red wine is beneficial in protecting against cognitive decline in AD, as well as cardiovascular disease, diabetes, and cancer.[130] The rationale is that red wine is highly enriched in polyphenol compounds including the epigenetic modulator, resveratrol. Critics of alcohol use in AD argue that moderate consumption of alcohol at the start may progress to impaired control over alcohol in the long run, hence counteracting the health benefits. This issue remains an open-ended question.

Adherence to the comprehensive MD pattern is preferred over individual diet components in reducing AD risks. It is likely that the individual components of the MD synergize with each other in reprogramming the chromatin complex within the context of hippocampal neurogenesis: upregulation of histone-3 and histone-4 were found with docosahexaenoic acid (DHA) in the presence of zinc in in vitro neuronal cell lines.[131] At the molecular level, eicosapentaenoic acid and DHA interact specifically with the nuclear transcriptional regulator, peroxisome proliferator receptor complex (PPAR-γ), binding with the histone protein within the epigenetics regulatory network.

In summary, preliminary evidence from a series of prospective studies suggests that an MD can slow the rate of age-related and AD-related cognitive decline and slow the progression from MCI to early AD. Most importantly, the MD is found to reduce the overall mortality related to AD.[132] Increased consumption of PUFA and MUFA from dietary sources of fish, vegetable oils, vegetables, and nuts is consistent with an evidence-based preventive strategy for AD, coupled with reducing the risks for cardiovascular disease, hypertension, obesity, and diabetes mellitus.

Chocolate, Coffee and Cocoa, Tea, and Red Wine

Dietary sources of flavonoids, the commonest group of polyphenolic compounds, can be found in fruits, vegetables, cereals, cocoa, chocolate, and spices. Structurally, flavonoids consist of 2 aromatic carbon rings, benzopyran (A and C rings) and benzene (B ring), with various substituents.[133] Recent interest has been directed toward characterizing the spectrum of neuroprotective actions of the family of flavonoids in models of AD.[133–136] Accumulating evidence suggests that dietary polyphenols play a significant role in preventing cognitive decline in aging through interacting specifically with the family of sirtuins.[135] Polyphenols exert pleiotropic CNS actions in antagonizing Aβ aggregation and interacting with signal cascade pathways involved in neurodegeneration and aging. Catechins enhanced expression of SIRT-1 and SIRT-3 in mice (reviewed in Ref.[136]). Within the tea family, green tea has the highest concentration of (+)-catechin, epigallocatechin gallate (EGCG), followed by oolong tea and black tea. In addition to catechins, fermented and nonfermented teas have various compositions of caffeine and the amino acid L-theanine.

Catechins and epigallocatechins play an important role in regulating gene expression, interacting with various transcription factors complexed with histone proteins.[137] In the human prostate cancer cells (−)-EGCG activated p53 through acetylation at the Lys373 and Lys382 residues by inhibiting class I HDACs. Treatment of cells with EGCG (5–20 μM) resulted in dose-dependent and time-dependent inhibition of class I HDACs (HDAC-1, -2, -3, and -8).[137]

Imaging studies show that activation of specific brain regions underlies the behavioral and cognitive effects of flavonoids. A functional MRI study found that green-tea extract increased the working memory–induced modulation of connectivity from the right superior parietal lobule to the middle frontal gyrus.[138] The magnitude of green tea–induced increase in parietofrontal connectivity positively correlated with improvement in task performance.[138] A PET study showed that in normal healthy subjects, caffeine displaced the radioactive ligand ^{18}F-CPFPX from labeled adenosine receptor (A-1) in a concentration-dependent manner. The half-maximal displacement was achieved at the plasma caffeine concentration of 67 μM, corresponding to 450 mg of caffeine (equivalent to 4.5 cups of coffee), in 70-kg human subjects.[139] The CNS pharmacology of caffeine (1-3,5-trimethylxanthine) has been well characterized.[133] Caffeine participates in the cyclic adenosyl monophosphate (AMP) signaling pathway coupled to phosphodiesterase-4 and behaves as an A-1 antagonist.[140] In the in vitro AD model, cocoa powder activates the BDNF cell survival pathway to counter Aβ aggregation, oligomer formation, and neurite dystrophy.[141]

A systematic review of 6 studies on the link between cognitive decline and the consumption of tea, coffee, or caffeine in the population or using case-control designs failed to find a robust dose-response relationship between tea, coffee, or caffeine consumption and protection against cognitive decline.[142] However, a positive trend was detected in the group of regular tea drinkers in terms of the rate of cognitive decline in the nondemented cohort. A recent Japanese study showed that in a large cohort of elderly residents (n = 732), the odds ratio for cognitive decline incidence (MCI or AD) was 0.32 for daily green-tea drinkers, compared with 0.47 for weekly green-tea drinkers.[143] Green tea may confer a reduced risk of cognitive decline among the elderly.

Clinical studies of caffeine in coffee and chocolates in age-related cognitive decline have met with mixed results. The Cardiovascular Health study (CHS) conducted in

United States found a gender-specific intervention of caffeine on cognitive decline in 4809 participants aged 65 years and older who were followed for at least 7 years to examine whether consumption of tea and coffee would alter the cognitive performance.[144] The investigators found modestly reduced rates of cognitive decline, as measured by the modified Mini-Mental State Examination (MMSE) for some, but not all, levels of coffee and tea consumption for women, whereas no consistent effect was found for men. Caffeine effect favoring the female gender has been confirmed in another prospective 10-year study of elderly women at high cardiovascular risk.[145] The cohort consisted of 2475 women aged 65 years and older in the Women's Antioxidant Cardiovascular Study, a randomized trial of the role of antioxidants and B vitamins as secondary prevention for cardiovascular disease. Results showed that slower rates of cognitive decline occurred with increasing caffeine intake (P-trend = .02). Caffeine's neuroprotective effect is specific for caffeinated coffee, but not for other caffeine-containing beverages (cola and chocolate). No adverse cardiac events were found in the study. The French Three-City study, recruiting a community sample of elderly subjects aged 65 years and older, reported similar gender-specific cognitive effects of caffeine.[146] Women with high rates of caffeine consumption (>3 cups per day) demonstrated less decline in verbal retrieval (odds ratio 0.67) over 4 years than women consuming 1 cup or less. It is noteworthy that a meta-analysis of 5 independent prospective studies found a J-shaped relationship of coffee consumption and heart failure.[147] The robust inverse relationship was found for a maximum of 4 servings of coffee per day. Higher levels of coffee consumption were associated with higher cardiac risks.

A recent 8-week randomized controlled trial of standardized cocoa flavanols[148] demonstrated for the first time that cocoa improved cognitive measures in elderly subjects (n = 90) diagnosed as MCI in a dose-dependent manner. The groups assigned to the high ($\approx$990 mg) and intermediate flavanols ($\approx$520 mg) did significantly better than the low flavanol ($\approx$45 mg) group in both the trail-making test and the verbal fluency test. The changes in cognitive function correlated with changes of insulin resistance as measured with the Homeostasis Model Assessment (HOMA), along with reduction in blood pressure and lipid peroxidation. The metabolic findings regarding cocoa flavanols are consistent with those of previous studies on the benefits of phyto-polyphenols in boosting vascular and metabolic health. In targeting insulin resistance in aging, flavonoids may represent a novel approach in delaying the onset of AD.

Emerging evidence suggests that cocoa's cognitive enhancing effect may be related to restoration of impaired neurovascular coupling (NVC). The metabolic demands of neuronal activities and related neuron-glial interactions have to match. In a randomized controlled study of NVC and cognition in response to cocoa consumption, elderly subjects showed that cocoa regimen had a dose-dependent, more being better, neuroprotective effect.[149] Emerging evidence suggests that cocoa's cognitive enhancing effect may be related to restoration of impaired NVC. The construct of NVC is fundamental to CNS neuronal functions. Under normal conditions, the metabolic demands of neuronal activities and related neuron-glial interactions must match with CBF regulated by the nitric oxide of cerebral microvasculature in the proximity of the BBB. The integral components of the NVC, namely endothelial cells, neurons, glia, and pericytes, are highly sensitive to the sporadic and chronic insults of oxidative stress and neuroinflammation, especially with advanced aging. In neurodegenerative disorders, impaired NVC with cerebral perfusion defects and reduced CBF can be the culprit in progressive cognitive changes.[58]

Accumulating evidence substantiates the cardiovascular and metabolic benefits of flavanols. A meta-analysis of 42 randomized controlled trials[150] comprising 1297 participants demonstrated that cocoa, chocolates, and flavanols improve insulin resistance as calculated with the HOMA–insulin resistance model, owing to a significant reduction in serum insulin. Flow-mediated dilation was also significantly improved after chronic (1.34%) and acute (3.19%) nutrient intake, independent of the "dose." Daily intake of 0.5 mg of flavan-3-ols (epicatechins) resulted in greater effects on systolic and diastolic pressure. No negative health effects were noted in any of the studies.

Fruits, Grapes, Red Wine, and Vegetables

The epigenetic impact of a wide array of fresh fruits, vegetables, spice, and related nutraceuticals in neurodegeneration has aroused equally intense interest in examining their actions in cognition. The discovery of the SRIT-1 modulator, resveratrol, as the principal polyphenol extracted from grape, has generated an unprecedented wave of excitement in finding the key to longevity. The health benefits of red wine with its high level of resveratrol for optimizing aging has been examined in detail. Resveratrol behaves as a multi-faceted target ligand, hitting multiple cellular footprints of AD. In vitro and in vivo studies[151] showed that resveratrol interferes with Aβ production and aggregation through the sirtuin-dependent activation of the crucial gene, encoding disintegrin and metalloproteinase domain-containing protein (ADAM-10). Resveratrol has also been found to facilitate Aβ clearance via the AMP-phosphokinase signal pathway, in addition to the lysosome and autophagy pathways. In aging, the progressive shortening of telomere length can make DNA highly vulnerable to cellular insults and stresses, hence accelerating cell death. Phyto-polyphenols can stabilize DNA through maintaining the length of telomeres by regulating telomerase catalytic activity. In addition, resveratrol may also do so by inducing SIRT-1 expression via PGC-1–dependent signal pathways.[136,152]

There is an ever growing body of evidence in support of the positive role of red wine in cognitive aging. In the Doetinchem Cohort Study, recruiting 2613 men and women aged 43 to 70 years at baseline (1995–2002), the outcome of the 5-year follow-up on red wine consumption was inversely associated with the decline in global cognitive function (P for trend <.01) as well as memory (P for trend <.01) and flexibility (P for trend = .03).[153] The threshold of red wine benefits was estimated to be at a daily intake of 1.5 glasses per day. None of the subjects progressed from the regulated use of red wine to alcohol abuse and dependence. The cognitive benefits are attributed primarily to the SIRT-1 modulator resveratrol, and not to ethanol. A recent randomized, placebo-controlled, double-blind trial with Concord grape juice supplementation, known for high content of polyphenols, for 12 weeks found that daily use of Concord grape juice resulted in verbal learning improvement.[154]

The antioxidant properties of many fruits containing carotenoids and polyphenols are likely to arise from their preferred epigenetics targets including the PPARγ forming complexes with histone proteins.[155] Fruits differ in their antioxidant potencies. Recently it was found that the pomegranate juice contains the highest content of polyphenols and antioxidant properties.[156] A recent RCT study of pomegranate juice in MCI subjects found preliminary evidence of cognitive enhancing effects.[157] The pomegranate-treated subjects significantly improved their verbal memory compared to the placebo control group, with increased fMRI activity during verbal and visual memory tasks. Blueberries contain numerous polyphenolic bioactive agents: anthocyanins have drawn increase attention in cognition.[158] A recent RCT trial found that daily consumption of blueberry juice significantly improved pair associated learning and word list recall when compared with placebo beverage.[159] Data from the Nurse's Health Study, a 6-yr longitudinal study, showed that regular daily consumption of a least 5 servings of nuts was associated with improvement in all the cognitive measures: verbal recall, category fluency and attention.[160] Synergy of berries and nuts has been suggested as dietary interventions to boost brain health in aging.[161]

Spices and Herbal Medicinal Foods

For the past decade, research in ED interventions have recently focused on the role of bioactive agents found in spices. Epidemiological evidence finds that the lower incidence of AD in Asia can be attributed in part to the common and regular consumption of spices.[162] Global history has authenticated records of spice use for enhancing flavor and color of foods. The chemicals derived from the wide array of spices (red pepper, black pepper, curry turmeric, licorice, clove, ginger, cinnamon, coriander, licorice) are now known to interact with multiple anti-inflammatory, antioxidant and vascular signal pathways relevant to AD.[163]

For many centuries curcumin, the bioactive component of turmeric, isolated from the rhizomes of *Curcuma longa* (Zingiberaceae), has been commonly used as a spice in India.[164,165] Curcumin is fully chemically identified to be [(1E,6E)-1,7-Bis(4-hydroxy-3-methoxyphenyl)-1,6-heptadiene-3,5-dione, and its neurotropic, antioxidant, and anti-inflammatory actions are well characterized. Curcumin inhibits amyloid oligomers and fibrils through binding to Aβ plaques. In AD models it has been fully characterized as a potent regulator of epigenetic signal pathways: curcumin inhibits HDAC isoforms 1, 3, 8 and histone acetyltransferase (HAT), and induces miRNA-22, miRNA-186a, and miRNA-199a. Curcumin participates in reprogramming of neural stem cell–directed neurogenesis through its pan-HDAC inhibitory effects.

Moving from preclinical pharmacology of curcumin to proof-of-concept clinical trials of curcumin presents unexpected challenges. Baum and colleagues[166] randomized 34 AD subjects in Hong Kong, China, to an active drug group (curcumin at oral dosages of 4 g/d and 1 g/d) and placebo group (4 g/d) over 6 months. The study protocol stipulated all the enrolled subjects were to receive standardized Gingko Biloba at 120 mg/d along with placebo or active curcumin. The results indicated that the serum Aβ levels remained unchanged, and no significant differences were observed between the curcumin and the placebo group with respect to the change in MMSE scores between baseline and follow-up sessions. An independent United States group of investigators[167] launched another randomized controlled trial using a different standardized formulation of curcumin: Curcumin C-3 complex. The study recruited 36 AD patients randomly assigned them to 2 g/d or 4 g/d or placebo for 24 weeks, followed by an open-label phase during which the placebo patients received either 2 g/d or 4 g/d of C-3 Complex while the active C-3 groups received the same dosage at baseline for another 24 weeks. The results did not demonstrate any significant difference between treatment groups of the primary efficacy measured by change in the Alzheimer's Disease Assessment scale: cognitive subscale (ASAS-cog). No serious adverse events were reported. However, no treatment effects were detectable with regard to the secondary outcome measures of MMSE, Neuropsychiatric Inventory (NPI), or the Alzheimer's Disease Cooperative study Activities of Daily Living (ADCS-ADL) scale. None of the plasma and CSF levels of Aβ40-42 or Tau changed. The study has methodological limitations such as the small sample size, the short duration of the study, and the poor bioavailability of oral curcumin. Hishikawa and colleagues,[168] in a case study of AD patients, observed a decrease in the NPI scores after 12 weeks of treatment with 100 mg/d curcumin. One patient experienced an increase in MMSE by 5 points from the baseline score of 12/30. All 3 patients were maintained on donepezil before starting curcumin. Curcumin most likely synergizes with acetylcholinesterase inhibitor in improving the cognitive decline in AD. Synergistic interaction of curcumin and donepezil is the most likely explanation. Our recent group has recently shown that liposomal formulated curcumin: LipocurcR was pharmacologically active in reducing apoptosis in the DJ-1 gene knockout model of Parkinson's disease.[169] No clinical trials have yet been conducted to evaluate LipocurcR (patented compound SignPath Pharmac, PA, USA) in AD.

Ginseng best exemplifies the cross roads of medicinal foods and nutraceuticals. In China and Korea, ginseng has been used for preparing soup and fermented with wine as a tonic for recovery from serious illnesses.[170] For many centuries, ginseng in Asia has been highly regarded as the phyto-chemical for many medical disorders ranging from diabetes, arthritis to cancer and stroke in Traditional Chinese and Korean Medicine.[171] Both Asian ginseng (Panax ginseng C. A. Meyer) and American ginseng (Panax quinquefolium) are the most popular ginsengs and belong to the chemical class of triterpine dammarrane glycosides with a 4-steroid- like ring with carbohydrate moieties labelled specifically as ginsenosides, or total ginseng saponins.[172] Panax ginseng comprises eight ginsenosides: Rb1, Rb2, Rc, Rd, Re, Rf, Rg1, Rg2. Ginseng exhibits multiple pharmacological actions in regulating immune systems, carbohydrate and lipid metabolism, cardiovascular system and modulating cognitive, affective and behavioral functions.

The neuroprotective and neurotrophic actions of ginseng have recently drawn much attention as possibly preventing cognitive decline. A recent RCT Korean study[173] found that AD patients treated with Korean Panax ginseng powder at the dosage of 4.5 g/day for 12 weeks improved significantly in two cognitive outcome measures: the Korean version of mini-mental state examination (K-MMSE) and Alzheimer Disease Assessment Scale (ADAS) ($P = 0.029$ and $P = 0.009$ vs. baseline, respectively) as compared with the placebo. However, the neuroprotection effects of ginseng were reversible upon 12-week discontinuation. Another open-label study in AD found that high-dose of Korean red ginseng (KRG) (9 g/day) augmented the effects of cholinesterase inhibitors in bringing about positive changes in the K-MMSE and ADAS.[174] Longer treatment with ginseng appears to be necessary for modifying the course of AD. A recent 24-month study reported that maintenance oral dosage of KRG at 4.5 g/day or 9.0 g/day improved both K-MMSE and ADAS with no further decline at the 48th and 96th week of the treatment period.[175]

Our research group has recently found that in the cohort of high cardiovascular risk cohort of patients diagnosed as schizophrenia, treatment with the standardized Panax ginseng extract, ginsana-115,R over 8-weeks at the oral dosage of 200 mg p.o. daily, significantly reduced insulin resistance (IR) as measured with (HOMA-IR).[176] The finding is relevant to AD and cognitive aging, since changes in insulin sensitivity contribute toward metabolic stress leading to epigenetic dysregulation in AD.[177] Interestingly enough, ginsenosides from Panax ginseng and American ginseng exhibit differential efficacies in interacting with the transcriptional regulator: PPARgamma and HDAC.[178,179]

Besides curcumin and grapes, spices, cruciferous vegetables, and citrus fruits of the family of berries display significant epigenetic activities.[152,168] The bioactive compound, sulforaphane isolated from Brussels sprouts, broccoli, and kale, is pharmacologically active in extending the life span and modifying epigenetics processes. The main components of the epigenetics diet are summarized in **Fig. 6**.

CONCLUSION AND FUTURE DIRECTIONS

In our study, we highlight recent developments in The pleiotropic CNS actions of the Epigenetics Diet and nutraceuticals in the context of aging and the phases of AD. We plan to link the different facets of the Epigenetics Diet to the regulation of the neural stem cells through the epigenetic regulatory network.[180]

In accelerated aging, the aberrant vascular signaling most likely interacts with defects in neural repair mechanisms in the hippocampus of the brain region.[181,182] The discovery of adult neural stem cells (NST) has challenged successfully the dogma "once neurons die, they cannot regenerate," because the NST possess the ability to self-renew and differentiate into multiple lineages (**Fig. 7**). Understanding the factors driving neurogenesis is critical in neural repair. Epigenetic control has been demonstrated to regulate NST renewal and pluripotency. Acetylation of the histone tails leads to access of transcription, streamlining gene activation and regulation. Whereas histone deacetylation catalyzed by HDACs favors gene repression, HDAC inhibition mediated through epigenetics diet and nutraceuticals facilitates gene expression. Hence, epigenetic reprogramming of NST through diet and chemical moieties can possibly delay the onset of AD. The NST-directed neural niche has been shown to be functionally linked with the vascular niche to form the neurogenesis coupled with angiogenesis. The combined vascular and cognitive benefits of nutraceuticals reflect an innovative intervention paradigm targeting specifically the coupled neurogenesis-angiogenesis.

SUMMARY AND FUTURE DIRECTIONS

The authors elaborate a novel model to explain how epigenetics regulatory networks can mediate the 4 pillars of stressors (metabolic stress, cardiovascular stress, psychosocial stress, and trauma stress) on cognition. The heuristic model known as stress-coupled-epigenetic dysregulation is compatible with what is known about the onset and progression of AD. It may be fortuitous that phytochemicals and dietary supplements have long been known as stress adaptogens to facilitate adaptive stress responses in aging. Epigenetics-driven nutraceuticals and diet in targeting impaired

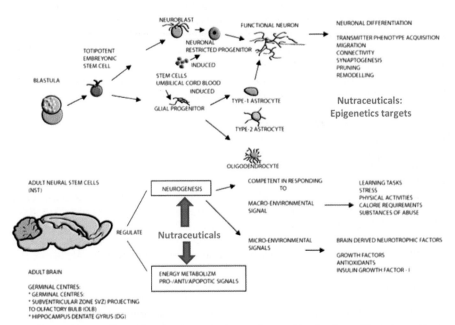

Fig. 7. Neural stem cell–mediated neurogenesis: regulatory role of epigenetics nutraceuticals. (*Adapted from* Chiu S, Husni M, Cernovsky Z, et al. New perspectives on gene-environment interactions in schizophrenia. Internet J Psychiatry 2010;1(1):4.)

epigenetics regulatory networks may be expected to be beneficial in preventing further cognitive decline and even in delaying and preventing AD. Despite promising leads, clinical evidence for the application of nutraceuticals in AD prevention remains inconclusive. This flux of prevention strategies lends itself to challenges and reevaluation of the scientific rationale behind the interventions. It is not too early, however, for health care providers in behavioral health for the aging population to be cognizant of the therapeutic windows that are open for AD prevention. The integrated care model is ideally suited to deliver diet interventions, especially when combined with enriched stress-management modalities. Multimodal lifestyle paradigms fusing exercise and cognitive stimulation with neuromodulation and brain games, coupled with an epigenetics diet, may open new frontiers in geriatric care. Furthermore, clinicians are on the cutting edge of personalizing interventions with epigenetics biomarkers. In this respect the clinical vision of personalized epigenomics-based nutrition across the life span to optimize cognitive aging can become a reality with advances in cutting-edge biotechnology in genomics and epigenomics. Transforming phytochemicals to anti-AD drugs is another fascinating area to be explored in the future.

REFERENCES

1. Thies W, Bleiler L, Alzheimer's Association. Alzheimer's Association report: 2013 Alzheimer's disease: facts and figures. Alzheimers Dement 2013;9:208–45.
2. Hugo J, Ganguli M. Dementia and cognitive impairment: epidemiology, diagnosis, and treatment. Clin Geriatr Med 2014;30(3):421–42. http://dx.doi.org/10.1016/j.cger.2014.04.001.
3. Reix Reitz C, Mayeux R. Alzheimer disease: epidemiology, diagnostic criteria, risk factors and biomarkers. Biochem Pharmacol 2014;88(4):640–51.
4. Schneider LS, Mangialasche F, Andreasen N, et al. Clinical trials and late-stage drug development for Alzheimer's disease: an appraisal from 1984 to 2014. J Intern Med 2014;275(3):251–83.
5. Cohen AD, Klunk WE. Early detection of Alzheimer's disease using PiB and FDG PET. Neurobiol Dis 2014. [Epub ahead of print].
6. Jiang T, Yu JT, Tian Y, et al. Epidemiology and etiology of Alzheimer's disease: from genetic to non-genetic factors [review]. Curr Alzheimer Res 2013;10(8): 852–67.
7. Sperling RA, Karlawish J, Johnson KA. Preclinical Alzheimer disease—the challenges ahead. Nat Rev Neurol 2013;9(1):54–8.
8. Frisoni GB, Bocchetta M, Chételat G, et al, ISTAART's Neuroimaging Professional Interest Area. Imaging markers for Alzheimer disease: which vs how. Neurology 2013;81(5):487–500.
9. Campbell NL, Unverzagt F, LaMantia MA, et al. Risk factors for the progression of mild cognitive impairment to dementia [review]. Clin Geriatr Med 2013;29(4): 873–93. http://dx.doi.org/10.1016/j.cger.2013.07.009.
10. Bihagi SW, Schumacher A, Maloney B, et al. Do epigenetic pathways initiate late onset Alzheimer disease (LOAD): towards a new paradigm. Curr Alzheimer Res 2012;9(5):574–88.
11. Mattson Mark P, Cheng A. Neurohormetic phytochemicals: low-dose toxins that induce adaptive neuronal stress response. Trends Neurosci 2008;29(11):631–9.
12. Berger SL, Kouzarides T, Shiekhattar R, et al. An operational definition of epigenetics. Genes Dev 2009;23:781–3.
13. Calabrese EJ, Baldwin LA. Defining hormesis. Hum Exp Toxicol 2002;21: 91–7.

14. Trollope AF, Gutièrrez-Mecinas M, Mifsud KR, et al. Stress, epigenetic control of gene expression and memory formation. Exp Neurol 2012;233(1):3–11.
15. McEwen BS. Central effects of stress hormones in health and disease: understanding the protective and damaging effects of stress and stress mediators. Eur J Pharmacol 2008;583:174–85.
16. Takeda S, Sato N, Rakugi H, et al. Molecular mechanisms linking diabetes mellitus and Alzheimer disease: beta-amyloid peptide, insulin signaling, and neuronal function. Mol Biosyst 2011;7(6):1822–7.
17. Yaffe K, Vittinghoff E, Lindquist K, et al. Posttraumatic stress disorder and the risk of dementia among US Veterans. Arch Gen Psychiatry 2010;67(6): 608–13.
18. Diniz BS, Butters MA, Albert SM, et al. Late-life depression and risk of vascular dementia and Alzheimer's disease: systematic review and meta-analysis of community-based cohort studies [review]. Br J Psychiatry 2013;202(5):329–35.
19. Kim DH, Yeo SH, Park JM, et al. Genetic markers for diagnosis and pathogenesis of Alzheimer's disease. Gene 2014;545(2):185–93.
20. Zannas AS, West AE. Epigenetics and the regulation of stress vulnerability and resilience. Neuroscience 2014;264:157–70.
21. Joëls M, Sarabdjitsingh RA, Karst H. Unraveling the time domains of corticosteroid hormone influences on brain activity: rapid, slow, and chronic modes. Pharmacol Rev 2012;64(4):901–38.
22. de Kloet ER. Functional profile of the binary brain corticosteroid receptor system: mediating, multitasking, coordinating, integrating. Eur J Pharmacol 2013;719(1–3):5.
23. Reul JM. Making memories of stressful events: a journey along epigenetic, gene transcription, and signaling pathways. Front Psychiatry 2014;5:5 eCollection 2014.
24. Stankiewicz AM, Swiergiel AH, Lisowski P. Epigenetics of stress adaptations in the brain. Brain Res Bull 2013;98:76–92. http://dx.doi.org/10.1016/j.brainresbull. 2013.07.003.
25. McGowan PO. Epigenomic mechanisms of early adversity and HPA dysfunction: considerations for PTSD research. Front Psychiatry 2013;4:110.
26. Klengel T, Pape J, Binder EB, et al. The role of DNA methylation in stress-related psychiatric disorders. Neuropharmacology 2014;80:115–32. http://dx.doi.org/ 10.1016/j.neuropharm.2014.01.013.
27. McGowan PO, Sasaki A, D'Alessio AC, et al. Epigenetic regulation of the glucocorticoid receptor in human brain associates with childhood abuse. Nat Neurosci 2009;12:342–8.
28. McGowan DP, Suderman M, Sasaki A, et al. Broad epigenetic signature of maternal care in the brain of adult rats. PLoS One 2011;6:e14739.
29. Oberlander TF, Weiberg J, Papsdorf M, et al. Prenatal exposure to maternal depression, neonatal methylation of human glucocorticoid receptor gene (NR3C1) and infant cortisol stress response. Epigenetics 2008;3:97–106.
30. Zhang TY, Labonté B, Wen XL, et al. Epigenetic mechanisms for the early environmental regulation of hippocampal glucocorticoid receptor gene expression in rodents and humans. Neuropsychopharmacology 2013;38(1):111–23.
31. Mifsud KR, Gutièrrez-Mecinas M, Trollope AF, et al. Epigenetic mechanisms in stress and adaptation. Brain Behav Immun 2011;25(7):1305–15.
32. Griffiths BB, Hunter RG. Neuroepigenetics of stress. Neuroscience 2014;275C: 420–4435.
33. Resick PA, Bovin MJ, Calloway AL, et al. A critical evaluation of the complex PTSD literature: implications for DSM-5. J Trauma Stress 2012;25(3):241–51.

34. Rusiecki JA, Byrne C, Galdzicki Z, et al. PTSD and DNA methylation in select immune function gene promoter regions: a repeated measures case-control study of U.S. Military Service Members. Front Psychiatry 2013;4:56.

35. Iraola-Guzmán S, Estivill X, Rabionet R. DNA methylation in neurodegenerative disorders: a missing link between genome and environment? Clin Genet 2011; 80(1):1–14.

36. Rusiecki JA, Chen L, Srikantan V, et al. DNA methylation in repetitive elements and post-traumatic stress disorder: a case-control study of US military service members. Epigenomics 2012;4(1):29–40.

37. Greenberg MS, Tanev K, Marin MF, et al. Stress, PTSD, and dementia. Alzheimers Dement 2014;10(Suppl 3):S155–65.

38. Golier JA, Harvey PD, Legge J, et al. Memory performance in older trauma survivors: implications for the longitudinal course of PTSD. Ann N Y Acad Sci 2006;1071:54–66.

39. Sibener L, Zaganjor I, Snyder HM, et al. Alzheimer's disease prevalence, costs, and prevention for military personnel and veterans. Alzheimers Dement 2014; 10(Suppl 3):S105–10.

40. Veitch DP, Friedl KE, Weiner MW. Military risk factors for cognitive decline, dementia and Alzheimer's disease [review]. Curr Alzheimer Res 2013;10(9): 907–30.

41. Noble JM, Hesdorffer DC. Sport-related concussions: a review of epidemiology, challenges in diagnosis, and potential risk factors. Neuropsychol Rev 2013; 23(4):273–84.

42. Costanza A, Weber K, Gandy S, et al. Review: contact sport-related chronic traumatic encephalopathy in the elderly: clinical expression and structural substrates. Neuropathol Appl Neurobiol 2011;37(6):570–84.

43. Stein TD, Alvarez VE, McKee AC. Chronic traumatic encephalopathy: a spectrum of neuropathological changes following repetitive brain trauma in athletes and military personnel. Alzheimers Res Ther 2014;6(1):4.

44. Fleminger S, Oliver DL, Lovestone S, et al. Head injury as a risk factor for Alzheimer's disease: the evidence 10 years on; a partial replication. J Neurol Neurosurg Psychiatry 2003;74:857–62.

45. Strong MJ, Volkening K, Hammond R, et al. TDP43 is a human low molecular weight neurofilament (hNFL) mRNA-binding protein. Mol Cell Neurosci 2007; 35:320–7.

46. Jordan BD. The clinical spectrum of sport-related traumatic brain injury. Nat Rev Neurol 2013;9(4):222–30.

47. Geuze E, Vermetten E, Bremner JD. MR-based in vivo hippocampal volumetrics: 2. Findings in neuropsychiatric disorders [review]. Mol Psychiatry 2005;10(2): 160–84.

48. Bauer ME, Wieck A, Lopes RP, et al. Interplay between neuroimmunoendocrine systems during post-traumatic stress disorder: a minireview. Neuroimmunomodulation 2010;17(3):192–5.

49. Pace TW, Heim CM. A short review on the psychoneuroimmunology of posttraumatic stress disorder: from risk factors to medical comorbidities. Brain Behav Immun 2011;25(1):6–13.

50. Schmidt U, Kaltwasser SF, Wotja CT. Biomarkers in posttraumatic stress disorder: overview and implications for future research. Dis Markers 2013;35(1):43–54.

51. Lu H, Freich J, Turtzo C, et al. Histone deacetylase inhibitors are neuroprotective and preserve NGF-mediated cell survival following traumatic brain injury. Proc Natl Acad Sci U S A 2013;110(26):10747–52.

52. Mahan AL, Ressler KJ. Fear conditioning, synaptic plasticity and the amygdala: implications for posttraumatic stress disorder. Trends Neurosci 2012;35(1): 24–35.
53. Sato N, Morishita R. Roles of vascular and metabolic components in cognitive dysfunction of Alzheimer disease: short and long-term modification by non-genetic risk factors. Front Aging Neurosci 2013;5(64):1–9.
54. Kelleher R, Soiza R. Evidence of endothelial dysfunction in the development of Alzheimer's disease: is Alzheimer's a vascular disorder? Am J Cardiovasc Dis 2013;394:197–226.
55. Binnewijzend MA, Kuijer JP, Benedictus MR, et al. Cerebral blood flow measured with 3D pseudocontinuous arterial spin-labeling MR imaging in Alzheimer disease and mild cognitive impairment: a marker for disease severity. Radiology 2013;267(1):221–30.
56. Wierenga CE, Hays CC, Zlatar ZZ. Cerebral blood flow measured by arterial spin labeling MRI as a preclinical marker of Alzheimer's disease. J Alzheimers Dis 2014. [Epub ahead of print].
57. Leszek J, Sochoka M, Gasioowski K. Vascular factors and epigenetic modifications in the pathogenesis of Alzheimer's disease. J Neurosci 2013;323:25–32.
58. Nicolakakis N, Hamel E. Neurovascular function in Alzheimer's disease patients and experimental models. J Cereb Blood Flow Metab 2011;31(6):1354–70.
59. Chen Z, Zhong C. Decoding Alzheimer's disease from perturbed cerebral glucose metabolism: implications for diagnostic and therapeutic strategies. Prog Neurobiol 2013;108:21–43.
60. Wolkowitz OM, Reus VI, Millon SH. Of sound mind and body: depression, disease and accelerated aging. Dialogues Clin Neurosci 2011;13(1):25–39.
61. Hermida AP, McDonald WM, Steenland K, et al. The association between late-life depression, mild cognitive impairment and dementia: is inflammation the missing link? Expert Rev Neurother 2012;12(11):1339–50.
62. Butterfield DA, Di Domenico F, Barone E. Elevated risk of type 2 diabetes for development of Alzheimer disease: a key role for oxidative stress in brain. Biochim Biophys Acta 2014;1842(9):1693–706.
63. Medhi B, Chakrabarty M. Insulin resistance: an emerging link in Alzheimer's disease. Neurol Sci 2013;34(10):1719–25.
64. Bekkering P, Jafri I, van Overveld FJ, et al. The intricate association between gut microbiota and development of type 1, type 2 and type 3 diabetes. Expert Rev Clin Immunol 2013;9(11):1031–41.
65. Felice FG, Lourenco MV, Ferreira ST. How does brain insulin resistance develop in Alzheimer's disease? Alzheimers Dement 2014;10:S26–32.
66. Pohanka M. Alzheimer's disease and oxidative stress: a review [review]. Curr Med Chem 2013;21(3):356–64.
67. Nguyen AD, Nguyen TA, Martens LH, et al. Progranulin: at the interface of neuro-degenerative and metabolic diseases. Trends Endocrinol Metab 2013;24(12): 597–606.
68. Srikanth V, Maczurek A, Phan T, et al. Advanced glycation endproducts and their receptor RAGE in Alzheimer's disease. Neurobiol Aging 2011;32(5):763–77.
69. Alagiakrishnan K, Sankaralingam S, Ghosh M, et al. Antidiabetic drugs and their potential role in treating mild cognitive impairment and Alzheimer's disease. Discov Med 2013;16(90):277–86.
70. Freiherr J, Hallschmid M, Frey WH 2nd, et al. Intranasal insulin as a treatment for Alzheimer's disease: a review of basic research and clinical evidence. CNS Drugs 2013;27(7):505–14.

71. Munir KM, Chandrasekaran S, Gao F, et al. Mechanisms for food polyphenols to ameliorate insulin resistance and endothelial dysfunction: therapeutic implications for diabetes and its cardiovascular complications. Am J Physiol Endocrinol Metab 2013;305(6):E679–86. http://dx.doi.org/10.1152/ajpendo.00377.2013.

72. Conreas D, Carvajal K, Toral-Rios D, et al. Oxidative stress and metabolic syndrome: cause or consequence of Alzheimer's disease? Oxid Med Cell Longev 2014;2014:497802, 1–11.

73. Paneni F, Costantino S, Volpre M, et al. Epigenetic signatures and vascular risk in type 2 diabetes: a clinical perspective. Atherosclerosis 2013;230:191–7.

74. Ryan JP, Fine DF, Rosano C. Type 2 diabetes and cognitive impairment: contributions from neuroimaging. J Geriatr Psychiatry Neurol 2014;27(1):47–55.

75. Yates KF, Sweat V, Yau PL, et al. Impact of metabolic syndrome on cognition and brain: a selected review of the literature. Arterioscler Thromb Vasc Biol 2012;32(9):2060–7.

76. Kovacic JC, Fuster V. Atherosclerotic risk factors, vascular cognitive impairment, and Alzheimer disease [review]. Mt Sinai J Med 2012;79(6):664–73. http://dx.doi.org/10.1002/msj.21347.

77. Tammen SA, Friso S, Choi SW. Epigenetics: the link between nature and nurture. Mol Aspects Med 2013;34(4):753–64.

78. Kavanagh DH, Dwyer S, O'Donovan MC, et al. The ENCODE project: implications for psychiatric genetics. Mol Psychiatry 2013;18(5):540–2.

79. Wright R, Saul RA. Epigenetics and primary care. Pediatrics 2013;132(Suppl 3):S216–23.

80. Wang J, Yu JT, Tan MS, et al. Epigenetic mechanisms in Alzheimer's disease: implications for pathogenesis and therapy. Ageing Res Rev 2013;12:1024–41.

81. Akbarian S, Beeri MS, Haroutunian V. Epigenetic determinants of healthy and diseased brain aging and cognition. JAMA Neurol 2013;70(6):711–8.

82. Telese F, Gamlie A, Skowronska-Krawczyk D, et al. "Seq-ing" insights into the epigenetics of neuronal gene regulation. Neuron 2013;77(4):606–23.

83. Walker MP, LaFeria F, Oddo SS, et al. Reversible epigenetic histone modifications and Bdnf Expression in neurons with aging and from the mouse model of Alzheimer's disease. Age 2013;35:519–31.

84. Adwan L, Zawia NH. Epigenetics: a novel therapeutic approach for the treatment of Alzheimer's disease. Pharmacol Ther 2013;139:41–51.

85. Vererappan C, Sleiman S, Coppola G. Epigenetics of Alzheimer's disease and frontotemporal dementia. Neurotherapeutics 2013;10:709–21.

86. Sultan F, Day J. Epigenetic mechanisms in memory and synaptic function. Epigenomics 2011;3(2):157–81.

87. Houston I, Pepter C, Mithell A, et al. Epigenetics in the human brain. Neuropsychopharmacology 2013;38:183–97.

88. Schonrock N, Götz J. Decoding the non-coding RNAs in Alzheimer's disease. Cell Mol Life Sci 2012;69(21):3543–59.

89. Mastroeni D, Grover A, Dalvaux E, et al. Epigenetic mechanisms in Alzhiemer's disease. Neurobiol Aging 2011;32(7):1161–80.

90. Tan L, Yu JT, Hu N, et al. Non-coding RNAs in Alzheimer's disease. Mol Neurobiol 2013;47(1):382–93.

91. Mill J. Toward an integrated genetic and epigenetic approach to Alzheimer's disease. Neurobiol Aging 2011;32(7):1188–91.

92. Lu H, Liu Z, Deng Y, et al. DNA methylation, a hand behind neurodegenerative diseases. Front Aging Neurosci 2013;5:85.

93. Madugundu GS, Cadet J, Wagner JR. Hydroxyl-radical-induced oxidation of 5-methylcytosine in isolated and cellular DNA. Nucleic Acids Res 2014; 42(11):7450–60.
94. Zawia NH, Lahiri DK, Cardozo-Pelaez F. Epigenetics, oxidative stress, and Alzheimer disease. Free Radic Biol Med 2009;46(9):1241–9.
95. Barrachina M, Gerrer L. DNA methylation of Alzheimer's disease and Taupathyl-related genes in postmortem brain. J Neuropathol Exp Neurol 2009;68:880–91.
96. Nicolia V, Fuso A, Cacallaro RA, et al. Vitamin B deficiency promotes tau phosphorylation through regulation of GSK3beta and PP2A. J Alzheimers Dis 2010; 19:895–907.
97. Fuso A, Scarpa S. One-carbon metabolism and Alzheimer's disease: is it all a methylation matter? Neurobiol Aging 2011;32(7):1192–5.
98. Cacciapuoti F. Lowering homocysteine levels with folic acid and B-vitamins do not reduce early atherosclerosis, but could interfere with cognitive decline and Alzheimer's disease. J Thromb Thrombolysis 2013;36(3):258–62.
99. Malouf R, Grimley Evans J. Folic acid with or without vitamin B12 for the prevention and treatment of healthy elderly and demented people. Cochrane Database Syst Rev 2008;(4):CD004514.
100. Peixoto L, Abel T. The role of histone acetylation in memory formation and cognitive impairments. Neuropsychopharmacology 2013;38:62–76.
101. Guan JS, Xie H, Ding X. The role of epigenetic regulation in learning and memory. Exp Neurol 2014. pii: S0014-4886(14)00147-2. [Epub ahead of print].
102. Jarome TJ, Lubin FD. Epigenetic mechanisms of memory formation and reconsolidation. Neurobiol Learn Mem 2014. pii: S1074-7427(14)00141-5. [Epub ahead of print].
103. Govindarajan N, Rao P, Burkhardt S, et al. Reducing HDAC6 ameliorates cognitive deficits in a mouse model for Alzheimer's disease. EMBO Mol Med 2013;5(1):52–63.
104. Agis-Balboa RC, Pavelka Z, Kerimoglu C, et al. Loss of HDAC5 impairs memory function: implications for Alzheimer's disease. J Alzheimers Dis 2013;33(1):35–44.
105. Graff J, Rei D, Guan JS, et al. An Epigenetic blockade of cognitive functions in the neuorodegenerative brain. Nature 2012;483(7388):222–6.
106. Stilling RM, Fischer A. The role of histone acetylation in age-associated memory impairment and Alzheimer's disease. Neurobiol Learn Mem 2011;96(1):19–26.
107. Coppedè F. The potential of epigenetic therapies in neurodegenerative diseases. Front Genet 2014;5:220. http://dx.doi.org/10.3389/fgene.2014.00220.
108. Raghavan A, Shah ZA. Sirtuins in neurodegenerative diseases: a biological-chemical perspective. Neurodegener Dis 2012;9(1):1–10.
109. Wang Y, Xu C, Liang Y, et al. SIRT1 in metabolic syndrome: where to target matters. Pharmacol Ther 2012;136(3):305–18.
110. Kugel S, Mostoslavsky R. Chromatin and beyond: the multitasking roles for SIRT6. Trends Biochem Sci 2014;39(2):72–81.
111. Mahlknecht U, Zschoernig B. Involvement of sirtuins in life-span and aging related diseases. Adv Exp Med Biol 2012;739:252–61.
112. Choi SE, Kemper JK. Regulation of SIRT1 by microRNAs. Mol Cells 2013;36(5): 385–92.
113. Poulsen MM, Jørgensen JO, Jessen N, et al. Resveratrol in metabolic health: an overview of the current evidence and perspectives. Ann N Y Acad Sci 2013; 1290:74–82.
114. Hubbard BP, Sinclair DA. Small molecule SIRT1 activators for the treatment of aging and age-related diseases. Trends Pharmacol Sci 2014;35(3):146–54.

115. Müller M, Kuiperij HB, Claassen JA, et al. MicroRNAs in Alzheimer's disease: differential expression in hippocampus and cell-free cerebrospinal fluid. Neurobiol Aging 2014;35(1):152–8.

116. Tiribuzi R, Crispoltoni L, Porcellati S, et al. miR128 up-regulation correlates with impaired amyloid β(1-42) degradation in monocytes from patients with sporadic Alzheimer's disease. Neurobiol Aging 2014;35(2):345–56.

117. Schmidt MV, Abraham WC, Maroun M, et al. Stress-induced metaplasticity: from synapses to behavior. Neuroscience 2013;250:112–20.

118. Hardy JM, Tollsfsbol T. Epigenetic diet: impact on the epigenome and cancer. Epigenomics 2011;3(4):503–18.

119. Ganguly R, Pierce GN. Trans fat involvement in cardiovascular disease. Mol Nutr Food Res 2012;56(7):1090–6.

120. Frisardi V, Panza F, Seripa D, et al. Nutraceutical properties of Mediterranean diet and cognitive decline: possible underlying mechanisms. J Alzheimers Dis 2010;22(3):715–40.

121. Berr C, Portet F, Carriere I, et al. Olive oil and cognition: results from the Three-City Study. Dement Geriatr Cogn Disord 2009;28(4):357–64.

122. Martínez-Lapiscina EH, Clavero P, Toledo E, et al. Virgin olive oil supplementation and long-term cognition: the PREDIMED-NAVARRA randomized, trial. J Nutr Health Aging 2013;17(6):544–52. http://dx.doi.org/10.1007/s12603-013-0027-6.

123. Féart C, Samieri C, Allès B, et al. Potential benefits of adherence to the Mediterranean diet on cognitive health. Proc Nutr Soc 2013;72(1):140–52.

124. Schwingshackl L, Missbach B, König J, et al. Adherence to a Mediterranean diet and risk of diabetes: a systematic review and meta-analysis. Public Health Nutr 2014;1–8 [Epub ahead of print].

125. Cederholm T, Salem N, Palmblad J. Omega-3 fatty acids in the prevention of cognitive decline in humans. Adv Nutr 2013;4:672–6.

126. Samieri C, Sun Q, Townsend MK, et al. The association between dietary patterns at midlife and health in aging: an observational study. Ann Intern Med 2013;159:159130.

127. Samieri C, Grodstein F, Rosner BA, et al. Mediterranean diet and cognitive function in older age. Epidemiology 2013;24(4):490–9.

128. Kesse-Guyot E, Andreeva VA, Lassale C, et al, SU.VI.MAX 2 Research Group. Mediterranean diet and cognitive function: a French study. Am J Clin Nutr 2013;97(2):369–76.

129. Loef M, Walach H. The omega-6/Omega-3 ratio and dementia or cognitive decline. J Nutr Gerontol Geriatr 2013;32:1–25.

130. Granzotto A, Zatta P. Resveratrol and Alzheimer's disease: message in a bottle on red wine and cognition. Front Aging Neurosci 2014;6:95.

131. Suphioglu C, Sadli N, Coonan D, et al. Zinc and DHA have opposing effects on the expression levels of histones H3 and H4 in human neuronal cells. Br J Nutr 2010;103(3):344–51.

132. Solfrizzi V, Panza F, Frisardi V, et al. A diet and Alzheimer's disease: risk factors or prevention: the current evidence. Expert Rev Neurthep 2011;11(5):677–708.

133. Nehlig A. The neuroprotective effects of cocoa flavanol and its influence on cognitive performance. Br J Clin Pharmacol 2013;75(3):716–27.

134. Sokolov AN, Pavlova MA, Klosterhalfen S, et al. Chocolate and the brain: neurobiological impact of cocoa flavanols on cognition and behavior. Neurosci Biobehav Rev 2013;37(10 Pt 2):2445–53.

135. Williams RJ, Spencer JP. Flavonoids, cognition, and dementia: actions, mechanisms, and potential therapeutic utility for Alzheimer disease. Free Radic Biol Med 2012;52(1):35–45.
136. Jayasena T, Poljak A, Smythe G, et al. The role of polyphenols in the modulation of sirtuins and other pathways involved in Alzheimer's disease. Ageing Res Rev 2013;12(4):867–83.
137. Thakur VS, Gupta K, Gupta S. Green tea polyphenols increase p53 transcriptional activity and acetylation by suppressing class I histone deacetylases. Int J Oncol 2012;41(1):353–61.
138. Schmidt A, Hammann F, Wölnerhanssen B, et al. Green tea extract enhances parieto-frontal connectivity during working memory processing. Psychopharmacology (Berl) 2014. [Epub ahead of print].
139. Elmenhorst D, Meyer PT, Matusch A, et al. Caffeine occupancy of human cerebral A1 adenosine receptors: in vivo quantification with ^{18}F-CPFPX and PET. J Nucl Med 2012;53(11):1723–9.
140. Costenla AR, Cunha RA, de Mendonça A. Caffeine, adenosine receptors, and synaptic plasticity. J Alzheimers Dis 2010;20(Suppl 1):S25–34.
141. Cimini A, Gentile R, D'Angelo B, et al. Cocoa powder triggers neuroprotective and preventive effects in a human Alzheimer's disease model by modulating BDNF signaling pathway. J Cell Biochem 2013;114(10):2209–20.
142. Arab L, Khan F, Lam H. Epidemiologic evidence of a relationship between tea, coffee, or caffeine consumption and cognitive decline. Adv Nutr 2013; 4:115–20.
143. Noguchi-Shinohara M, Yuki S, Dohmoto C, et al. Consumption of green tea, but not black tea or coffee, is associated with reduced risk of cognitive decline. PLoS One 2014;9(5):e96013.
144. Arab L, Biggs ML, O'Meara ES, et al. Gender differences in tea, coffee, and cognitive decline in the elderly: the Cardiovascular Health Study. J Alzheimers Dis 2011;27(3):553–66.
145. Vercambre MN, Berr C, Ritchie K, et al. Caffeine and cognitive decline in elderly women at high vascular risk. J Alzheimers Dis 2013;35(2):413–21.
146. Ritchie K, Carrière I, de Mendonca A, et al. The neuroprotective effects of caffeine: a prospective population study (the Three City Study). Neurology 2007;69(6):536–45.
147. Mostofsky E, Rice MS, Levitan EB, et al. Habitual coffee consumption and risk of heart failure: a dose-response meta-analysis. Circ Heart Fail 2012;5(4):401–5.
148. Desideri G, Kwik-Uribe C, Grassi D, et al. Benefits in cognitive function, blood pressure, and insulin resistance through cocoa flavanol consumption in elderly subjects with mild cognitive impairment: the Cocoa, Cognition, and Aging (CoCoA) study. Hypertension 2012;60(3):794–801.
149. Sorond FA, Hurwitz S, Salat DH, et al. Neurovascular coupling, cerebral white matter integrity, and response to cocoa in older people. Neurology 2013; 81(10):904–9.
150. Hooper L, Kay CO, Abdelhamid A, et al. Effects of Chocolate, cocoa and Flavan-3-ols on cardiovascular health: a systematic review and meta-analysis of randomized trials. Am J Clin Nutr 2012;95:740–51.
151. Pasinetti GM. Novel role of red wine-derived polyphenols in the prevention of Alzheimer's disease dementia and brain pathology: experimental approaches and clinical implications. Planta Med 2012;78(15):1614–9.
152. Martin SL, Hardy TM, Tollefsbol TO. Medicinal chemistry of the epigenetic diet and caloric restriction. Curr Med Chem 2013;20(32):4050–9.

153. Nooyens AC, Bueno-deMesquita HB, van Gelder BM, et al. Consumption of alcoholic beverages and cognitive decline at middle age: the Doetinchem Cohort Study. Br J Nutr 2014;111(4):715–23.

154. Krikorian R, Nash TA, Shidler MD, et al. Concord grape juice supplementation improves memory function in older adults with mild cognitive impairment. Br J Nutr 2010;103(5):730–4.

155. Devore EE, Kang JH, Breteler MM, et al. Dietary intakes of berries and flavonoids in relation to cognitive decline. Ann Neurol 2012;72(1):135–43.

156. Cherniack EP. A berry thought-provoking idea: the potential role of plant polyphenols in the treatment of age-related cognitive disorders. Br J Nutr 2012; 108(5):794–800.

157. Bookheimer SY, Renner BA, Ekstrom A, et al. Pomegranate juice augments memory and FMRI activity in middle-aged and older adults with mild memory complaints. Evid Based Complement Alternat Med 2013;946298.

158. Shukitt-Hale B. Blueberries and neuronal aging. Gerontology 2012;58(6): 518–23.

159. Krikorian R, Shidler MD, Nash TA, et al. Blueberry supplementation improves memory in older adults. J Agric Food Chem 2010;58(7):3996–4000.

160. O'Brien J, Okereke O, Devore E, et al. Long-term intake of nuts in relation to cognitive function in older women J Nutr Health Aging 2014;18(5):496–502.

161. Joseph JA, Shukitt-Hale B, Willis LM. Grape juice, berries, and walnuts affect brain aging and behavior. J Nutr 2009;139(9):1813S–7S.

162. Panickar KS. Beneficial effects of herbs, spices and medicinal plants on the metabolic syndrome, brain and cognitive function. Cent Nerv Syst Agents Med Chem 2013;13(1):13–29.

163. Kannappan R, Chandra Gupta S, Kim JH, et al. Neuroprotection by Spice Derived Nutraceuticals: You are what you eat. Mol Neuorol 2011;44(2):142–59.

164. Chin D, Huebbe P, Pallauf K, et al. Neuroprotective properties of curcumin in Alzheimer's disease—merits and limitations [review]. Curr Med Chem 2013; 20(32):3955–85.

165. Brondino N, Re S, Boldrini A, et al. Curcumin as a therapeutic agent in dementia: a mini systematic review of human studies. ScientificWorldJournal 2014;174282. http://dx.doi.org/10.1155/2014/174282.

166. Ringman JM, Frautschy SA, Teng E, et al. Oral curcumin for Alzheimer's disease: tolerability and efficacy in a 24-week randomized, double blind, placebo-controlled study. Alzheimers Res Ther 2012;4(5):43. http://dx.doi.org/10.1186/alzrt146 eCollection 2012.

167. Baum L, Lam CW, Cheung SK, et al. Six-month randomized, placebo-controlled, double-blind, pilot clinical trial of curcumin in patients with Alzheimer disease. J Clin Psychopharmacol 2008;28(1):110–3.

168. Kannappan R, Chandra Gupta S, Kim J, et al. Neuroprotection by spice-derived nutraceuticals: you are what you eat. Mol Neurobiol 2011;44:144–59.

169. Chiu S, Terpstra KJ, Bureau Y, et al. Liposomal-formulated curcumin [Lipocurc™] targeting HDAC (histone deacetylase) prevents apoptosis and improves motor deficits in Park 7 (DJ-1)-knockout rat model of Parkinson's disease: implications for epigenetics-based nanotechnology-driven drug platform. J Complement Integr Med 2013;7:10–6.

170. Jesky R, Hailong C. Are herbal compounds the next frontier for alleviating learning and memory impairments? An integrative look at memory, dementia and the promising therapeutics of traditional Chinese medicines. Phytother Res 2011;25(8):1105–11.

171. Shergis JL, Zhang AL, Zhou W, et al. Panax ginseng in randomised controlled trials: a systematic review. Phytother Res 2013;27(7):949–65.

172. Radad K, Moldzio R, Rausch WD. Ginsenosides and their CNS targets. CNS Neurosci Ther 2011;17(6):761–8.

173. Heo JH, Lee ST, Oh MJ, et al. Improvement of cognitive deficit in Alzheimer's disease patients by long term treatment with Korean red ginseng. J Ginseng Res 2011;35(4):457–61.

174. Lee ST, Chu K, Sim JY, et al. Panax ginseng enhances cognitive performance in Alzheimer disease. Alzheimer Dis Assoc Disord 2008;22(3):222–6.

175. Heo JH, Lee ST, Chu K, et al. An open-label trial of Korean red ginseng as an adjuvant treatment for cognitive impairment in patients with Alzheimer's disease. Eur J Neurol 2008;15(8):865–8.

176. Chiu S, Lalone S, Cernovsky Z, et al. Effects of standardized Panax Ginseng extract : Ginsana-115 on insulin resistance in Clozapine-treated treatment resistant schizophrenia: posthoc analysis of RCT study. American Psychiatric Association annual meeting Poster 2012.

177. Kang KA, Piao MJ, Kim KC, et al. Compound K, a metabolite of ginseng saponin, inhibits colorectal cancer cell growth and induces apoptosis through inhibition of histone deacetylase activity. Int J Oncol 2013;43(6):1907–14.

178. Mucalo I, Rahelić D, Jovanovski E, et al. Effect of American ginseng (Panax quinquefolius L.) on glycemic control in type 2 diabetes. Coll Antropol 2012; 36(4):1435–40.

179. Yuan HD, Kim JT, Kim SH, et al. Ginseng and Diabetes: The Evidences from in vitro, animal and human studies. J Ginseng Res 2012;36(1):27–39.

180. Maruszak A, Pilarski A, Murphy T, et al. Hippocampal neurogenesis in Alzheimer's disease: is there a role for dietary modulation? J Alzheimers Dis 2014;38(1):11–38. http://dx.doi.org/10.3233/JAD-131004.

181. Silva-Vargas V, Crouch EE, Doetsch F. Adult neural stem cells and their niche: a dynamic duo during homeostasis, regeneration, and aging [review]. Curr Opin Neurobiol 2013;23(6):935–42. http://dx.doi.org/10.1016/j.conb.2013.09.004.

182. Devore EE, Kang JH, Breteler MM, et al. Dietary intakes of berries and flavonoids in relation to cognitive decline. Ann Neurol 2012;72(1):135–43.

Dermatological Manifestations of Stress in Normal and Psychiatric Populations

Edgardo Rodriguez-Vallecillo, MD, FAAD[a,b,*],
Michel A. Woodbury-Fariña, MD, DFAPA, FAIS[c]

KEYWORDS

- Psychodermatology • Psychosomatic • Stress • Mind • NICS • Psoriasis • Acne
- Vitiligo

KEY POINTS

- Stress is a key factor that affects all organs including the skin.
- Stress has been associated with premature aging of the skin and neoplasia.
- Psychological stress takes its own toll on the skin, being a known trigger for several dermatological disorders.
- Stress may be the result of how a person deals with dermatological disorders that affect the skin from the cosmetic and functional standpoints.
- Diseases that affect the skin have important effects on the emotional well-being and quality of life of the individual.
- The dermatologist, psychiatrist, psychologist, and family physician need to become familiar with this subject so as to be able to provide a proper bio-psycho-social approach to the patient with a skin disease or the cutaneous manifestations of a psychiatric disorder.

INTRODUCTION

The skin is the largest organ of the body, and one that is constantly challenged by our environment. It is well adapted to serve as the first line of defense against invading microbes and penetration of toxic substances and irritants. It allows us to regulate our body temperature through the microcirculation of the skin and perspiration.

Disclosure Statement: Woodbury-Fariña is Speaker for Pfizer.
[a] Private Practice, 29 Washington Street, Suite 507, San Juan, PR 00907, USA; [b] Dermatology, HIMA San Pablo Hospital, Sta. Cruz Street, Bayamon, PR 00961, USA; [c] Department of Psychiatry, University of Puerto Rico School of Medicine, 307 Calle Eleonor Roosevelt, San Juan, PR 00918-2720, USA
* Private Practice, 29 Washington Street, Suite 507, San Juan, PR 00907.
E-mail address: derm507@gmail.com

Psychiatr Clin N Am 37 (2014) 625–651
http://dx.doi.org/10.1016/j.psc.2014.08.009
0193-953X/14/$ – see front matter © 2014 Elsevier Inc. All rights reserved.

Abbreviations	
ACTH	Adrenocorticotropic hormone (corticotropin)
BDD	Body dysmorphic disorder
CRH	Corticotropin-releasing hormone
CSE	Cigarette smoke extract
DRES	Drug rash with eosinophillia and systemic symptoms
DSM-V	*Diagnostic and Statistical Manual of Mental Disorders*, 5th edition
DSM-IV-TR	*Diagnostic and Statistical Manual of Mental Disorders*, 4th edition text revision
HCP	Health care professional
HPA	Hypothalamic-pituitary axis
HRQoL	Health-related quality of life
HSV	Herpes simplex virus
IL	Interleukin
NE	Neurotic excoriations
NICS	Neuro-immuno-cutaneous system
OCD	Obsessive-compulsive disorder
PSP	Pathological skin picking
QoL	Quality of life
RAAS or RAS	Renin-angiotensin-aldosterone system
ROS	Reactive oxygen species
SAM	Sympathetic-adrenal-medullary system
SJS	Stevens-Johnson syndrome
SPD	Skin-picking disorder
TEN	Toxic Epidermal Necrolysis
Th	T-helper cell
TTM	Trichotillomania
UVR	Ultraviolet radiation

The skin is also a sensory organ that allows us to perceive subtle changes in our environment, both pleasurable and noxious, and to react to them accordingly. It allows us to communicate socially and sexually. It is intricately involved with the immune, endocrine, and neural systems, resulting in the ability to elaborate important hormones, peptides, neuromediators, and other important immunomodulators.

The intact skin is perfectly designed to provide mechanical support for proper function. It is thicker on acral areas and very delicate on the eyelids. It can be moist when and where needed and lubricated where necessary. Its sensory nerves, which vary according to anatomical region, provide us proprioception and protection from noxious stimuli and enjoyment from pleasurable stimuli.

Despite all these blessings in health, from the psychological standpoint the skin may become a curse in disease. Whereas internal organs may malfunction in a way that may not be readily apparent to others, the skin is noticed immediately in the setting of social interactions. When it becomes scarred, scaly, blistered, excoriated, or inflamed, the person may be subjected to stigma and rejection, which can be devastating to the self-esteem of the individual and a great a source of significant distress, resulting in impairments in social, occupational, or other areas of functioning.

As discussed herein, many dermatological diseases can be triggered or exacerbated by emotional stress. In other cases the disease process itself may provoke cutaneous changes that can affect the cosmetic and/or functional level to such an extent that it becomes a source of stress, anxiety, depression, and shame.

The skin is an excellent barometer of these stressors because it is clearly visible to the naked eye for clinical observation. Biopsies may be readily taken for further histopathological, immunological, or biochemical studies. Moreover, it is easily accessible not only in humans but also in experimental animals.

STRESS AND THE SKIN

There exist both intrinsic and extrinsic factors that act as stressors on the integumentary system, the most important ones being ultraviolet radiation (UVR), mechanical and psychological stress, poor eating habits, smoking, alcohol intake, ionizing radiation, sound stress, and environmental pollution.[1] It is estimated that UVR contributes up to 80% of the environmental stress[2] that can translate clinically into premature aging, photoaging, or skin cancer.

UVR damage is produced by the generation of free radicals and reactive oxygen species (ROS).[3] Free radicals are chemical species possessing an unpaired electron, also viewed as a fragment of a molecule,[1,4] and will try to take away electrons from their surroundings, which can include the DNA. The cells of the skin have to provide electrons that will neutralize the free radicals. When the formation of ROS in the skin exceeds the capacity of the target cell to produce the extra electron, oxidative stress develops.[5] Normally much of the damage of ROS is corrected by the various antioxidants (enzymatic and nonenzymatic) and repair mechanisms of the skin cells.[1] However, as we age these endogenous repair mechanisms begin to fail, resulting in oxidative stress overwhelming the cell's repair capacities and leading to oxidative damage that can result in immunotoxicity, premature skin aging, skin cancer, cell damage, and death.[5,6]

The skin is equipped with a network of protective antioxidants; these include enzymatic antioxidants such as glutathione peroxidase, superoxide dismutase and catalase, and nonenzymatic low molecular weight antioxidants such as vitamin E isoforms, vitamin C, glutathione, uric acid, and ubiquinol.[4] The 2 main categories of antioxidant defenses are those whose role is to prevent the generation of ROS and those that intercept any free radicals generated.[7] The epidermis contains a higher concentration of antioxidants than the dermis.[8]

It is estimated that a human cell sustains an average of 10,000 oxidative hits per day as a result of cellular oxidative metabolism.[1,9,10] Taking into account the large amount of damage the skin receives each day, especially via UVR, it is surprising that the incidence of skin cancer is not higher.[5] This evidence favors the idea that DNA is functionally stable because of the efficient and redundant repair mechanisms.[5] Moreover it is thought that, because the epidermis is a fairly rapid-turnover epithelium, cells with damage to the DNA may be shed more rapidly in comparison with the status of mutations on other organs such as the liver, which has a slower turnover of cells.[5,11]

Cigarette smoking is an independent risk factor for premature facial wrinkling and skin aging in general.[12] It produces vasoconstriction and delayed wound healing, among other deleterious effects.[13] It may also be indirectly linked to psychological stress, as smokers habitually increase their consumption when stressed, creating further oxidative stress on the skin. The classical facial features of smokers have been described since 1985 as "smoker's face" and include wrinkling (especially perioral wrinkles) and sallow facial coloration.[13]

In a recent in vitro study using human fibroblasts from preputial skin, a cigarette smoke extract (CSE) induced morphological and ultrastructural changes of senescence in the fibroblasts, key cells in skin integrity and collagen production, by augmenting ROS levels of superoxide, hydrogen peroxide, and hydroxyl radicals.[14] Whether similar changes occur in vivo or whether CSE affects all cell types to the same degree will need to be further studied.[14]

PSYCHOLOGICAL STRESS

There is still no definitive evidence directly linking psychological stress to skin aging.[6] However, psychological stress produces a wide spectrum of physiological responses that can be harmful at times to the skin. These changes contribute to inflammation, oxidative stress, and DNA damage, all of which are associated with aging.[6]

Psychological stress is ubiquitous and is usually triggered by a noxious stimulus or a stressor. When submitted to stressors, the skin reacts by activating multiple pathways, which create diverse peptides at the local level that attenuate or mediate the cutaneous immunologic response. This process allows for responses not only at the central level but also at a peripheral level, which permit a more precise multidirectional response from this local neuroendocrine system.[15] Through its effectors, this peripheral control axis is capable of regulating skin pigmentary, immune, epidermal, dermal, and adnexal systems.[15]

Psychological stress activates the sympathetic-adrenal-medullary (SAM) system, renin-angiotensin-aldosterone system (RAAS or RAS), hypothalamic-pituitary-adrenal (HPA) axis, and cholinergic system, all of which can not only contribute to immune dysfunction, and possible disease states,[16] but also ROS formation and DNA damage. Thus, psychological stress may trigger or exacerbate immune-mediated dermatological disorders.

Psychological stress activates the autonomic nervous system, which involves triggering the release of catecholamines (epinephrine and norepinephrine) from the adrenal glands.[17] Initially epinephrine and norepinephrine increase the pulse, respiratory rate, and blood pressure, which is appropriate and beneficial in the short term. Over the long term, however, catecholamines can have many deleterious effects on the body.[6,18] Among other adverse effects, long-term increases in catecholamines can cause DNA damage, immunosuppression, tumor growth, dementia, and cardiovascular disorders.[6,19–23]

The RAS is one of the most important hormonal systems in the body. It oversees the functions of the cardiovascular, renal, and adrenal glands by regulating blood pressure, fluid volume, and sodium and potassium balance.[24] While RAS is activated primarily in response to decreased renal blood flow, it is also stimulated by upright posture, sodium depletion, or potassium infusion. It is also activated by signals generated from the sympathetic and HPA systems in response to physical or psychosocial stressors.[25,26] Prolonged or repetitive stress-induced activation of RAS, through its physiological effects, may lead to vascular inflammation and atherosclerosis.[25] RAS has been demonstrated to have proinflammatory and profibrotic effects at the cellular and molecular levels.[27] Prolonged activation of the RAS may also lead to oncogenesis.[28]

The HPA axis responds to stress, be it physiological or psychological, by secreting corticotropin-releasing hormone (CRH) and adrenocorticotropic hormone (ACTH). In turn this stimulates the release of glucocorticoids from the adrenal cortex.[6] As is well known, excess glucocorticoids have many adverse effects on all tissues, including the skin. The more prominent effects are tissue atrophy, impaired wound healing, and acceleration of the aging process.[29,30]

The brain and the skin have the same ectodermal origin, and are affected by similar hormones and neurotransmitters.[31] To help maintain global homeostasis the skin has a parallel, complex network of communication between it and the neuroendocrine and immune system, which has been described as the neuro-immuno-cutaneous system (NICS).[32]

NICS uses mediators similar to those involved in the classical HPA axis. This cutaneous NICS is also regulated via feedback inhibition.[15] Thus, the skin and its adnexa, that is, the hair follicles and the sebaceous and sudoriparous glands, are not only prominent targets of key stress mediators (such as CRH, ACTH, cortisol, prolactin, epinephrine, norepinephrine, substance P, and nerve growth factor) but also are a potent source of prototypic, immunomodulatory mediators of the stress response.[33,34]

There is evidence that the skin also produces other neuroendocrine signals such as CRH as well as precursor proteins/peptides used to make ACTH. Thus the skin has its own HPA axis that can coordinate with the central HPA axis. The skin also produces prolactin, melatonin, and catecholamines, in addition to neurotrophins and neuropeptides from its sensory nerves.[16] It also synthesizes or metabolizes androgens or estrogens in addition to being a target for these hormones.[15]

ACUTE VERSUS CHRONIC STRESS

Stress can either increase or decrease the body's defenses, depending on various factors such as the duration of the stressful condition.[35] Acute and chronic stress are distinguished in terms of how it affects homeostasis; acute stress may be considered beneficial, whereas chronic stress is thought to be noxious to the body's ability to maintain homeostasis, fight infections, and decrease aging.[6,34–39]

Acute stress mobilizes both cellular and humoral adaptive immunity responses that increase the migration of effector cells to damaged tissues to fight infection or respond to trauma.[6,34–36,38–40] Epinephrine, released as a response to acute stress, has a stimulatory effect on chemotaxis,[40] allowing the immune system to respond to infections appropriately and in a timely fashion.[34]

Chronic stress, however, has the opposite effect, namely, immunosuppression, which may lead to increased risk of infections or diseases.[2,34,35,41–43] In this environment of prolonged stress, persistent adrenergic stimulation is continuously mobilizing immune cells. When there is an added acute stress event, no reserves are available that could further boost chemotaxis, leading to a faulty immune response.[25,35,44]

There is also evidence that prolonged stress may lead to DNA damage[21] which, in turn, may promote aging,[17,19] oncogenesis,[17,22] neuropsychiatric conditions,[17,23,45] and spontaneous abortions.[17,46] Cumulative damage to DNA and its repair system plays a role in the ability of the body to repair itself, maintain homeostasis, and decrease the rate of aging.[6] The end result of the persistent activation of these pathways is an imbalance of oxidative free radicals with resultant DNA damage and an increase of inflammatory cytokines, which contribute to atherosclerosis, aging, and oncogenesis.[6]

Thus far this brief review has covered the main effects of stress in terms of its basic physiology and how it relates to immunity. How stress manifests clinically, in relation to dermatological diseases and cutaneous disorders in psychiatric patients, is now discussed.

PSYCHODERMATOLOGY

Psychological stress may be sustained or composed of many overlapping stressful events that may trigger persistent secretions of stress hormones.[17] Over time, the physiological response to these stressors may have serious adverse effects for the individual.

Today's stressors, such as divorce, death of loved ones, examinations, unemployment, or relocation, to name a few, are far different from those of our ancestors. The classical fight-or-flight response, with its well-known sympathetic effects (increased circulation to the heart, lungs, and striated muscle of the extremities, increased cardiac strength, perspiration, increased glycemia, and reduced activity of the gastrointestinal tract),[16,47] evolutionarily convenient for the individual to survive predators, is perhaps no longer needed in the same way if one lives in a safe environment. It may at times be overused resulting in malfunction, serving as a trigger for many immune, inflammatory, neuropsychiatric, or allergic diseases, many of which involve the skin.

The concept of psychodermatology describes the interaction between the mind and the skin,[48] and relates to the interaction between dermatology and psychiatry/psychology. Because any physiological, pathological, or self-induced change of the skin is frequently visible to others, the sufferer will be subjected to being judged, increasing the possibility of being stigmatized in addition to having a personal reaction to such change.

The incidence of psychiatric disorders in patients with skin disease is estimated to be between 30% and 60%.[49,50] Nonetheless, most dermatologic patients, probably because of the social stigma of being mentally ill or "crazy," resist being referred to a mental care professional, even in cases where dermatological treatment alone has proved to be ineffective or suboptimal.

CLASSIFICATION

While there is no perfect classification for these dermatological diseases or conditions because of some apparent overlap, the most uniformly accepted classification is that by Koo and Lee (**Box 1**).[50]

To keep within the scope of this article there follows a discussion of those conditions in which stress plays a major role in triggering or perpetuating the dermatological condition, and those in which the psychiatric condition drives patients to damage their skin, creating stress from the cosmetic standpoint. Other studies address a wider view of these disorders based on the same classification.[24,50,51]

PSYCHOPHYSIOLOGICAL DISORDERS

These groups of diseases are not caused by stress but are generally worsened or triggered by it. The influence of stress on each disease may vary significantly, and has been reported from 50% for acne to greater than 90% for rosacea, alopecia areata, neurotic excoriations, lichen simplex chronicus, and hyperhidrosis.[52]

Acne Vulgaris

The spectrum of acne vulgaris (hereafter referred to as acne) varies widely, from mild cases consisting mostly of open or closed comedones to very severe cystic acne, which may affect not only the face but also the trunk and buttocks. For many patients, acne resolves gradually in their early twenties but for many individuals, it may extend well into their adult lives.

Box 1
Classification of psychocutaneous disorders

1. Dermatoses of primary psychological/psychiatric genesis, responsible for self-induced dermatological disorders (dermatitis artefacta, trichotillomania, delusional parasitosis, body dysmorphic disorders)

2. Dermatoses with a multifactorial basis whose course is subjected to emotional influences-psychosomatic diseases (psoriasis, atopic dermatitis, acne, chronic forms of urticaria, lichen simplex chronicus, hyperhidrosis)

3. Psychiatric disorders secondary to serious or disfiguring dermatoses/somatopsychic illnesses (adjustment disorders with depression or anxiety seen in conditions like alopecia areata or vitiligo)

From Koo JY, Lee CS. General approach to evaluating psycho-dermatologic disorders. In: Koo JY, Lee CS, editors. Psychocutaneous medicine. New York: Marcel Dekker Inc; 2003. p. 1–29

Acne has been associated with impaired health-related quality of life (HRQoL), at times with negative impacts as great as that of severe and even life-threatening diseases.[53] Facial acne, being an external, clearly visible ailment, impairs self-image, affects psychological well-being, and may interfere with the ability to develop social relationships.[54] Acne is flared by emotional stress, depression, and hormonal changes, as seen by the premenstrual cluster of emotional and physiological symptoms.[55]

Nodulocystic acne (acne grade IV or acne conglobata) can have devastating psychological effects because permanent scarring is generally present. Young men with such severe acne scarring are at particular risk of depression and even suicide.[56–58]

Adult acne is a more prevalent condition than previously thought,[59] and is one of the most visible skin problems in adults in the United States. Women have a higher incidence than men. Goulden and colleagues[60] report that approximately 12% to 22% of women in the United States suffer from adult acne, compared with 3% of men. Adult female acne, according to an Acne-specific Quality of Life questionnaire, made women feel less confident, more self-conscious around other people, frustrated, and embarrassed.[61]

Many acne patients and even normal individuals will occasionally pick at their skin, but most do so to deal with clearly visible lesions and, after it resolves when better, the picking stops. Only a small fraction of patients, independent of acne severity, will pick persistently to the point of erosions and crusting, which is then termed acne excoriée.[51,62] Because this can leave significant dyspigmentation and scarring, more embarrassment and anxiety is created. As the acne and general appearance worsen, the individual becomes more stressed, creating a vicious cycle.[63]

Acne excoriée is more prevalent in women with late-onset acne.[63] Patients with acne excoriée may present other psychiatric comorbidities such as depression, anxiety, obsessive-compulsive disorder (OCD), trichotillomania (TTM), body dysmorphic disorder (BDD), delusional disorders, personality disorders, and social phobias.[52,64–66]

It has more recently been recognized that patients with acne excoriée fall within the spectrum of BDD rather than OCD, the confusion arising because there are many clinical similarities.[67–71] Acne patients, in general, may exhibit aspects of BDD in 14% to 21%[72] of cases. BDD patients are more commonly females and may have other grooming disorders such as TTM and oncyhophagia.[73]

Psoriasis

Psoriasis is a common, chronic, genetically determined inflammatory skin disease that affects 2% of the United States population,[74] usually starting before the age of 30 years.[75] Psoriasis is a multifactorial disease with both genetic and environmental factors[75] and a strong T-cell component.[16] T cells play a significant role in disease pathogenesis, particularly T cells expressing IL-17.[16]

In recent years it has been shown that psoriasis has been associated with many comorbidities including depression, anxiety, cardiovascular disease, obesity, diabetes, hypertension, dyslipidemia, metabolic syndrome, nonalcoholic fatty liver disease, cancer, and inflammatory bowel disease.[75]

There is a large body of medical literature on the psychological aspects of psoriasis.[76–80] Stress has been reported to precede the onset of psoriasis in 44% of patients and to initiate recurrent skin flares in 88% of psoriatics.[75–77,81] Psoriasis is associated with substantial impairment of HRQoL, negatively affecting psychological, vocational, social, and physical functioning.[57,82]

Psoriasis patients suffer from poor self-esteem, sexual dysfunction, anxiety, and depression, and may have suicidal ideation.[83–86] Suicidal ideation rates tend to correlate with a higher self-rating of disease severity.[83,87] Regarding sexual dysfunction,

30% to 70% of patients report a decline in sexual activity, particularly when there is scaling affecting the groin.[86,88]

Some studies have shown that the emotional effects and functional impact of the disease are not necessarily proportionate to the clinical severity of psoriasis.[89] However, other studies have found higher levels of depression in patients with a greater percentage of their skin affected by psoriasis.[90] Pruritus in psoriasis may vary among patients and is often not proportional to the disease severity. In a study by Remröd and colleagues of 101 patients with plaque psoriasis,[91] those with severe pruritus were associated with higher scores for depression and anxiety. Pruritus severity in psoriasis and perhaps in other dermatological disorders is a factor that can help select subsets of patients that may benefit from supplemental psychological interventions. In a study by Sampogna and colleagues,[86] the frequency of psychiatric disturbances decreased with improvements in the clinical severity and symptoms of psoriasis. Psoriatic women have been reported to have higher degrees of depression than psoriatic men.[86,92]

Quality of life (QoL) is mostly affected by the visibility of the disease, its chronicity, and the need for lifelong adherence to treatment regimens.[93] It is frequently a vicious cycle for the patient, as psoriasis causes stress and stress exacerbates psoriasis[75] to the point that psoriasis may exacerbate depression, which in turn may increase the perception of pruritus. Severe scratching may induce skin trauma which, in turn, may exacerbate psoriasis. When psoriasis appears exactly where the patient has been scratching or where the skin has been traumatized in any form, including surgically, it is called an isomorphic response or Koebner phenomenon, which is any skin phenomenon that only appears secondary to scratching or trauma and is not attributable to an infective or chemical cause.[94]

Psoriasis patients often report having high levels of stress, social stigmatization, and physical limitations from their disease.[57] In one study, more than half of the patients with psoriasis reported being self-conscious around strangers.[95] Weiss and colleagues[57] reported that more than three-fourths of those surveyed would often avoid activities like swimming and sports because of their psoriasis and one-third of patients were often inhibited in their sexual relationships because of their psoriasis.[96]

It is therefore important to recognize that the cosmetic disfigurement that psoriasis produces has a profound effect in the overall perception of QoL as measured by the current scales of well-being. The treatment approach to the psoriatic patient with so many comorbidities, including the psychological ones, must therefore be multidisciplinary.

Atopic Dermatitis

Atopic dermatitis, one of the main causes of eczema, is a common inflammatory disease that affects 6% of the United States population.[16,97]

Atopic dermatitis is characterized by intensely pruritic eczematous patches and frequent lichenification of the skin. Genetic, environmental, psychological and pharmacological factors may play a role in its pathogenesis.[98]

Stress plays a significant role in exacerbating and perpetuating the itch-scratch cycle in atopic dermatitis. Psychological stress triggers the HPA axis and the SAM system, which in turn produces inflammatory mediators that play a role in affecting the skin barrier.[16,99] Among other effects, it creates increased transepidermal water loss and increased susceptibility to exogenous irritants such as detergents, contaminants, occupational chemicals, or other irritants. Atopics have a blunted HPA response and an overactive SAM system that may exacerbate the disease.[16]

Studies in stress-aggravated mice have demonstrated the role of mast cell degranulation in inflammatory skin diseases.[100–102] These results suggest a role for neurogenic inflammation in psychological stress that is independent of the HPA axis.[99]

Using mice stressed by electric foot shock, Shimoda et al[102] showed an inhibition of the dermal mast cell response due to a reduced degranulation of dermal mast cells seen when pre-treated with chlorpromazine, an antipsychotic drug, and anxiolytic agents (tandospirone and CRA1000), suggesting that in those skin conditions that are associated with inflammation, these kinds of medications might be an appropriate approach via this inhibition of mast cell degranulation.[102]

The impact of psychological stress on barrier recovery has been studied in humans.[103] Individuals with high levels of perceived psychological stress had significantly delayed barrier recovery rates in comparison with those reporting low perceived stress levels. These investigators concluded that stress-induced changes in epidermal function may serve as precipitators of inflammatory dermatoses.[6,93,99] These results strengthen the concept that release of glucocorticoids during psychological stress affects homeostasis in the stratum corneum, which may worsen atopic dermatitis. Glucocorticoids can cause atrophy and impaired wound healing (after scratching) by interfering with keratinocyte and fibroblast function.[6,104]

Stratum corneum barrier recovery, after its removal by tape stripping, has also been studied in rats submitted to immobilization and crowding stress. In this study by Denda et al., the use of the tranquillizers diazepam and chlorpromazine hastened the rate of barrier recovery, which suggests that pharmacologic reduction of emotional stress may play a role in promoting a faster healing of the normal stratum corneum barrier.[16,105] Owing to factors such as skin barrier malfunction and transepidermal water loss, atopic skin becomes so dry that it can be a trigger for inducing pruritus, which can start a repetitive cycle of scratching inducing further irritation, more pruritus, and more scratching. The inflamed and excoriated appearance of their skin may provoke social phobia, depression, and anxiety, leading to further scratching, perpetuating the cycle even more.

Although the disease tends to improve over time, with the disease becoming inactive in many adults, some do persist having repeated exacerbations that interfere with their QoL. Children with severe atopic dermatitis have been reported to have a QoL impairment equal or greater to that of bronchial asthma or diabetes mellitus.[100]

Adults who have suffered atopic dermatitis during childhood may see their condition persist into adulthood, with more localized disease resulting in areas of lichenification of the skin that patients cannot resist scratching or picking at. In less severe forms this is called lichen simplex or lichen simplex chronicus. However, this falls under the larger scope of what has been termed neurodermatitis, a "wastebasket" term encompassing an overlap of several skin disorders that may seem confusing, especially for nondermatologists.

Neurodermatitis

To begin with, the term neurodermatitis stigmatizes the patients themselves, as does other terms such as neurotic excoriations (NE), which many abbreviate as N-excoriations, a euphemism that creates a more palatable term for the patient. The term psychogenic pruritus has been suggested as a replacement, particularly since in the *Diagnostic and Statistical Manual of Mental Disorders*, 5th edition (DSM-V)[65] the term neurosis has been discontinued. Some have argued that the word "psychogenic" may be misinterpreted by the patient as "psychotic."[101] Psychogenic pruritus may occur in patients with depression, anxiety, aggression, obsessional behavior, and alcoholism.[51,102]

When the areas of lichenification and excoriation are widely distributed but exist as localized nodules, usually within the patient's reach, the term prurigo nodularis is used. The extensor surfaces of the arms and the anterior aspects of the thighs are usually affected. Women are more commonly affected than men.[106]

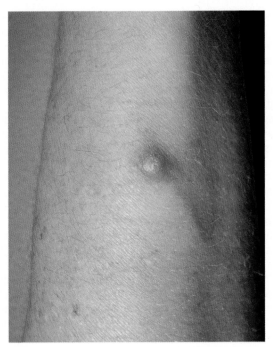

Fig. 1. Prurigo nodularis in a patient with atopic dermatitis.

Prurigo nodularis may develop in atopics (**Fig. 1**) but has also been described in other pruritic dermatoses such as scabies, xerosis cutis, and bullous pemphigoid.[107] In these cases, the prurigo nodularis occurs as a result of a primary dermatological disease. This condition should be differentiated from the usually more severe, primary type of prurigo nodularis, which is actually a primary psychiatric condition that may also include dermatitis artefacta, TTM, and NE.[105]

Prurigo nodularis may be grouped within the spectrum of skin-picking disorders (SPD), also termed pathological skin picking. This body-focused, repetitive, and compulsive picking of the skin leads to excoriation, oozing, crusting, lichenification, dyspigmentation, and scarring. These patients have little or no insight into the psychological basis of their cutaneous problem.[105]

SPD was not explicitly listed in the *Diagnostic and Statistical Manual of Mental Disorders*, 4th edition text revision (DSM-IV-TR),[108,109] but has been added to DSM-V. NE, in general, have also been associated with depression, bipolar disorder, anxiety, OCD, BDD, borderline personality disorder, delusions of parasitosis, and dermatitis artefacta.[93,105,107] Their prevalence in a dermatologic clinic has been estimated at 2%.[110,111] There are no studies of its prevalence in the general population, but in a study of a group of college students the prevalence was even higher, at 3.8%.[112,113]

Grant and colleagues[73] have proposed the following criteria to help differentiate other causes of persistent scratching and trauma:

1. Recurrent skin picking resulting in skin lesions
2. Repeated attempts to decrease or stop skin picking
3. The skin picking causes clinically significant distress or impairment in social, occupational, or other important areas of functioning

4. The skin picking is not attributable to the direct physiological effects of a substance (eg, cocaine) or another medical condition (eg, scabies)
5. The skin picking is not better accounted for by symptoms of another DSM-V disorder

SPD is often misdiagnosed as either OCD or BDD.[113] The patient with prurigo nodularis does not seem to fall into the category of SPD associated with BDD because they do not seem to be trying to improve or correct any perceived imperfection. As compared with atopic dermatitis patients with lichen simplex, these patients are very difficult to improve with topical corticosteroids, emollients, or antihistamines. This evidence strengthens the concept that these patients have a primary psychiatric disorder.

The triggers to pick can vary greatly and may be multiple. Stress, anxiety, boredom, anger, and not being engaged in any activity are all well-known triggers.[73] SPD patients usually pick at areas they can reach with their hands or nails, usually sparing the middle back. Many report using common household objects such as tweezers, scissors, and knives.[114] Although scarring and dyspigmentation are most commonly seen, infections are encountered at times, and serious bleeding has also been reported.[115,116]

SPD tends to run a protracted course and, if untreated, may lead to psychosocial dysfunction and serious medical and cosmetic complications.[69,73] A close collaboration is required between the fields of psychiatry, dermatology, and general medicine to deal with the various aspects of the disease spectrum and its potential complications.

Psychogenic Pruritus

There are also cases described as psychogenic pruritus whereby the patient scratches, especially when under stress, but does not develop tissue damage, at least not to a degree that would cause depression or social phobia because of the appearance. This diagnosis must always be one of exclusion because there may be other causes of pruritus that may not provoke primary lesions, ranging from adverse effects of drugs or drug interactions, mild contact allergy or irritation, scabies, metabolic disorders, and even internal malignancies.

The French psychodermatology group, using the term "functional itch disorder," has published specific criteria to support this diagnosis.[117] It consists of 3 compulsory criteria, namely:

1. Local or generalized pruritus without primary skin lesions
2. Chronicity lasting longer than 6 weeks
3. No somatic cause

The diagnosis must also meet 3 of the following 7 optional criteria:

1. Chronological relationship of the pruritus with 1 or several life events that could have psychological repercussions
2. Intensity variations in association with stress
3. Nocturnal variations
4. Predominance during rest or inaction
5. Associated psychological disorder
6. Pruritus that may be improved by psychotropic drugs
7. Pruritus that could be improved by psychotherapies

Some researchers use a wider definition of psychogenic pruritus that includes lichen simplex chronicus, neurotic excoriation, prurigo nodularis, and pruritus that is intermittent, short-term, severe, and without tissue damage such as excoriations or abrasions. In a study on patients with this wider definition of psychogenic pruritus, Radmanesh and Shafiei[118] found that all patients had affective disorders (depressions, anxieties, and mixed anxiety and depressive disorders) and 18% (12 of 65) also had associated personality disorders.

Body Dysmorphic Disorder

BDD, or dysmorphophobia, is a frequent but commonly overlooked gamut of diverse clinical presentations whereby the patients are stressed and inappropriately concerned about 1 or more of their body parts having an abnormality or are dissatisfied with it/them, for which there appears to be minimal, if any, objective findings. Patients may describe this body area or defect as being deformed, ugly, or disfigured.[67,69] Most individuals with this disorder have poor or absent insight regarding the true nature of their problem.[68,119]

Depending on the gender of the individual, they may complain of problems on their faces or hair, minuscule imperfections that they visualize as a major defect. Some present to the dermatologist or a plastic surgeon as their last resort for help. It is estimated that 7% to 15% of patients seeking cosmetic surgery and 12% of patients seeking dermatological treatment may have some form of BDD.[120–122]

BDD usually starts in adolescence and affects both men and women, being slightly more common in the latter.[65] Women may complain of the size or shape of their hips or breasts, facial marks, or scars. Male patients may be dissatisfied with facial features such as the size or shape of their nose or their genitals, thinning hair, acne scars, or overall body build. Patients may spend many hours a day thinking about their perceived flaw or looking in the mirror often, in addition to camouflaging their problem with makeup or clothing.[67,71]

There may be other comorbidities in BDD that include depression, OCD, skin picking, TTM, social phobias, marital difficulties, and substance abuse.[51,71] Anxiety is very common in these patients. In one study, 60% of BDD patients were reported to have a lifetime history of an anxiety disorder.[123] Suicidal tendencies have also been reported, especially in cases related to facial complaints.[124] Overall, BDD causes significant distress and impairment in functioning, and is associated with an unusually poor QoL.[67,125]

Alopecia Areata

Although the exact mechanism by which stress induces the hair loss in alopecia areata has still not been clearly elucidated, acute emotional stress has long been a well-recognized trigger in its development. Stress can initiate or worsen alopecia areata.[63,126] Depending on the size and location of the alopecic patches and the capacity to be camouflaged or covered, the disease creates anxiety and feelings of social rejection, which may worsen the underlying condition. Depression has also been reported to worsen alopecia areata.[124]

Other comorbidities reported in these patients are major depression, generalized anxiety disorder, phobic states, and paranoid disorder.[127,128] Higher rates of anxiety disorder (58%), affective disorder (35%), and substance abuse (35%) have been reported in first-degree relatives of patients with alopecia areata.[51,129]

In diseases characterized by disfigurement leading to stigmatization, such as severe atopic dermatitis, psoriasis, acne vulgaris, and alopecia areata, psychiatric manifestations such as depression and social phobia likely occur as sequelae of the dermatological illnesses rather than preceding them.[48]

Trichotillomania

TTM is a condition in which individuals pull their own hair, creating irregular bald patches. It is more common in females and tends to start before puberty.[65] Hair may be pulled from the scalp, especially parietal and vertex areas, but areas such as eyebrows and eyelashes and the pubic area are commonly affected.[65] Pediatric patients mostly pull from their scalp.[108] Patients may refer to the act as gratifying because it reduces tension, anger, depression, and anxiety.[108]

The most common psychopathology associated with TTM is obsessive-compulsive behavior.[130] TTM has also been associated with other psychiatric conditions such as anxiety, depression, dementia, mental retardation, mood disorders, substance abuse, and eating disorders.[131–133]

In TTM, hairs may be of varying lengths representing broken hairs. There may be small black dots at the surface, and the patches are more irregular in shape in comparison with the more circular type in alopecia areata. A pull test is negative; that is, hair does not come out easily on traction.[108] Although there is no inflammation on the scalp, the scalp may feel rough especially when compared with the very smooth alopecic patches of alopecia areata. Patients may attempt to conceal or camouflage hair loss by using caps, hats, wigs, and so forth.[65]

TTM may be associated with distress in addition to social and occupational impairment. Most individuals admit the picking yet claim that they cannot stop the urge to pick. The DSM-IV-TR diagnosis of TTM or hair-pulling disorder has been moved from a DSM-IV classification of impulse-control disorders, not elsewhere classified, to obsessive-compulsive and related disorders in DSM-V.

Among the diagnostic criteria for TTM, the DSM-V states that this condition cannot be better explained as being a part of another psychiatric disorder, such as BDD.

As may be ascertained from the foregoing discussion, there may be some overlap in these conditions, and when the conduct, be it hair pulling or skin picking, is directed toward the goal of improving or correcting a perceived flaw, both diagnoses should be classified as BDD.[65]

Rosacea

In rosacea, facial flushing and papular inflammation both tend to flare with stress.[134] In a survey of the National Rosacea Society of 1066 rosacea patients, 79% reported stress as a factor that triggers their disease.[135] However, in a study by Cotterill,[52] more than 90% of the patients reported emotional triggers.

The role of microorganisms has been studied in many diseases including rosacea. How the microbiome affects or modulates inflammatory diseases is an area of active research and one that still raises more questions than answers. The results of different studies that have evaluated the role of both *Demodex folliculorum*, a human commensal mite that lives in hair follicles, and *Helicobacter pylori* in possible associations with rosacea suggest that these microorganisms do not play a central role in the pathogenesis of rosacea, but may act as trigger factors or potentiators of inflammation in an undefined subset of predisposed patients.[136]

Vitiligo

Vitiligo is a depigmentary disorder of the skin of probable autoimmune origin.[137] Psychological stress has been associated with its onset. Vitiligo can also initiate or exacerbate depression, especially in darker-skinned individuals in whom the disease is most noticeable.[138] Approximately one-third of patients may have psychiatric comorbidity. The prevalence of depression in vitiligo patients was 39% in a QoL study.[63,86]

Vitiligo may also affect sexual relationships, especially in single patients and men, mostly because of embarrassment.[139] In a study by Porter and colleagues,[139] the patients felt more general embarrassment in nonsexual interpersonal encounters than in more intimate sexual/social relationships.

In another study of vitiligo patients, 57% said people stared at them, 20% had been the victims of rude remarks, and 8% encountered job discrimination as a result of their disease.[140] In fact, vitiligo is associated with more psychosocial embarrassment than is any other skin condition.[51]

Herpes Simplex

Herpes simplex, both orofacial and genital, is well known to be triggered by anxiety, sun exposure (**Fig. 2**), and repeated trauma during intercourse, all sharing in common a stress factor on the skin. Experimentally induced emotional stress has been reported to lead to herpes simplex virus (HSV) reactivation.[51,141] It has also been suggested that stress-induced release of immunomodulating signal molecules (eg, catecholamines, cytokines, and glucocorticoids) compromises the host's cellular immune response, leading to reactivation of HSV.[51,142]

Other Dermatological Conditions Triggered by Stress

Several other dermatological diseases have been reported to be frequently triggered by stress, including seborrheic dermatitis, dyshidrosis, telogen effluvium, urticaria, recurrent aphthous stomatitis, hyperhidrosis, perioral dermatitis, and lichen planus (**Box 2**).[51,63,143] Pruritus as a symptom is also worsened by stress.[51]

CAN MEDICATIONS GIVEN TO DECREASE STRESS CAUSE SKIN RASHES?

Any medication or combinations of medications used in psychiatry have the potential to cause allergic or adverse drug events, frequently so benign that treatment may be antihistamines or simple discontinuation of the offending agent(s). Rarely, a life-threatening reaction called Toxic Epidermal Necrolysis (TEN) can occur, which is a medical emergency that needs to be treated in a hospital setting. At present, the general consensus is that TEN is the most severe presentation of the spectrum of Stevens-Johnson Syndrome (SJS) - Toxic Epidermal Necrolysis (TEN)[144]

There is also another severe drug reaction called drug rash with eosinophilia and systemic symptoms (DRESS) syndrome which would appear to be a form of SJS, also triggered by drugs such as carbamazepine and phenytoin, among others. These

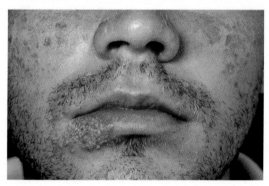

Fig. 2. Recurrent herpes simplex virus type 1 after severe sunburn.

Box 2
Common psychodermatological diseases
Psoriasis
Acne vulgaris
Vitiligo
Hyperhidrosis
Seborrheic dermatitis
Atopic dermatitis
Rosacea
Alopecia areata
Herpes simplex
Urticaria

cases also present with fever, eosinophilia, leukocytosis, lymphadenopathy and hepatic manifestations in conjunction with a generalized exfoliative dermatitis.[145]

SJS-TEN is frequently associated with anticonvulsants, especially the combination of lamotrigine and divalproex sodium.[155] The likelihood of any benign rash occurring with lamotrigine is around 10%[147] and increases when the dose of lamotrigine is increased too quickly, especially if combined with divalproex sodium. Divalproex sodium increases plasma levels of lamotrigine when the two are given concomitantly,[148] due to divalproex sodium inhibiting the metabolic pathway of lamotrigine,[149] which is glucuronidation. This increased level of lamotrigine will slightly increase the likelihood of a drug reaction with this combination due to lamotrigine being associated with rash. The slower the dose increase of the lamotrigine, with or without divalproex sodium, the less likely any rash will occur.[150]

SJS/TEN is rare, being seen in one of 300 adults and one of 100 children in patients starting antiepileptic medications, especially if increased too rapidly.[147] With lamotrigine, following the new dosing strategies, the rate of serious rash was 0.08% in adults in monotherapy and 0.13% when used as adjunctive therapy.[151] In the case that it does occur, Mockenhaupt et al. reported that more than 90% of SJS/TEN cases occurred during the first 63 days of therapy.[152] Because of these concerns lamotrigine has a black box warning concerning this reaction.

The spectrum of SJS-TEN is an allergic idiosyncratic reaction that is unpredictable.[153] It is more frequent in patients with HIV, in those younger than 13,[147] in the elderly or in patients with renal or hepatic insufficiency. In these patients, there is a build-up of chemically reactive metabolites which may trigger the reaction.[154]

Genetic factors are also related to these severe hypersensitivity reactions. Inquiry into the family history is useful in assessing potential risk. If a first-degree relative has had a serious drug reaction to a particular medication, especially another antiepileptic medication,[155] the patient will be at a higher risk.[154] Hung et al[156] reported that carbamazepine-induced SJS/TEN is strongly associated with the HLAB*1502 gene in the Han Chinese. In milder morbilliform or hypersensitivity reactions the association was not observed.[157]

The second author uses lamotrigine extensively with a pediatric population who are even more susceptible to developing a rash because of their age.[147,155] In this population, he is very conservative with the lamotrigine dose increase, adhering to the dosing guidelines in monotherapy of giving 0.2 mg/kg a day for the first two weeks, followed by 0.5 mg/kg a day for the next 2 weeks, and increasing thereafter by 0.5-1 mg/kg every other week to a maximum of 200 mg/day.[147] However, when the goal of 50mg/day is reached, as there is evidence that this dose can be effective,[157] the patient stays at that dose for two weeks to evaluate response. If there are no signs of an adequate response, the titration is continued. (For more complete dosing guidelines, including the recommendations in combination therapy with divalproex sodium, please refer to the package insert on Lamictal® by GlaxoSmithKline, Research Triangle Park, NC 27709.)

Since steroids have been found to be effective in treating allergic rashes, he always gives the parents/guardian a prescription for dexamethasone 4mg for the parents/guardians to fill in case of an eruption and the instructions to call him immediately when there is the suspicion of a rash to assess its severity. He has had success treating mild to moderate rashes with dexamethasone 4mg/day until the rash subsides and then 2mg/d for the same number of days that it took to eliminate the rash.

Early discontinuation of the offending drug is a priority in any case of rash especially if one wants to try to avoid the development of blistering drug reactions because the earlier the discontinuation, the more likely one will decrease morbidity/mortality.[158] The most severe allergic reaction seen in his clinic was aborted with immediate identification, discontinuation of medication and dexamethasone. It is of note that while early intervention with steroids has been shown to be helpful,[146] if the condition develops into a full blown SJS/TEN, steroids are usually contraindicated.[153]

Dermatological medications can cause psychiatric symptoms. The most notorious of these are isotretinoin and interferon alpha (IFNα) treatment. Isotretinoin is an oral medication used for the treatment of severe nodulocystic acne, mostly given to teenagers, in whom it has been associated with the development of depression.[159] IFNα treatment, a proinflammatory cytokine, also causes depression and this observation has been instrumental in fomenting the view of this psychiatric disease as being the result of an inflammatory process.[160]

PSYCHOLOGICAL TREATMENT

Since there are many stress-related phenomena that affect the skin, the use of conventional psychological techniques is a logical choice to help these patients. In fact, when such therapy is suggested, this mind-skin link should be mentioned to the patient to dullen the impact of having to accept the psychological component of their illness. Thus, one can say that we have the fight/flight response in our skin and that we need the help of our brain to calm it down. If the patient has some psychological insight and accepts help, psychotherapy,[161] mindfulness-based[161] therapies, counselling,[161] habit reversal training, cognitive behavioral therapy,[161,162] biofeedback[162] and even hypnosis[162,163] have been used with success. If there is a psychological component to the dermatological disease, such as all of the neurogenic dermatoses, any single or combination of the aforementioned psychological techniques will help.

Since hypnosis is a much underused and misunderstood therapy technique, and simplified versions are within the reach of any health care professional (HCP), including dermatologists, more information will be given. Its underuse is unfortunate because many medical and dermatological conditions have responded to this treatment. In a Medline search done by Shenefelt,[163] there was documented evidence that the following dermatological conditions were found to respond to hypnosis, in no particular order: vitiligo, acne excoriée, verruca vulgaris, urticaria, trichotillomania, rosacea, psoriasis, pruritus, postherpetic neuralgia, nummular dermatitis, neurodermatitis, lichen planus, ichthyosis vulgaris, hyperhidrosis, herpes simplex, glossodynia, furuncles, erythromelalgia, dyshidrotic dermatitis, congenital ichthyosiform erythroderma, atopic dermatitis and alopecia areata.[164]

The point must be made that there are no placebo-controlled studies to actually verify whether or when hypnosis is going to be helpful. The recommendation is to identify those who are susceptible to being hypnotized and suggest this as a treatment.[163] Any suggestion from the HCP that hypnosis is beneficial increases the placebo response. In fact, there are some conditions, such as verruca vulgaris, that may be cured with the simple suggestion from the doctor that the warts will go away,[163] which is why this condition is notoriously known to respond to placebo.[164]

While hypnosis has been compared to placebo and seen by some as being similar except that hypnosis does not meet its goal by deception,[165,166] hypnosis has been found to have different effects than the placebo response. One study by McGlashan et al. pointed out that the results from hypnotic analgesia are very different from placebo analgesia.[167] In fact, there are more and more neuroimaging studies that are showing definite changes in the brain during hypnosis.[168]

If hypnosis is to be recommended, the selected patient should be emotionally and mentally stable, be cooperating with the treatment, be giving a sense of wanting to make the doctor happy and be motivated to try this modality. If treatment is to be undertaken, the selection of patients can be made even easier by using rating scales that can be used to rate hypnotisability,[169,170] choosing those patients that are medium or highly hypnotizable. For just self-guided imagery that can be used to relax and decrease discomfort, it is not necessary to have them rated at these levels.[171]

Physicians and nurses should learn the basics of hypnosis to help the uncomplicated patient relax in general or to help prepare for a painful treatment. Usually the light or medium hypnotic state is enough to help. Deep hypnotic states are needed for surgery and would require much more experience. Shenenfelt has developed a protocol to help the practitioner with using hypnosis in pain prevention.[172] With more complicated patients, referral to a hypnotherapist should be made as hypnotherapists have their own protocols, for example see the Hypnosis Academy's Scope of Practice.[173]

When hypnosis is to be performed, informed consent should be obtained, at least verbally. It should be presented as a technique whereby the patient will be highly concentrated on the thoughts that are being presented, be totally oblivious of any other distractions, be in a state of tranquility, be in control, be highly suggestible[174] and be able to remember all that was discussed. Suffice it to say that the patient can be told that the immediate goal in hypnosis is to be able to relax and enter into a deeper relaxation state that should be referred to as such or as the hypnotic state, avoiding calling this state a "trance," as this word has negative connotations. The patient can be told that the long term goal of hypnosis is to take advantage of the suggestible state to internalize more adaptive ways of dealing with stress in the future.

The challenge of the hypnotherapist is to help the patient reach this hypnotic state and does so using various techniques that are collectively called induction. It should be noted that the second author has avoided the need to measure hypnotizability due to the success of using a cranial-electric stimulation device, with a FDA-indication for anxiety, depression, insomnia and pain,[175] to help with the induction and is successful in almost all but the most severe cases. This device has made the deep relaxation part of induction extremely easy for the patient to achieve and maintain.

However, many feel hypnosis is simply this relaxed, trance-like state that comes after a successful induction. The actual state of hypnosis is a set-up to start the actual therapy.[163] Once the patient is in the state of hypnosis or hypnotic state, actual therapeutic work can commence, this aspect being known as hypnotherapy. There are various techniques available that can help eliminate the patient's dysfunctional behaviors, the most common being direct suggestion,[176–178] which is helpful in dealing with compulsive behaviors such as scratching, picking, nail biting and hair pulling.[176]

In addition, the patient can be taught self-hypnosis[172] which usually consists of guided imagery that helps the patient deal with stress. The simplest way to do so is a four step approach that the second author uses that has its origins in anger management techniques. (See http://www.mindtools.com/pages/article/newTCS_97.htm[179] for further short pointers if anger needs to be managed). The first step is to close the eyes, covering them if necessary. The second step is to inhale quickly and exhale very slowly, taking up to 20 seconds. These two steps are continued throughout the exercise. The third step is to think of a favorite place and think of all the positive qualities that one has. As can be perceived, these first three steps are to obtain a quick induction. The final step consists of the therapeutic work which is usually centered on trying to identify and control the primitive, dysfunctional impulses. This last step is where the health professional can be of great help in identifying ways to understand the progression of the stress response and how to abort it. Basic cognitive-behavioral techniques can be successfully applied during this latter step.

For more information on these cognitive techniques, refer to the classic reference by Beck[180] and the more popular version by Burns.[181,182] The self-help book by Burns is especially helpful for patients[182] who are motivated to learn and treat their mood disorders on their own. For further information on the application of hypnosis in dermatology, see Shenefelt.[171] For information on hypnotherapists, one can refer to the American Society of Clinical Hypnosis or any other well established professional organization dedicated to hypnotherapy.

There are also references that are helpful for the practitioner who would like to learn about hypnosis, including a review of the use of hypnosis in skin diseases[176,183] as well as one excellent reference book that can help patients understand the role of hypnosis in the mind-skin problem.[184]

SUMMARY

Stress, whether it be physical, across the ample spectrum that has been considered, or psychological, which may either trigger or modify a disease or be caused by the emotional effects of a disease, is a common pathway for the deterioration of skin. It may induce premature aging and skin cancer, but may also be at the heart of serious emotional reactions that interfere with QoL and, in severe cases, may end in suicide.

In many instances, vicious cycles are established in which stress triggers or worsens a skin disorder and, as it worsens even further, the cosmetic appearance is even more affected, increasing the anxiety the individual suffers, completing the vicious cycle.

Frequently, much of the suffering either may go unnoticed or is not properly recognized. Therefore, a good liaison between psychiatrists, dermatologists, and primary care physicians is critical to provide these patients a more holistic bio-psycho-social approach for the care of their skin.[185] It is important that mental health professionals and primary care physicians understand the same terminology and what it represents so that subtle dermatologic clues do not go undetected.

Unfortunately, the evaluation of stress in medical practices is not commonly done as many medical doctors, including dermatologists, do not really have a psychologically based practice.[186] In this kind of practice the HCP/dermatologist has advanced communication skills and can identify and convince patients to receive some sort of psychological support, even if it is only from the doctors themselves. At the very least the HCP should at least point out that stress is expressed in the skin. The goal of this attitude is to accept stress as being part of the mind-body-skin connection and to present it as an aspect of any skin problem.

The easiest intervention, with a patient who might have psychological issues, is to recommend a self-help book such as the one by Burns.[182] A very quick solution would involve the teaching of the four step relaxation technique as part of the treatment of skin disorders so that the patients can learn what to do when faced with "skin-stress." If interested, an even more advanced procedure would be the teaching of self-hypnosis that could be coordinated by the physician's nurse. All these do not entail referral to an outside specialist. Of course, if the mental condition is more complicated, attempts should be made to convince the patient that in order to understand their skin they need to understand their mind, thus diplomatically identifying the problem area as being the skin and not the mind.

In summary, psychological issues cannot be seen as taboo and the influence of stress should be seen as a common everyday occurrence and not as a sign of mental illness. Every patient should hear that the skin is part of the stress response and that the result of any treatment will be enhanced if stress is kept to a minimum. This is not an easy task, but the goal of any doctor-patient interaction should be to acquire a more comprehensive understanding of the underlying psychological/psychiatric problems which may easily go unnoticed in a busy, problem-oriented dermatology practice. Even with time constraints, with this orientation, it is hoped that more appropriate psychological interventions can be made that will not take much time out of busy medical practices.

Likewise, it behooves dermatologists to acquire a more comprehensive understanding of the underlying psychiatric problems that may easily go unnoticed in a busy, problem-oriented dermatological practice. Dermatologists must also become familiar with the pharmacological armamentarium of psychiatry, because dermatologists may provide basic care to those patients who cannot be persuaded for referral to a psychiatrist and may become otherwise lost to treatment.

REFERENCES

1. Poljšak B, Dahmane R. Free radicals and extrinsic skin aging. Dermatol Res Pract 2012;2012:135206. http://dx.doi.org/10.1155/2012/135206.
2. Poljšak B. Decreasing oxidative stress and retarding the aging process. Hauppauge, New York: Nova Science; 2010.
3. Hanson KM, Clegg RM. Observation and quantification of ultraviolet-induced reactive oxygen species in ex vivo human skin. Photochem Photobiol 2002; 76(1):57–63.
4. Shindo Y, Witt E, Packer L. Antioxidant defense mechanisms in murine epidermis and dermis and their responses to ultraviolet light. J Invest Dermatol 1993;100(3):260–5.
5. Godic A, Poljšak B, Adamic M, et al. The role of antioxidants in skin cancer prevention and treatment. Oxid Med Cell Longev 2014;2014:860479. http://dx. doi.org/10.1155/2014/860479.
6. Dunn JH, Koo J. Psychological stress and skin aging: a review of possible mechanisms and potential therapies. Dermatol Online J 2013;19(6):1.
7. Cheeseman KH, Slater TF. An introduction to free radical biochemistry. Br Med Bull 1993;49(3):481–93.
8. Shindo Y, Witt E, Han D, et al. Enzymic and non-enzymic antioxidants in epidermis and dermis of human skin. J Invest Dermatol 1994;102(1):122–4.

9. Fraga CG, Motchnik PA, Shigenaga MK, et al. Ascorbic acid protects against endogenous oxidative DNA damage in human sperm. Proc Natl Acad Sci U S A 1991;88(24):11003–6.

10. Poljšak B, Dahmane RG, Godić A. Intrinsic skin aging: the role of oxidative stress. Acta Dermatovenerol Alp Pannonica Adriat 2012;21:33–6.

11. Fuchs J, Huflejt ME, Rothfuss LM, et al. Acute effects of near ultraviolet and visible light on the cutaneous antioxidant defense system. Photochem Photobiol 1989;50(6):739–44.

12. Chung JH, Lee SH, Youn CS, et al. Cutaneous photodamage in Koreans: influence of sex, sun exposure, smoking, and skin color. Arch Dermatol 2001;137: 1043–51.

13. Model D. Smokers' faces: who are the smokers? Br Med J 1985;291:1760–2.

14. Yang G, Zhang CL, Liu XC, et al. Effects of cigarette smoke extracts on the growth and senescence of skin fibroblasts in vitro. Int J Biol Sci 2013;9(6): 613–23. http://dx.doi.org/10.7150/ijbs.6162.

15. Slominski A. Neuroendocrine system of the skin [review]. Dermatology 2005; 211(3):199–208.

16. Hall JM, Cruser D, Podawiltz A, et al. Psychological stress and the cutaneous immune response: roles of the HPA axis and the sympathetic nervous system in atopic dermatitis and psoriasis. Dermatol Res Pract 2012;2012:403908. http://dx.doi.org/10.1155/2012/403908.

17. Hara MR, Kovacs JJ, Whalen EJ, et al. A stress response pathway regulates DNA damage through β[2]-adrenoreceptors and β-arrestin-1. Nature 2011. http://dx.doi.org/10.1038/nature10368. pii:nature10368.

18. Flint MS, Budiu RA, Teng PN, et al. Restraint stress and stress hormones significantly impact T lymphocyte migration and function through specific alterations of the actin cytoskeleton. Brain Behav Immun 2011;25(6):1187–96. http://dx.doi. org/10.1016/j.bbi.2011.03.009. pii:S0889-1591(11)00077-8.

19. Lu T, Pan Y, Kao SY, et al. Gene regulation and DNA damage in the ageing human brain. Nature 2004;429(6994):883–91. pii:nature02661.

20. Charmandari E, Tsigos C, Chrousos G. Endocrinology of the stress response. Annu Rev Physiol 2005;67:259–84. http://dx.doi.org/10.1146/annurev.physiol. 67.040403.120816.

21. Flint MS, Baum A, Chambers WH, et al. Induction of DNA damage, alteration of DNA repair and transcriptional activation by stress hormones. Psychoneuroendocrinology 2007;32(5):470–9. http://dx.doi.org/10.1016/j.psyneuen.2007.02. 013. pii:S0306-4530(07)00054-6.

22. Thaker PH, Han LY, Kamat AA, et al. Chronic stress promotes tumor growth and angiogenesis in a mouse model of ovarian carcinoma. Nat Med 2006;12(8): 939–44. http://dx.doi.org/10.1038/nm1447. pii:nm1447.

23. Fratiglioni L, Paillard-Borg S, Winblad B. An active and socially integrated lifestyle in late life might protect against dementia. Lancet Neurol 2004;3(6):343–53. http:// dx.doi.org/10.1016/S1474-4422(04)00767-7. pii:S1474442204007677.

24. Korabel H, Dudek D, Jaworek A, et al. Psychodermatology: psychological and psychiatrical aspects of aspects of dermatology. Przegl Lek 2008;65:244–8.

25. Groeschel M, Braam B. Connecting chronic and recurrent stress to vascular dysfunction: no relaxed role for the renin-angiotensin system. Am J Physiol Renal Physiol 2011;300(1):F1–10. http://dx.doi.org/10.1152/ajprenal.00208. 2010. pii:ajprenal.00208.2010.

26. Dimsdale JE, Ziegler M, Mills P. Renin correlates with blood pressure reactivity to stressors. Neuropsychopharmacology 1990;3(4):237–42.

27. Pacurari M, Kafoury R, Tchounwou PB, et al. The renin-angiotensin-aldosterone system in vascular inflammation and remodeling. Int J Inflam 2014;2014: 689360. http://dx.doi.org/10.1155/2014/689360.
28. Rodrigues-Ferreira S, Abdelkarim M, Dillenburg-Pilla P, et al. Angiotensin II facilitates breast cancer cell migration and metastasis. PLoS One 2012;7(4):e35667. pii:PONE-D-12-02354.
29. Boscaro M, Barzon L, Fallo F, et al. Cushing's syndrome. Lancet 2001; 357(9258):783–91. pii:S0140-6736(00)04172-6.
30. Kahan V, Andersen ML, Tomimori J, et al. Can poor sleep affect skin integrity? Med Hypotheses 2010;75(6):535–7. http://dx.doi.org/10.1016/j.mehy.2010.07. 018. pii:S0306-9877(10)00246-X.
31. Koblenzer CS. Psychosomatic concepts in dermatology. Arch Dermatol 1983; 119:501–12.
32. Misery L. Neuro-immuno-cutaneous system (NICS). Pathol Biol (Paris) 1996;44: 867–74.
33. Arck PC, Slominski A, Theoharides TC, et al. Neuroimmunology of stress: skin takes center stage. J Invest Dermatol 2006;126:1697–704.
34. Dhabhar FS. Enhancing versus suppressive effects of stress on immune function: implications for immunoprotection and immunopathology. Neuroimmunomodulation 2009;16(5):300–17. http://dx.doi.org/10.1159/000216188. pii: 000216188.
35. Dragoş D, Tǎnǎsescu MD. The effect of stress on the defense systems. J Med Life 2010;3(1):10–8.
36. Dhabhar FS, Saul AN, Daugherty C, et al. Short-term stress enhances cellular immunity and increases early resistance to squamous cell carcinoma. Brain Behav Immun 2010;24(1):127–37. http://dx.doi.org/10.1016/j.bbi.2009.09.004. pii:S0889-1591(09)00426-7.
37. Dhabhar FS. A hassle a day may keep the pathogens away: the fight-or-flight stress response and the augmentation of immune function. Integr Comp Biol 2009;49(3):215–36. http://dx.doi.org/10.1093/icb/icp045. pii:icp045.
38. Viswanathan K, Dhabhar FS. Stress-induced enhancement of leukocyte trafficking into sites of surgery or immune activation. Proc Natl Acad Sci U S A 2005;102(16):5808–13. http://dx.doi.org/10.1073/pnas.0501650102. pii:0501650102.
39. Dhabhar FS. Stress, leukocyte trafficking, and the augmentation of skin immune function. Ann N Y Acad Sci 2003;992:205–17.
40. Redwine L, Snow S, Mills PJ, et al. Acute psychological stress: effects on chemotaxis and cellular adhesion molecule expression. Psychosom Med 2003;65:598–603.
41. Glaser R, Kiecolt-Glaser JK. Stress-induced immune dysfunction: implications for health. Nat Rev Immunol 2005;5(3):243–51. http://dx.doi.org/10.1038/nri1571. pii: nri1571.
42. Reiche EM, Nunes SO, Morimoto HK. Stress, depression, the immune system, and cancer. Lancet Oncol 2004;5(10):617–25. http://dx.doi.org/10.1016/S1470-2045(04)01597-9. pii:S1470204504015979.
43. Zorrilla EP, Luborsky L, McKay JR, et al. The relationship of depression and stressors to immunological assays: a meta-analytic review. Brain Behav Immun 2001;15(3): 199–226. http://dx.doi.org/10.1006/brbi.2000.0597. pii:S0889-1591(00)90597-X.
44. Bosch JA, Ring C, de Geus EJ, et al. Stress and secretory immunity. Int Rev Neurobiol 2002;52:213–53.
45. Kinney DK, Munir KM, Crowley DJ, et al. Prenatal stress and risk for autism. Neurosci Biobehav Rev 2008;32:1519–32.

46. Nepomnaschy PA, Welch KB, McConnell DS, et al. Cortisol levels and very early pregnancy loss in humans. Proc Natl Acad Sci U S A 2006;103:3938–42.

47. McLeod SA. What is the stress response. 2010. Available at: http://www.simplypsychology.org/stressbiology.html.

48. Ghosh S, Behere RV, Sharma PS, et al. Psychiatric evaluation in dermatology: an overview. Indian J Dermatol 2013;58(1):39–43.

49. Shenefelt PD. Psychodermatological disorders: recognition and treatment. Int J Dermatol 2011;50(11):1309–22.

50. Koo JY, Lee CS. General approach to evaluating psycho-dermatological disorders. In: Koo JY, Lee CS, editors. Psychocutaneous medicine. New York: Marcel Dekker Inc; 2003. p. 1–29.

51. Jafferany M. Psychodermatology: a guide to understanding common psychocutaneous disorders. Prim Care Companion J Clin Psychiatry 2007;9:203–13.

52. Cotterill JA. Psychophysiological aspects of eczema. Semin Dermatol 1990;9:216–9.

53. Mallon E, Newton JN, Klassen A, et al. The quality of life in acne: a comparison with general medical conditions using generic questionnaires. Br J Dermatol 1999;140(4):672–6.

54. Dreno B. Assessing quality of life in patients with acne vulgaris: implications for treatment. Am J Clin Dermatol 2006;7(2):99–106.

55. Lucky AW. Quantitative documentation of a premenstrual flare of facial acne in adult women. Arch Dermatol 2004;140:42–4.

56. Cotterill JA, Cunliffe WJ. Suicide in dermatological patients. Br J Dermatol 1997;137:246–50.

57. Weiss SC, Kimball AB, Liewehr DJ, et al. Quantifying the harmful effect of psoriasis on health-related quality of life. J Am Acad Dermatol 2002;47(4):512–8.

58. Ginsburg IH, Link BG. Feelings of stigmatization in patients with psoriasis. J Am Acad Dermatol 1989;20:53–63.

59. Silverberg NB, Weinberg JM. Rosacea and adult acne: a worldwide epidemic. Cutis 2001;68:85.

60. Goulden V, Stables GI, Cunliffe WJ. Prevalence of facial acne in adults. J Am Acad Dermatol 1999;41(4):577–80.

61. Tanghetti EA, Kawata AK, Daniels SR, et al. Understanding the burden of adult female acne. J Clin Aesthet Dermatol 2014;7(2):22–30.

62. Gupta MA, Gupta AK, Schork NJ. Psychological factors affecting self-excoriative behavior in women with mild-to-moderate facial acne vulgaris. Psychosomatics 1996;37:127–30.

63. Shenefelt PD. Psychological interventions in the management of common skin conditions. Psychol Res Behav Manag 2010;3:51–63.

64. Koo JY, Smith LL. Psychologic aspects of acne. Pediatr Dermatol 1991;8:185–8.

65. American Psychiatric Association. Diagnostic and statistical manual of mental disorders. 5th edition. Washington, DC: American Psychiatric Association; 2013.

66. Bach M, Bach D. Psychiatric and psychometric issues in acne excoriee. Psychother Psychosom 1993;60:207–10.

67. Grant JE, Phillips KA. Recognizing and treating body dysmorphic disorder. Ann Clin Psychiatry 2005;17:205–10.

68. Phillips KA, Dufresne RG, Wilkel CS, et al. Rate of body dysmorphic disorder in dermatology patients. J Am Acad Dermatol 2000;42:436–41.

69. Phillips KA, McElroy SL, Keck PE, et al. Body dysmorphic disorder: 30 cases of imagined ugliness. Am J Psychiatry 1993;150:302–8.

70. Phillips KA. The broken mirror: understanding and treating body dysmorphic disorder. New York: Oxford University Press; 1996.
71. Phillips KA, Dufresne RG Jr. Body dysmorphic disorder: a guide for primary care physicians. Prim Care 2002;29:99–111.
72. Bowe WP, Leyden JJ, Crerand CE, et al. Body dysmorphic disorder symptoms among patients with acne vulgaris. J Am Acad Dermatol 2007;57:222–39.
73. Grant JE, Odlaug BL, Chamberlain SR, et al. Skin picking disorder. Am J Psychiatry 2012;169(11):1143–9. http://dx.doi.org/10.1176/appi.ajp.2012.12040508.
74. Sander HM, Morris LF, Phillips CM, et al. The annual cost of psoriasis. J Am Acad Dermatol 1993;28(3):422–5.
75. Ni C, Chiu MW. Psoriasis and comorbidities: links and risks [review]. Clin Cosmet Investig Dermatol 2014;7:119–32 eCollection 2014.
76. Al'Abadie MS, Kent GG, Gawkrodger DJ. The relationship between stress and the onset and exacerbation of psoriasis and other skin conditions. Br J Dermatol 1994;130(2):199–203.
77. Griffiths CE, Richards HL. Psychological influences in psoriasis. Clin Exp Dermatol 2001;26(4):338–42.
78. Heller MM, Lee ES, Koo JY. Stress as an influencing factor in psoriasis. Skin Therapy Lett 2011;16(5):1–4.
79. Faber EM, Nall L. Psoriasis: a stress-related disease. Cutis 1993;51:322–6.
80. Gaston L, Lassonde M, Bernier-Buzzanga J, et al. Psoriasis and stress: a prospective study. J Am Acad Dermatol 1987;17(1):82–6.
81. Devrimci-Ozguven H, Kundakci TN, Kumbasar H, et al. The depression, anxiety, life satisfaction and affective expression levels in psoriasis patients. J Eur Acad Dermatol Venereol 2000;14(4):267–71.
82. Skevington SM, Bradshaw J, Hepplewhite A, et al. How does psoriasis affect quality of life. Assessing an Ingram-regimen outpatient programme and validating the WHOQOL-100? Br J Dermatol 2006;154:680–91.
83. Gupta MA, Gupta AK. Depression and suicidal ideation in dermatology patients with acne, alopecia areata, atopic dermatitis and psoriasis. Br J Dermatol 1998;139:846–50.
84. Schmitt JM, Ford DE. Role of depression in quality of life for patients with psoriasis. Dermatology 2007;215:17–27.
85. Esposito M, Saraceno R, Giunta A, et al. An Italian study on psoriasis and depression. Dermatology 2006;212:123–7.
86. Sampogna F, Tabolli S, Abeni D. The impact of changes in clinical severity on psychiatric morbidity in patients with psoriasis: a follow-up study. Br J Dermatol 2007;157:508–13.
87. Gupta MA, Schork NJ, Gupta AK, et al. Suicidal ideation in psoriasis. Int J Dermatol 1993;32(3):188–90.
88. Gupta MA, Gupta AK. Psoriasis and sex: a study of moderately to severely affected patients. Int J Dermatol 1997;36:259–62.
89. Russo PA, Ilchef R, Cooper AJ. Psychiatric morbidity in psoriasis: a review. Australas J Dermatol 2004;45:155–9.
90. Scharloo M, Kaptein AA, Weinman J, et al. Patients' illness perceptions and coping as predictors of functional status in psoriasis: a 1-year follow-up. Br J Dermatol 2000;142(5):899–907.
91. Remröd C, Sjöström K, Svensson A. Pruritus in Psoriasis: A Study of Personality Traits, Depression and Anxiety. Acta Dermato-Venereologica 2014. [Epub ahead of print].

92. Akay A, Pekcanlar A, Bozdag KE, et al. Assessment of depression in subjects with psoriasis vulgaris and lichen planus. J Eur Acad Dermatol Venereol 2002; 16(4):347–52.

93. Basavaraj KH, Navya MA, Rashmi R. Relevance of psychiatry in dermatology: present concepts. Indian J Psychiatry 2010;52(3):270–5. http://dx.doi.org/10. 4103/0019-5545.70992.

94. Alolabi N, White CP, Cin AD. The Koebner phenomenon and breast reconstruction: Psoriasis eruption along the surgical incision. Can J Plast Surg 2011;19(4):143–4.

95. Gupta MA, Gupta AK. The Psoriasis Life Stress Inventory: a preliminary index of psoriasis-related stress. Acta Derm Venereol 1995;75(3):240–3.

96. Ramsay B, O'Reagan M. A survey of the social and psychological effects of psoriasis. Br J Dermatol 1988;118:195–201.

97. Hanifin JM, Reed ML, Drake LA, et al. A population based survey of eczema prevalence in the United States. Dermatitis 2007;18(2):82–91.

98. Grewe M, Bruijnzeel-Koomen CA, Schöpf E, et al. A role for Th1 and Th2 cells in the immunopathogenesis of atopic dermatitis. Immunology Today 1998;19(8):359–61.

99. Garg A, Chren MM, Sands LP, et al. Psychological stress perturbs epidermal permeability barrier homeostasis: implications for the pathogenesis of stress-associated skin disorders. Arch Dermatol 2001;137(1):53–9.

100. Lewis-Jones S. Quality of life and childhood atopic dermatitis: the misery of living with childhood eczema. Int J Clin Pract 2006;60(8):984–92.

101. Brodin MB. Neurotic excoriations. J Am Acad Dermatol 2010;63(2):341–2.

102. Shimoda T, Liang Z, Suzuki H, et al. Inhibitory effects of antipsychotic and anxiolytic agents on stress-induced degranulation of mouse dermal mast cells: experimental dermatology. Clin Exp Dermatol 2010;35(5):531–6.

103. Berger A. Science commentary. Th1 and Th2 responses: what are they? BMJ 2000;321(7258):424.

104. Boumpas DT, Chrousos GP, Wilder RL, et al. Glucocorticoid therapy for immune-mediated diseases: basic and clinical correlates. Ann Intern Med 1993;119(12): 1198–208.

105. Wong JW, Nguyen TV, Koo JY. Primary psychiatric conditions: dermatitis artefacta, trichotillomania and neurotic excoriations. Indian J Dermatol 2013;58(1): 44–8. http://dx.doi.org/10.4103/0019-5154.105287.

106. Koblenzer CS. Psychocutaneous disease. Orlando (FL): Grune and Stratton; 1987.

107. Staender S, Luger T, Metze D. Treatment of prurigo nodularis with topical capsaicin. J Am Acad Dermatol 2001;44(3):471–8.

108. American Psychiatric Association. Diagnostic and statistical manual of mental disorders. 4th edition text revision. Washington, DC: Author; 2000.

109. Mutasim DF, Adams BB. The psychiatric profile of patients with psychogenic excoriation. J Am Acad Dermatol 2009;61(4):611–3.

110. Arnold LM, Auchenbach MB, McElroy SL. Psychogenic excoriation: clinical features, proposed diagnostic criteria, epidemiology and approaches to treatment. CNS Drugs 2001;15:351–9.

111. Heller MM, Koo JM. Neurotic excoriations, acne excoriée, and factitial dermatitis. In: Heller MM, Koo JY, editors. Contemporary diagnosis and management in psychodermatology. 1st edition. Newton (PA): Handbooks in Health Care Co; 2011. p. 37–44.

112. Keuthen NJ, Deckersbach T, Wilhelm S, et al. Repetitive skin-picking in a student population and comparison with a sample of self-injurious skin-pickers. Psychosomatics 2000;41:210–5.

113. Grant JE, Menard W, Phillips KA. Pathological skin picking in individuals with body dysmorphic Disorder. Gen Hosp Psychiatry 2006;28(6):487–93.

114. Neziroglu F, Rabinowitz D, Breytman A, et al. Skin picking phenomenology and severity comparison. Prim Care Companion J Clin Psychiatry 2008;10:306–12.
115. Weintraub E, Robinson C, Newmeyer M. Catastrophic medical complication in psychogenic excoriation. South Med J 2000;93:1099–101.
116. Kim DI, Garrison RC, Thompson G. A near fatal case of pathological skin picking. Am J Case Rep 2013;14:284–7.
117. Misery L, Alexandre S, Dutray S, et al. Functional itch disorder or psychogenic pruritus: suggested diagnosis criteria from the French psychodermatology group. Acta Derm Venereol 2007;87:341–4.
118. Radmanesh M, Shafiei S. Underlying psychopathologies of psychogenic pruritic disorders. Dermatol Psychosom 2001;2:130–3.
119. Conrado LA, Hounie AG, Diniz JB, et al. Body dysmorphic disorder among dermatologic patients: Prevalence and clinical features. J Am Acad Dermatol 2010;63(2):235–43.
120. Raman K, Ponnudurai R, Ravindran OS. Body dysmorphic disorder: borderline category between neurosis and psychosis. Indian J Psychiatry 2014;56(1):84–6.
121. Phillips KA. The obsessive-compulsive spectrums. Psychiatr Clin North Am 2002;25:791–809.
122. Phillips KA, Siniscalchi JM, McElroy SL. Depression, anxiety, anger, and somatic symptoms in patients with body dysmorphic disorder. Psychiatr Q 2004;75(4):309–20.
123. Phillips KA, Coles ME, Menard W, et al. Suicidal ideation and suicide attempts in body dysmorphic disorder. J Clin Psychiatry 2005;66:717–25.
124. Hughes H, Brown BW, Lawlis GF, et al. Treatment of acne vulgaris by biofeedback relaxation and cognitive imagery. J Psychosom Res 1983;27:185–91.
125. Grant JE, Phillips KA. Captive of the mirror: I pick at my face all day, every day. Curr Psychiatr 2003;2:45–52.
126. Gupta MA, Gupta AK, Watteel GN. Stress and alopecia areata: a psychodermatologic study. Acta Derm Venereol 1997;77:296–8.
127. Garcia-Hernandez MJ, Ruiz-Doblado S, Rodriguez-Pichardo A, et al. Alopecia areata, stress and psychiatric disorders: a review. J Dermatol 1999;26:625–32.
128. Koo JY, Shellow WV, Hallman C, et al. Alopecia areata and increased prevalence of psychiatric disorders. Int J Dermatol 1994;33:849–50.
129. Colon EA, Popkin MK, Callies AL, et al. Lifetime prevalence of psychiatric disorders in patients with alopecia areata. Compr Psychiatry 1991;32:245–51.
130. McElroy SL, Phillips KA, Keck PE. Obsessive compulsive spectrum disorder. J Clin Psychiatry 1994;55:33–53.
131. Schlosser S, Black DW, Blum N, et al. The demography, phenomenology, and family history of 22 persons with compulsive hair pulling. Ann Clin Psychiatry 1994;6:147–52.
132. Mittal D, O'Jite J, Kennedy R, et al. Trichotillomania associated with dementia: a case report. Gen Hosp Psychiatry 2001;23:163–5.
133. Stein DJ, Gardner JP, Keuthen NJ, et al. Trichotillomania, stereotypic movement disorder, and related disorders. Curr Psychiatry Rep 2007;9:301–2.
134. Garnis-Jones S. Psychological aspects of rosacea. J Cutan Med Surg 1998;2(Suppl 4):9–16.
135. Available at: http://www.rosacea.org/patients/materials/triggersgraph.php.
136. Holmes AD. Potential role of microorganisms in the pathogenesis of rosacea. J Am Acad Dermatol 2013;69(6):1025–32.
137. Lotti T, D'Erme AM. Vitiligo as a systemic disease. Clin Dermatol 2014;32(3):430–4. http://dx.doi.org/10.1016/j.clindermatol.2013.11.011.

138. Dogra S, Kanawar AJ. Skin diseases: psychological and social consequences. Indian J Dermatol 2002;47:197–201.

139. Porter JR, Beuf AH, Aaron B, et al. The effect of vitiligo on sexual relationships. J Am Acad Dermatol 1990;22(2):221–2.

140. Porter J, Beuf A, Lerner A, et al. Response to cosmetic disfigurement patients With Vitiligo. Cutis 1987;39:493–4.

141. Buske-Kirschbaum A, Geiben A, Wermke C, et al. Preliminary evidence for herpes labialis recurrence following experimentally induced disgust. Psychother Psychosom 2001;70:86–91.

142. Sainz B, Loutsch JM, Marquart ME, et al. Stress-associated immunomodulation and herpes simplex virus infection. Med Hypotheses 2001;56:348–56.

143. Guarneri F, Marini H. An unusual case of perioral dermatitis: possible pathogenic role of neurogenic inflammation. J Eur Acad Dermatol Venereol 2007;21:410–2.

144. Ghislain P, Roujeau JC. Treatment of severe drug reactions: Stevens-Johnson syndrome, toxic epidermal necrolysis and hypersensitivity syndrome. Dermatol Online J 2002;8(1):5.

145. Allam J, Paus T, Reichel C, et al. DRESS syndrome associated with carbamazepine and phenytoin. Eur J Dermatol 2004;14:339–42.

146. Chang C, Shiah IS, Chang HA, et al. Toxic epidermal necrolysis with combination lamotrigine and valproate in bipolar disorder. Prog Neuropsych. Biol Psychiatry 2006;30(1):147–50.

147. Guberman A, Besag FM, Brodie MJ, et al. Lamotrigine-associated rash: risk/benefit considerations in adults and children. Epilepsia 1999;40(7):985–91.

148. Pisani F, Di Perri R, Perucca E, et al. Interaction of lamotrigine with sodium valproate. Lancet 1993;341(8854):1224.

149. Yuen A, Land G, Weatherley BC, et al. Sodium valproate acutely inhibits lamotrigine metabolism. Br J Clin Pharmacol 1992;33(5):511–3.

150. Zaccara G, Franciotta D, Perucca E. Idiosyncratic adverse reactions to antiepileptic drugs. Epilepsia 2007;48:1223–44.

151. Kanner A. Lamotrigine-induced rash: can we stop worrying? Epilepsy Curr 2005;5(5):190–1.

152. Mockenhaupt M, Messenheimer J, Tennis P, et al. Risk of Stevens-Johnson syndrome and toxic epidermal necrolysis in new users of antiepileptics. Neurology 2005;64(7):1134–8.

153. Yi Y, Lee JH, Suh ES. Toxic epidermal necrolysis induced by lamotrigine treatment in a child. Korean J Pediatr 2014;57(3):153–6.

154. Pereira FA, Mudgil AV, Rosmarin DM. Toxic epidermal necrolysis. J Am Acad Dermatol 2007;56:181–200.

155. Hirsch L, Weintraub DB, Buchsbaum R, et al. Predictors of lamotrigine-associated rash. Epilepsia 2006;47(2):318–22.

156. Hung S, Chung WH, Liou LB, et al. HLA-B*5801 allele as a genetic marker for severe cutaneous adverse reactions caused by allopurinol. Proc Natl Acad Sci U S A 2005;102(11):4134–9.

157. Calabrese JR, Bowden CC, Sachs GS, et al. A double-blind placebo-controlled study of lamotrigine monotherapy in outpatients with bipolar I depression. Lamictal 602 Study Group. J Clin Psychiatry 1999;60(2):79–88.

158. Garcia-Doval I, LeCleach L, Bocquet H, et al. Toxic epidermal necrolysis and Stevens-Johnson syndrome: does early withdrawal of causative drugs decrease the risk of death? Arch Dermatol 2000;136(3):323–7.

159. Goodfield M, Cox NH, Bowser A, et al. Advice on the safe introduction and continued use of isotretinoin in acne in the U.K. 2010. Br J Dermatol 2010;162(6):1172–9.

160. Friebe A, Horn M, Schmidt F, et al. Dose dependent development of depressive symptoms during adjuvant interferon Alpha treatment of patients with malignant melanoma. Psychosomatics 2010;51:466–73.

161. de Zoysa P. Psychological interventions in dermatology. Indian J Dermatol 2003; 58(1):58–60.

162. Shenefelt PD. Biofeedback, cognitive-behavioral oral methods, and hypnosis in dermatology: is it all in your mind? Dermatol Ther 2003;16(2):114–22.

163. Shenefelt PD. Hypnosis in dermatology. Arch Dermatol 2000;136(3):393–9.

164. Sulzberger MB, Wolf J. The treatment of warts by suggestion. Med Rec 1934; 740:552–6.

165. Kirsch I. Clinical hypnosis as a nondeceptive placebo: Empirically derived techniques. Am J Clin Hypn 1994;37(2):95–106.

166. Kirsch I. Clinical hypnosis as a nondeceptive placebo. Washington, DC: American Psychological Association; 1999.

167. McGlashan TH, Evans FH, Orne MT. The nature of hypnotic analgesia and placebo response to experimental pain. Psychosom Med 1969;31(3):227–46.

168. Raz A, Fan J, Posner MA. Hypnotic suggestion reduces conflict in the human brain. Proc Natl Acad Sci U S A 2005;102(28):9978–83.

169. Spiegel H, Spiegel D. Trance and treatment: clinical uses of hypnosis. The hypnotic induction profile. New York: Basic Books; 1978.

170. Hilgard ER, Weitzenhoffer AM, Landes J, et al. Stanford hypnotic susceptibility scale. Psychological Monographs: General and Applied 1961;75(8):1–22.

171. Shenefelt PD. Applying hypnosis in dermatology. Dermatol Nurs 2003;15:6.

172. Shenefelt PD. Hypnosis-facilitated relaxation using self-guided imagery during dermatologic procedures. Am J Clin Hypn 2003;45:225–32.

173. Scope of practice. Available at: http://www.hypnotherapyacademy.com/combined_for_web_Scope_of_Practice.pdf.

174. Brink TL. Psychology: a student friendly approach. Unit 5: perception. 2008.

175. Kirsch DL, Francine-Nichols F. Cranial electrotherapy stimulation for treatment of anxiety, depression, and insomnia. Psychiatr Clin N Am 2013;36:169–76.

176. Scott M. Hypnosis in skin and allergic diseases. Springfield (IL): Charles C Thomas Publisher; 1960.

177. Scott M. Hypnosis in dermatology. Springfield (IL): Charles C Thomas; 1963.

178. Hartland J. Hypnosis in dermatology. Br J Clin Hypn 1969;1:2–7.

179. Available at: http://www.mindtools.com/pages/article/newTCS_97.htm. Accessed August 22, 2014.

180. Beck AT. Cognitive therapies and emotional disorders. New York: New American Library; 1976.

181. Burns DD. Feeling good: the new mood therapy. New York: New American Library; 1980.

182. Burns DD. The feeling good handbook. Revised and updated, 1999 edition. New York: William Morrow and Co; 1999.

183. Crasilneck HB, Hall JA. Clinical hypnosis. 2nd edition. Orlando (FL): Grune & Stratton; 1985.

184. Grossbart TA, Sherman C. Skin deep: a mind/body program for healthy skin. Revised edition. Santa Fe (NM): Health Press; 1992.

185. Shenefelt PD. Psychological interventions in the management of common skin conditions. Psychol Res Behav Manag 2010;3:51–63.

186. Poot F, Sampogna F, Onnis L. Basic knowledge in psychonur. J Eur Acad Dermatol Venereol 2007;21:227–34.

The Role of Glia in Stress

Polyamines and Brain Disorders

Serguei N. Skatchkov, PhD[a,b,*], Michel A. Woodbury-Fariña, MD, DFAPA, FAIS[c],
Misty Eaton, PhD[a]

KEYWORDS

- Stress • Brain disorders • Glia • Polyamines

KEY POINTS

- Polyamines (PAs) are one of the principal differences between glia and neurons, because they are stored, but not synthesized, almost exclusively in glial cells, from which they can be released to regulate neuronal synaptic activity.
- PAs have not yet been a focus of much glial research.
- PAs affect many neuronal and glial receptors, channels, and transporters.
- PAs are key elements in the development of many diseases and syndromes, thus forming the rationale for PA-focused and glia-focused therapy for these conditions.

GLIA VERSUS NEURONS

Ramón y Cajal[1] predicted how glia could help in health and disease by saying that glia are "insulating the neurons and switching their signaling." His work has been analyzed by many scientists.[2–9] Ramón y Cajal knew that glia were more than just connective tissue but could never prove this. He was able to highlight novel features of glial cells. These observations can be considered to be the discovery of the importance of glia as the second brain. Ramón y Cajal, who has been considered by many to be the father of modern neuroscience, made a principal glial discovery: he visualized what are now known as radial glial cells (RGCs). Recent studies have shown that these cells are of ectodermic origin, which means that RGCs are universal precursors for both neurons and glia. This finding broke the dogma that glia and neurons have separate origins and lineages.[10] Then came the studies that neurogenesis was observed in adult human[11] and rat[12] brains, shattering yet another dogma, that neurogenesis was absent in the mature brain.

The authors have nothing to disclose.
[a] Department of Biochemistry, School of Medicine, Universidad, Central del Caribe, PO Box 60-327, Bayamón, PR 00960-6032, USA; [b] Department of Physiology, School of Medicine, Universidad, Central del Caribe, PO Box 60-327, Bayamón, PR 00960-6032, USA; [c] Department of Psychiatry, University of Puerto Rico School of Medicine, 307 Calle Eleonor Roosevelt, San Juan, PR 00918-2720, USA
* Corresponding author. Departments of Biochemistry and Physiology, School of Medicine, Universidad Central del Caribe, PO Box 60-327, Bayamón, PR 00960-6032.
E-mail addresses: sergueis50@yahoo.com; serguei.skatchkov@uccaribe.edu

Abbreviations	
A/N ratio	Ratio of astrocytes to neurons
AChR	Acetylcholine receptor
AMPAR	α-Amino-3-hydroxy-5-methyl-4-isoxazolepropionic acid receptor
ATP	Adenosine triphosphate
Ca	Calcium
CA	Cornu ammonis area
Ca^{2+}	Extracellular calcium
Cl^{+}	Extracellular chloride
CNS	Central nervous system
CSF	Cerebral spinal fluid
Cx	Connexin
G/N ratio	Ratio of glial cells to neurons
Glu	Glutamate
H^{+}	Extracellular hydrogen
Ir K = Kir	Inwardly rectifying potassium
K^{+}	Extracellular potassium
Na^{+}	Extracellular sodium
NMDA	N-Methyl-D-aspartate
NMDAR	N-Methyl-D-aspartate receptor
OCT	Organic cation transporter
ODC	Ornithine decarboxylase
Panx	Pannexin
PAs	Polyamines
PUT	Putrescine
RGCs	Radial glial cells
SPD	Spermidine
SpdS	Spermidine synthase
SPM	Spermine
TRPV1	Transient receptor potential cation channel, subfamily V, member 1

There is increasing evidence that RGCs build the brain by accommodating in the inner and outer subventricular zone to send their processes into the ventricular zone. RGCs show polarity and are the stem cells of the developing brain.[13–16] Several morphologically distinct subtypes of RGCs in fetal macaque neocortex produce neurons and are guides for the migration of neural progenitors.[17]

Therefore, there are many different types of glial cells that are of RGC origin: NG-2, astrocytes, oligodendrocytes, tanycytes (in whole brain), Müller glia (in retina), and Bergmann glia (in cerebellum), as well as ependymal cells (in the ventricular surface). These cells represent the major neuroglial population in the adult central nervous system (CNS). On the other hand, peripheral glial cells, such as Schwann cells, satellite glia (in the sympathetic, parasympathetic, and sensory ganglia), enteric glia (in the ganglia of the digestive system), and pituicytes (astrocytic glia in the posterior pituitary), are also types of neuroglia. Although there are the microglia (mesodermal origin), which are macrophages in the brain, in this review, the microglia are not discussed. One of the major differences between glia and neurons is accumulation of biogenic polyamines; astrocytes expressing arginine decarboxylase can produce agmatine, a principal element in brain PA-exchange, and therefore, glial cells can be agmatine reservoirs.[18] In general, the ratio of astrocytes to neurons (A/N) increases in evolution with increasing brain size,[19] and the highest glial cell (G) to neuron (G/N) ratio is found in brainstem,[20] where the most important controls of body functions occur, for example control of respiration.[21,22] On the other hand, there is also evidence that the frontal cortex has the highest G/N ratio. RGCs, as well as astrocytes, are filled with the

PAs spermine (SPM) and spermidine (SPD).[23–25] One surprising function of RGCs was recently discovered, which is that in the adult retina, RGCs provide photon signaling and serve as light guiding fibers.[26,27]

INTERACTION OF POLYAMINES WITH RECEPTORS AND ION CHANNELS

PAs such as SPD and SPM are involved in glial-neuronal communication, especially during periods of stress, such as during ischemia and trauma; the mechanisms of storage and release are not well known. Because neurodegeneration is a major problem during stress, ischemia, and CNS diseases, identifying potential neuroprotective mechanisms could provide new targets for therapeutic interventions. In the 1980s, it was discovered that the PA SPM was a principal radical group in spider venom,[28–31] and the SPM portion of the venom could insert itself into and block glutamate receptors.[30] In the late 1990s, PAs were brought to the attention of neuroscientists. However, the sources of PAs in the brain were not known.

PAs affect glial inwardly rectifying potassium (Kir)4.1 channels[25,32,33] and most of the known neuronal receptors and channels.[34] In the brain and peripheral nervous system, SPM and SPD are known to have specific intracellular and extracellular actions. SPM affects numerous receptors and channels in neurons with differing affinities ranging from ~ 10 nM to 200 μM.[35–38] Intracellular SPM/SPD induces voltage-dependent block of Kir channels,[25,39,40] as well as neuronal nicotinic acetylcholine receptor (AChR) channels,[35,41] glutamate (Glu)A-2 lacking α-amino-3-hydroxy-5-methyl-4-isoxazolepropionic acid receptor (AMPAR) channels,[42] N-methyl-D-aspartate receptors (NMDARs),[34,43] olfactory cyclic nucleotide-gated cation channels,[44] and voltage-gated sodium channels.[45] In addition, some NMDAR and AMPAR channels show rectification in the presence of PAs or their derivatives.[31,36,42,46–50] PAs are the strongest blockers of Kir channels, glutamate receptor channels (such as AMPAR, NMDAR, KainateR) and AChR channels[31,35,36,39,51–53] and also act as the calcium (Ca)-sensing receptors agonists[54] and antagonists of transient receptor potential cation channel, subfamily M, member 7 and transient receptor potential cation channel, subfamily V member 1 (TRPV1) channels.[38,55] Also relevant are the extracellular actions of PA on GluA-2-lacking and GluA5/6-enriched AMPA/Kainate receptor channels in interneurons,[56–58] because glial cells may release PAs to control synaptic activity. These receptor channels have an affinity for SPM in the micromolar range.

Spermine/Spermidine Localization in Central Nervous System: Bidirectional Polyamine Signaling Between Glia and Neurons

The PAs SPD and SPM are accumulated in glia (**Fig. 1**), and their distribution is clearly evolutionarily determined; it is found throughout the brain,[23] retina,[24,25] peripheral nervous system,[59] and in glial-neuronal cocultures[60] of multiple species, including man.[24] This phenomenon raises key questions: (1) What are the mechanisms that underlie such uneven distribution, accumulation, and release from glia?; (2) What are the consequences of PA fluxes within the brain on neuronal function?; (3) What are the roles of PAs in brain disorders and diseases?

Astrocytes enwrap presynaptic and postsynaptic neuronal terminals, generating a tripartite synapse.[61–63] Failure of synaptic transmission[64,65] and vasodilation[66,67] has been ascribed to the malfunction of perisynaptic and perivascular astrocytes, respectively. Neuronal damage is evident after glial depletion in hepatic encephalopathy,[68] and neuronal degeneration can occur after apoptosis of glial cells.[69] It has long been accepted that glia provide a support function to neurons by buffering

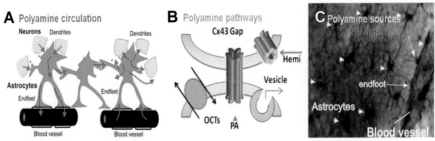

Fig. 1. Circulation of PAs in brain. (*A*) Suggested interaction between astrocytes, neuronal dendrites, and synapses and blood vessels based on bidirectional PA fluxes (1) between neurons and astrocytes, (2) between astrocytes in their syncytium, and (3) between astrocytes and blood vessels. PAs are taken up and released from glia to neurons as well as propagated distantly through the syncytium (*red arrows*). (*B*) Suggested PA pathways (uptake and release) in glia via connexin 43 (Cx43) hemichannels, Cx43 gap junctions, reverse organic cation transporters (OCTs), and vesicular release. (*C*) Accumulation of spermine (SP) in astrocytes shown by immunocytochemical method in rat hippocampus. Astrocytes enwrap blood vessels and connect to each other. Note: no SPM and SPD labels found in neurons in this stratum radiatum area of CA1 rat hippocampus.

extracellular K$^+$ and glutamate.[70–74] However, potential signal functions of glia are less studied and understood.

Glial cells release signaling molecules such as arachidonate, glutamate, adenosine triphosphate (ATP), D-serine, tumor necrosis factor α, which regulate neurons and blood vessels.[61,66,75–86] Thus, finding the signaling functions of glial cells and potential endogenous glial transmitters is one of the frontiers of glial research. Although such gliotransmitters may be PAs, they are mostly underestimated and less studied; yet, in the context of stress and glial function, they might be a key element in helping to modulate neurons.

PAs may have harmful or neuroprotective effects via multiple pathways. For example, blocking Ca^{2+}-permeable GluR2-lacking AMPA receptor channels by SPM[42,56,87,88] reduces Ca^{2+} influx and prevents excitotoxicity.[89] Furthermore, potentiation by SPM of GluR-6 kainate receptors on inhibitory neurons[58,90] inhibits the activity of downstream pyramidal cells, which can result in a neuroprotective effect. Ischemia, glucose deprivation, or mild mechanical trauma all can result in neuronal death because of Ca^{2+} overload, followed by apoptosis,[91,92] if not protected by PAs.[89] The primary pathway for Ca^{2+} entry under these conditions is via fast GluR2-lacking AMPA receptors as well as slow N-methyl-D-aspartate (NMDA) receptors.[50,93–95] Therefore, the amount of PAs stored and released from glia may underlie the strength of neuroprotection. There might be an aging effect, because the amount of PAs stored in the brain declines with age.[96–101] PA-sensitive interneurons (lacking GluR2 subunits) within the brain, but not pyramidal neurons (expressing GluR2 subunits), are enveloped by PA-filled astrocytes (eg, in the hippocampus). During ischemic conditions, there is a striking disparity in the rate of neuronal death in this region of the brain. Interneurons are spared, whereas pyramidal neurons are susceptible.[89] This observation can be explained by the proximity of astrocytes, because they take better care of their direct neighbors, the interneurons. By contrast, the cortex interneurons and pyramidal cells are less formally organized. Glial cells are unevenly distributed between the 2 cell types, making the neuronal sensitivity to ischemia less for interneurons than for pyramidal cells.[102] We suggest that the resistance of hippocampal interneurons to ischemia and apoptosis is a result of localized SPM/SPD release from the surrounding glia and the subsequent block of GluR2-lacking AMPA receptors. In support of this theory, there is compelling evidence for a protective role of exogenous PAs in brain ischemia and neurotransmitter-induced excitotoxicity: for instance, the application of naphthylacetyl-SPM or SPM/SPD in vitro or in vivo dramatically protects cornu ammonis area 1 (CA1) neurons under these conditions.[89,91,92,103] So, we suggest that when experiments are performed with brain slices that might have their endogenous PAs washed out of the astrocytes by being disconnected from the blood circulation (a source of PAs), there should be supplementation with external PAs to keep PAs buffering the astrocytes which improve neuronal survival and function.[104] This situation can be directly related to stress and neuroprotection. Another observed phenomenon is that PAs can be oxidized, which results in the production of toxic compounds that can be captured by glial cells. When cultured in the absence of glia, neurons show a delayed death in response to exogenous PAs.[105,106] Even although extracellular PAs are present in physiologic tissues,[107] the healthy brain clearly avoids significant PA toxicity, probably because extracellular levels in the cerebrospinal fluid are buffered by the astrocytes. Consistent with this finding, and in contrast to the findings in pure neuronal cultures, 50 μM SPM applied exogenously in cortical brain slices is well tolerated, and neuronal death is not observed.[56] We, therefore, hypothesize that, in the intact brain, glial cells provide protection against trauma and excitotoxicity at least in part by using PAs as a buffer, thereby, preventing oxidation. PAs can then be released at appropriate sites with the potential to block inappropriate Ca permeability through glutamate receptor regulation. Indirect support for this hypothesis is the observation that in perfused brain slices, excitotoxicity induced by anoxia and toxic chemicals (eg, NMDA) in hippocampal slices was prevented if SPM was used.[108] If PAs may be considered as neuroprotective agents, then what are the physiologic ranges of PA concentrations and what are the free versus bound forms of PAs in the brain?

The total concentration of intracellular SPM in nonneuronal cells is high (3–10 mm),[96,109–113] although SPM is greatly buffered in the cells by negatively charged phosphates, ATP, guanosine-5'-triphosphate, DNA, RNA, membrane proteins, and other polypeptides.[110,114–118] Because SPM and SPD are not synthesized in glia,[119,120] but instead are accumulated in glia[23–25,60] (see **Fig. 1**C), the PAs putrescine (PUT), SPD, and SPM may be exchanged during different conditions, such as development, membrane depolarization, substrate cotransport, or metabolic downregulation. Our immunolocalization data show preferential SPM/SPD accumulation in glia that enwrap blood vessels (see **Fig. 1**). SPM and SPD were not found in most neurons of the retina[24,25] and in brain.[23] This finding is consistent with our recent studies suggesting that the free SPM concentration in glia (≤800 μM[33]) may be higher than estimated in neurons ~10 nM to 80 μM.[35–38] In the brain, PAs show a strikingly uneven distribution. Using radioactive PAs[59,115,116] and polyclonal antibodies specific for PUT[60] or SPM/SPD,[23–25] we and others have shown that PAs are taken up in brain,[109,121] and astrocytes are capable of taking up PAs (see **Fig. 1**B).[60,112,122–126]

Therefore, if PAs were to be synthesized in some neurons,[127–130] then, they would be released from those neurons, possibly from synaptic neuronal vesicles, to the extracellular space. A vesicular transport system was found.[131,132] This finding leads to an immediate accumulation and storage of PAs in glial cells (see **Fig. 1**A). An alternative source of PAs could be from the blood vessels, with which astrocytes maintain intimate contact, wrapping the vascular interface by endfoot processes (see **Fig. 1**A, C). Here, glial cells may use several uptake pathways, such as transporters and large pores (see **Fig. 1**B), which are discussed later.

Brain Disorders and Glia

Global amnesia, depression, stress, anxiety, autism, glioblastoma multiforme, glaucoma, migraines, neuropathic pain, sleeplessness, and drug addiction are among a host of devastating neurologic diseases or disorders for which prevention or a cure must be found.[133–150] The later discussion shows that these disorders can be tightly linked with the PA machinery.

Since their original discovery by Leeuwenhoek,[151] the PAs SPM and SPD have attracted the attention of scientists and clinicians.[118,152,153] In the middle of the twentieth century, there was great interest in their role in maintaining DNA structure and the possibility of treating cancer by blocking PA synthesis. In part because of neurologic complications in anticancer treatment, this approach failed.[154] Later studies showed that this situation could have been predicted, because of the existence of multiple effects of PAs on receptors and channels in the brain.

Multiple biological effects of PAs have been reported, including increasing longevity,[96,100,155,156] cell proliferation and differentiation,[157] receptor and channel regulation,[29,34,158–160] modulation of behavior, learning, and memory,[103,161–164] as well as antinociceptive,[38,165,166] neuroprotective,[167–169] antidepressant,[170,171] and antioxidant effects.[96,172]

Although PAs are still a mystery in the brain,[18,60,109,113,121,130,155,173–182] they are known to be tightly associated with glial cells. Altered PA metabolism may underlie certain brain disorders,[183,184] including depression with suicidal tendency.[185] Endogenous depletion of SPD and SPM by dietary means[107,186] or by genetic activation of SPD/SPM-acetyl transferase results in the loss of PAs and a loss of neuroprotection.[187,188] Although SPM/SPD are involved in the pathology of neurodegenerative diseases, they predominantly accumulate in glia and not in neurons.[23–25] However, SPD is not synthesized in glial cells,[119,120,176,189] and thus, SPM cannot be synthesized without SPD, because it is the precursor. A solution to their origins comes from the idea that PAs are probably taken up from external sources by glial cells.[113,124,190] It has been hypothesized that PAs are taken up by glia from the blood circulation, cerebral spinal fluid (CSF), or macrophages penetrating the blood-brain barrier. One of the possible pathway is the organic cation transporter (OCT) system, which is expressed in glia.[191,192]

Several CNS diseases have been shown to be associated with neuroglia, such as astrocytes, oligodendrocytes, ependyma, and other glial cells. Neurodegenerative diseases in which glia play a key role are Alzheimer disease,[141,193–196] amyotrophic lateral sclerosis,[197–199] Alexander disease,[200] Parkinson disease,[201] Huntington disease,[202–204] multiple sclerosis,[205,206] and others.

Still other brain disorders and syndromes in which glial cells play a pivotal role have been recognized. One of them is directly related to stress and epilepsy, in which (1) PA-dependent glial Kir4.1 channels are involved[74,207–210] together with (2) glial connexin (Cx) gap junctions,[211,212] and (3) downregulation of adenosine signaling.[149,213–215] In addition, there are severe disorders such as ischemia and stroke in which reactive gliosis and an inability to regulate pH, K^+ buffering, glutamate homeostasis, and water exchange were found to result in the release of cytotoxic molecules, glial swelling, and neuronal death.[216–220] The study of both physical[217,221] and chemical brain trauma resulting in the depression of glial metabolism[65] or reconstitution after brain edema and inflammation[222,223] showed that reactive glia were no longer supporting neurons.

The PA-regulated Kir4.1 channels[224,225] and a PA transporter OCT SLC22A subfamily, OCT3, are mislocalized[226] in glial cells involved in brain cancer genesis (gliomas). These tumors produce increased intracranial pressure, metabolic deficiencies, toxicity, and cell death.[227] Down syndrome and Snyder-Robinson syndrome have malfunction of PA homeostasis.[143,228–230] The neurologic manifestations of EAST/SeSAME syndrome with glial Kir4.1 mutations[208,210,231] is solely of glial origin, and blood-brain circulation disorders are seen when astrocytes cannot regulate vasodilation.[67,194,232] All of these recent findings show the unique role of glial cells and PAs in CNS disorders.

By What Mechanisms Do Glia Accumulate and Release Polyamines?

The enzymes ornithine decarboxylase (ODC) and SPD synthase (SpdS) synthesize PUT and SPD, respectively, which are the precursors of SPM. In the normal brain, ODC and SpdS expression is typically found only in a few neurons, without any being detectable in glia.[119,120,176,233] In addition, we found that SPM synthase is also absent in glia. This finding suggests that under normal conditions, PAs may be synthesized outside glia in some neurons.[119,128,129,176,234] By unknown mechanisms, PAs accumulate in glia.[23–25,60] Strong evidence for this theory is the finding that injections of radioactive PUT into axons result in the transfer of the radioactive label to surrounding glial cells.[59] Even in brain areas in which many adult neurons lack SpdS activity[119] and show low levels of SPM/SPD,[23] there are still robust and potential sources of PAs in blood capillaries, because PAs can permeate the walls of blood vessels[18] to which glial cells are attached to by endfeet (see **Fig. 1**A, C). Therefore, accumulation of PAs in the glial cytoplasm is not primarily caused by SPD/SPD synthesis, but instead by either passive or active transport (fluxes) of PAs (see **Fig. 1**).

There are several potential pathways for exchange of SPM/SPD among glia, neurons, and blood vessels, such as the following:

1. Large pores, including Cx or pannexin (Panx) hemichannels
2. Ion channels
3. Exocytotic vesicular release and endocytotic uptake.

All of these candidate pathways have been identified in glial cells for different molecules, but not yet for SPM/SPD.[9,78,80,235–240] It was suggested that PAs could be taken up from external sources by glial cells via hypothetical transporters, which would bring PAs into the cells[113,124,190,191] by transporters localized at the endfeet that are attached to blood vessels and brain ventricles. According to this view, the blood circulation and CSF would be the major sources of PA uptake. The macrophages that penetrate the blood-brain barrier and enter the brain may be additional sources.

Recent data show that SPD may be taken up by transporters such as polyspecific electrogenic OCTs SLC22A subfamily,[192] which were suggested as a pathway for monoamines such as dopamine, tetraethylammonium, and others,[124,125,190,191] which are also well suited for PAs.[192] Such transporters may function in a reverse mode, releasing PAs by exchanging with other OCT substrates,[241] or, as was shown for glutamate reverse transport[242] or dopamine reverse transport[243,244] with similar and different mechanisms. Therefore, transporters may fulfill the function of regulating the PA content in the extracellular cleft and thus can regulate neuronal activity.

There may be other minor pathways for PAs; SPM permeates glutamate receptor channels,[52,53] TRPV1 channels,[38] and glial Kir4.1 channels.[245] These are most likely negligible pathways for SPM flux, because the channel pores (6–9Å) are comparable in size with SPM (4Å diameter and 16Å long). In addition, although exocytotic release as described for glutamate[78] and ATP[246] may be applicable to PAs, there is no still evidence suggesting SPM release via this vesicular pathway.

The most likely major pathways for SPM/SPD exchange are via the large pores such as Cx and Panx hemichannels and transporters such as OCTs. SPM/SPD may pass through Cx gap junctions and fill the astrocytic syncitium.[104] Although several studies suggest that unpaired Cx43 hemichannels are present in the plasma membrane of astrocytes[80,236,247] and in cell lines,[248] Cx hemichannels are normally closed, because of the blocking effects of external divalent cations and voltage. When external Ca is decreased[80] or internal Ca is increased[248] Cx43 hemichannels open, forming large nonselective pores. Glial cells express several Cxs, the most prevalent is Cx43, which together with Cx26, Cx30, and Cx45, forms glial hemichannels and gap junctions with a large pore diameter (10–15Å),[249,250] which SPM can readily pass through. Because Cx38 hemichannels in *Xenopus* oocytes are permeable to SPD[251] and there are hemichannels in rat cortical astrocytes, most probably Cx43, permeable to PAs,[104] then, this makes the Cx pathway a likely candidate to be where uptake and release of SPM are regulated. Consistent with this possibility is the finding that gap junctions comprising Cx43 are not blocked by PAs, whereas others made from neuronal Cx40 are blocked by SPM.[252,253] An alternative potential pathway for SPM/SPD fluxes are Panx hemichannels, 3 of which (Panx1–3) are expressed in glia. These are nonselective pores that can open with normal external Ca levels.[239,247] However, Panx is not blocked by gadolinium,[254] whereas SPM flux in astrocytes is blocked by gadolinium, making Panxs an unlikely pathway.[255] In support of a direct exchange of SPM between the neuronal and glial cytoplasm via Cx hemichannels is the finding that larger dye molecules can pass between astrocytes, but not between oligodendrocytes or neurons or between neurons.[256] We have found that SPM/SPD fluxes are sensitive to Ca^{2+} and gadolinium (Gd^{3+}), favoring the possibility that Cx hemichannels rather than Panx hemichannels are the relevant pathway.[255–258]

As mentioned earlier, another potential mechanism for SPM/SPD fluxes in glial cells is through polyspecific cation transporters (OCTs).[192] These transporters can translocate monovalent, divalent, and even polyvalent cations such as SPM and SPD.[192,259] Polyspecific cation transporters (which include OCT1, OCT2, OCT3, and OCTN2, multidrug and toxin extrusion protein) are present in astrocytes and control signal transmission and energy homeostasis by removing released transmitters and substrates, such as dopamine, norepinephrine, epinephrine, 5-hydroxytryptamine, carnitine, and histamine, from the extracellular space.[260–263] OCT transporter messenger RNA has been found in cultured astrocytes[191,264,265] and has been well described.[192,266]

GLIA-CONTROLLED POLYAMINE REGULATION IN THE NEURONAL NETWORK

There should be a mechanistic basis to explain diseases, disorders, and syndromes that are associated with glia and with PAs. The glial membrane potential ($\sim$−85 mV) is typically 20 to 30 mV more hyperpolarized than resting neurons, therefore, polyvalent cations SPM^{4+} and SPD^{3+} are concentrated in glia by electrodiffusion via large pores (like Cx43) or OCTs (which require electrical transmembrane potential), because of this hyperpolarization. Once inside the cell, PAs are buffered by polyanions (eg, RNA, ATP, acid proteins) in the cytosol. When neurons are generating action potentials, there can be large transient decreases in extracellular Ca ($[Ca^{2+}]_o$)[267,268] and sodium ($[Na^+]_o$) levels, and an increase of potassium ($[K^+]_o$),[269] all of which accelerate both glial depolarization and hemichannel opening. With a delay of only a few minutes during ischemia, there is a dramatic increase of $[K^+]_o$ ($\leq$55 mM) and a lowering of $[Na^+]_o$, $[Cl^-]_o$, $[H^+]_o$ and $[Ca^{2+}]_o$ to 60 mM, 75 mM, pH = 6.5, and 0.08 mM from normal levels, respectively.[270–273] This situation provides favorable conditions for

Cx43 hemichannel opening that do not block OCTs. Normally, $[Ca^{2+}]_o$ can block Cx43 hemichannels.[80,248] During epilepsy, ischemia, spreading depression, or trauma, the activity of $[Ca^{2+}]_o$ is decreased by an order of magnitude from 1.2 to 0.06 mM.[270–273] This is a condition under which Cx43 hemichannels can open,[274,275] potentially allowing PAs to be released outside glia, where they may help to remove the external H^+ block of Cx43. Also, during ischemia, pH may reach acid levels of ~6.5 to 6.1,[270,272] and OCTs are depressed by acid pH and depolarization.[259,266,276] Therefore, the Cx43 and OCT pathways function differently: at normal conditions, OCTs are a major PA pathway, then, with excessive neuronal activation or ischemia, there is a stimulation that opens Cx43 hemichannels that allow the release of PAs, thus, conferring neuroprotection, as mentioned earlier, by blocking Ca^{2+}-permeable neuronal channels and preventing apoptosis.

Selective depolarization of astrocytes with aminoadipic acid changes the neuronal firing rate; this is blocked by carbenoxolone, a nonselective blocker of hemichannels.[256] This finding is consistent with the idea that hemichannels are key players in neuronal regulation. SPM/SPD release via hemichannels from astrocytes may be induced by depolarization (see **Fig. 1**B). The consequences of such release depend critically on which neuronal receptors are exposed to the potentially high localized release.

POLYAMINES: ROLE IN THE CENTRAL NERVOUS SYSTEM DISORDERS

Although previously unrecognized, recent data highlight dynamic signaling within glia and between glia and neurons via PAs. Many studies have reported neuroprotective effects of PAs.[91,108,120,172,184,277,278] Under pathologic conditions, PAs may be oxidized and converted to cytotoxic aldehydes and reactive oxygen species, which may be responsible for subsequent neurotoxic damage.[193,277] The downregulation of the synthesis of SPM caused by a mutation in the X chromosome causes Snyder-Robinson syndrome, which so severely affects human brain function that the result is mental retardation, hypotonia, and cerebellar dysfunction.[229,230] Conversely, unmodified PAs may block Ca^{2+}-permeable receptors and channels, which is critical in protecting neurons from apoptosis (see earlier discussion). Despite these recognized modifications and potential targets, the localization and dynamics of PAs in the brain are largely unknown.

What is important to know is that many of these disorders show a tight link between PAs and glia. SPM/SPD levels decline with age[96,100,156] and are involved in Parkinson disease.[279,280] These reports clearly show a vital role for PAs in brain plasticity. For instance, there is evidence that in brain diseases, PAs play a principal role in restoring age-related memory impairment,[100] because PA depletion stops mammalian cell growth and PA supplementation reverses the effect.[281] Treatments with SPD, agmatine, and by genetic modulation that increase endogenous PA levels resulted in not only an increase in life span[96] but also in memory restoration.[96,100,195] PA-rich nutrition increased the life span of aging mice,[97–99,282] whereas some amines and PAs (such as agmatine, arginine, PUT, SPD, SPM) are lost during aging and in the diseased CNS.[96,101,155,176–179,282] Also, PAs inhibit age-associated changes in global DNA methylation as well as dimethylhydrazine-induced tumor genesis.[99] It has been hypothesized that information in the brain can be stored (memory) in the chromatin (a complex of DNA-proteins-PAs) and can be changed during epigenetic chromatin modifications, as in Alzheimer disease, in which macrophages penetrate the brain via the leaky blood-brain barrier and probably cleave up memory proteins in chromatin.[283] Because glia (G) outnumber neurons (N) in the human brain (the G/N ratio reaches 11.35 in brainstem and 3.76 in cortex[20]), glia can represent a substantial source of memory capacity, especially given that PAs are bound to DNA in chromatin, to RNA, and to acid proteins.[110,164,284] There are severe psychiatric disorders directly linked with neuroglia and PA dysfunction, such as schizophrenia and mood disorders, in which failure of PA exchange is seen,[176–179] autism with disorders in the PA and Na-H exchange,[147,285] depression, which is associated with decreased glial cell mass, OCTs, and PA levels,[170,286] suicide, which correlates with PA homeostatic imbalances,[287] aging, in which glial cells lose PAs[98,99,282] and downregulate Ca^{2+} signaling,[232] and fear extinction, in which PAs reinforce extinction via NMDAR regulation.[288] Recently, many human CNS diseases have been linked with PA levels, including Alzheimer disease,[101,289,290] Parkinson disease,[126,291–293] Huntington disease,[164,294–297] and amyotrophic lateral sclerosis.[183,184,298] Despite a broad phenomenological description in the literature, there still remain functional links between PAs and glia in the brain that have not been mechanistically deciphered. However, what is known is that PAs are stored in glial cells, with the level of storage and PA buffering capacity depending solely on glial cells.

Therefore, research is focusing on glial-based PA-related CNS problems for several reasons. First, PAs are powerful modulators of the neuronal-glial network.[56,299] Second, PAs are accumulated preferentially in glial cells, not in neurons.[23–25] Third, PA homeostasis is critical for life.[96,100,181,182,300] Fourth, PA exchanges play a principal role in brain disorders, including inflammation,[220,222,223] depression,[286] and anxiety[301,302] (see earlier discussion). Fifth, PA-sensitive glial Kir4.1, Cx43/Cx30, and OCTs are fundamental for survival of the cells and whole brain.[29,73,74,124,125,205,209,211,219,226,245,255,266] Sixth, Cx43 and OCTs are candidates for PA uptake and release.[104,192,241,255,257,258] Because CNS disorders are closely related to PA exchange in stress and aging,[101,155,167,176–179] therapeutic supplement by PAs or their precursors have been suggested for neuroprotective treatment.[18,97–101,109,163,282,303] As for the supplemental therapy, attention should also be focused on PA carriers such as Cx43 and OCT proteins. Although there has been an increase in the research on PAs, the mechanisms of glial-dependent PA actions in the CNS are just beginning to be elucidated, and it seems that the glial-PA avenue for research has not yet been blueprinted; more work needs to be done.

SUMMARY

PAs are stored in glia[23–25] and together with their derivatives and precursors have been suggested as neuroprotective agents.[18,60,92,108,109,121,172,174,190,278,303] However, the oxidation of PAs results in toxic products such as aldehydes, which may be harmful for brain cells.[106] Lower-molecular-weight PAs have less toxicity. One of the PA precursors, agmatine (decarboxylated arginine or 1-(4-aminobutylguanidine)), is a natural product discovered more than 100 years ago in herring sperm,[304] and research indicates its exceptional modulatory action at multiple molecular targets, including neurotransmitter systems, nitric oxide, and PA production, therefore providing bases for current therapeutic applications. A triamine (SPD) and a diamine (PUT; 1,4-diaminobutane) were isolated from prokaryotic and eukaryotic systems, thereby showing that there are many sources of different PAs in any diet.[97–100,305,306] Recent preclinical and initial clinical evidence shows a positive effect of agmatine treatment,[18] making for challenging research opportunities for the use of agmatine in treating diabetes, neurologic trauma, neurodegeneration, different types of addictions, mood disorders, cancer, and cognitive and memory disorders. It seems that agmatine (aminoguanidine), guanidine-based drugs, and synthetic amines are examples of the best substrates for OCTs of the SLC22A subfamily,[192,307,308] which have been found and characterized in astrocytes and other glial cells in the brain.[259–266,276] Specifically, recent data show that a polymorphism of OCT1 is directly related to Parkinson disease,[309] and OCT3 is a key modulator of neurodegeneration in the nigrostriatal dopaminergic pathway.[310]

Therefore, not only should agmatine, SPD, and other PAs be a focus in designing future pharmaceutical tools to treat psychiatric disorders but also the PA transporter systems (eg, OCTs,[309,310] Cx43[104]) and buffering agents for Pas, such as acid proteins, ATP, and phosphates,[110] should be considered.

Targeting of certain disorders with PAs needs to be taken with great care, as, for example, in the case of gliomas, in which translocation of glial Kir4.1 and OCT3 from the glioma cell plasma membrane to the nuclear membrane[224–226] makes these important glial proteins unreachable by drugs from the extracellular space. The future challenge is to find drugs that are able to reach these crucial areas and modulate the PA system. Only this way will it be known if the modulation of the PA system can give us another tool in the fight against brain dysfunction.

REFERENCES

1. Ramón y Cajal S. Sobre un nuevo proceder de impregnación de la neuroglia y sus resultados en los centros nerviosos del hombre y animales. Trab Lab Invest Biol Univ Madrid 1913;11:219–37 [in Spanish].
2. Somjen GG. Nervenkitt: notes on the history of the concept of neuroglia. Glia 1988;1(1):2–9.
3. Beatty JT. The human brain: essentials of behavioral neuroscience. 1st edition. Thousand Oaks (CA): Sage Publications Inc; 2001.
4. Berlucchi G. The origin of the term plasticity in the neurosciences: Ernesto Lugaro and chemical synaptic transmission. J Hist Neurosci 2002;11(3): 305–9.
5. García-Marín V, García-López P, Freire M. Cajal's contributions to glia research. Trends Neurosci 2007;30(9):479–87.
6. García-Marín V, García-López P, Freire M. Cajal's contributions to the study of Alzheimer's disease. J Alzheimers Dis 2007;12(2):161–74.
7. DeFelipe J. Cajal and the discovery of a new artistic world: the neuronal forest. Prog Brain Res 2013;203:201–20.
8. Chvátal A, Anderová M, Neprasová H, et al. Pathological potential of astroglia. Physiol Res 2008;57(Suppl 3):S101–10.
9. Parpura V, Verkhratsky A. Neuroglia at the crossroads of homoeostasis, metabolism and signalling: evolution of the concept. ASN Neuro 2012;4(4):201–5.
10. Malatesta P, Hartfuss E, Götz M. Isolation of radial glial cells by fluorescent-activated cell sorting reveals a neuronal lineage. Development 2000;127(24): 5253–63.
11. Eriksson PS, Perfilieva E, Bjork-Eriksson T, et al. Neurogenesis in the adult human hippocampus. Nat Med 1998;4:1313–7.
12. Kaplan MS. Neurogenesis in the 3-month-old rat visual cortex. J Comp Neurol 1981;195(2):323–38.
13. Kriegstein A, Alvarez-Buylla A. The glial nature of embryonic and adult neural stem cells. Annu Rev Neurosci 2009;32:149–84.
14. Spassky N, Merkle FT, Flames N, et al. Adult ependymal cells are postmitotic and are derived from radial glial cells during embryogenesis. J Neurosci 2005;25(1):10–8.

15. Pilz GA, Shitamukai A, Reillo I, et al. Amplification of progenitors in the mammalian telencephalon includes a new radial glial cell type. Nat Commun 2013;4: 2125.

16. Hagemann TL, Paylor R, Messing A. Deficits in adult neurogenesis, contextual fear conditioning, and spatial learning in a Gfap mutant mouse model of Alexander disease. J Neurosci 2013;33(47):18698–706.

17. Betizeau M, Cortay V, Patti D, et al. Precursor diversity and complexity of lineage relationships in the outer subventricular zone of the primate. Neuron 2013;80(2): 442–57.

18. Piletz JE, Aricioglu F, Cheng JT, et al. Agmatine: clinical applications after 100 years in translation. Drug Discov Today 2013;18(17–18):880–93.

19. Reichenbach A. Glia: neuron index: review and hypothesis to account for different values in various mammals. Glia 1989;2:71–7.

20. Lent R, Azevedo FA, Andrade-Moraes CH, et al. How many neurons do you have? Some dogmas of quantitative neuroscience under revision. Eur J Neurosci 2012;35(1):1–9.

21. Erlichman JS, Leiter JC, Gourine AV. ATP, glia and central respiratory control. Respir Physiol Neurobiol 2010;173(3):305–11.

22. Gourine AV, Kasymov V, Marina N, et al. Astrocytes control breathing through pH-dependent release of ATP. Science 2010;329(5991):571–5.

23. Laube G, Veh RW. Astrocytes, not neurons, show most prominent staining for spermine/spermidine-like immunoreactivity in adult rat brain. Glia 1997;19(2):171–9.

24. Biedermann B, Skatchkov SN, Bringmann A, et al. Spermine/spermidine is expressed by retinal glial (Müller) cells, and controls distinct K+ channels of their membrane. Glia 1998;23:209–20.

25. Skatchkov SN, Eaton MJ, Krušek J, et al. Spatial distribution of spermine/spermidine content and K^+- current rectification in frog retinal glial (Müller) cells. Glia 2000;31:84–90.

26. Franze K, Grosche J, Skatchkov SN, et al. Müller cells are living optical fibers in the vertebrate retina. PNAS 2007;104:8287–92.

27. Reichenbach A, Franze K, Agte S, et al. Live cells as optical fibers in the vertebrate retina. In: Yasin M, Harun SW, Arof H, editors. Selected topics on optical fiber technology. InTech; 2012. p. 247–70.

28. Grishin EV, Volkova TM, Arsen'ev AS, et al. Structural-functional characteristics of argiopine–the ion channel blockers from the spider Argiope lobata venom. Bioorg Khim 1986;12(8):1121–4 [in Russian].

29. Grishin EV, Volkova TM, Arsen'ev AS. Glutamate receptor antagonists from the spider Argiope lobata venom. Bioorg Khim 1988;14(7):883–92.

30. Antonov SM, Grishin EV, Magazanik LG, et al. Argiopin blocks the glutamate responses and sensorimotor transmission in motoneurones of isolated frog spinal cord. Neurosci Lett 1987;83(1–2):179–84.

31. Frølund S, Bella A, Kristensen AS, et al. Assessment of structurally diverse philanthotoxin analogues for inhibitory activity on ionotropic glutamate receptor subtypes: discovery of nanomolar, nonselective, and use-dependent antagonists. J Med Chem 2010;53(20):7441–51.

32. Skatchkov SN, Rojas L, Eaton MJ, et al. Functional expression of Kir 6.1/SUR1-Katp channels in frog retinal Müller glial cells. Glia 2002;38:256–67.

33. Kucheryavykh YV, Shuba YM, Antonov SM, et al. Complex rectification of Müller cell Kir currents. Glia 2008;56:775–90.

34. Williams K. Modulation and block of ion channels: a new biology of polyamines. Cell Signal 1997;9:1–13.

35. Haghighi AP, Cooper E. Neuronal nicotinic acetylcholine receptors are blocked by intracellular spermine in a voltage-dependent manner. J Neurosci 1998;18: 4050–62.
36. Bowie D, Mayer ML. Inward rectification of both AMPA and kainate subtype glutamate receptors generated by polyamine-mediated ion channel block. Neuron 1995;15:453–62.
37. Fakler B, Brandle U, Glowatzki E, et al. Strong voltage-dependent inward rectification of inward rectifier K^+ channels is caused by intracellular spermine. Cell 1995;13:149–54.
38. Ahern GP, Wang X, Miyares RL. Polyamines are potent ligands for the capsaicin receptor TRPV1. J Biol Chem 2006;281:8991–5.
39. Lopatin AN, Makhina EN, Nichols CG. Potassium channel block by cytoplasmic polyamines as the mechanism of intrinsic rectification. Nature 1994;372:366–9.
40. Fakler B, Brandle U, Bond C, et al. A structural determinant of differentially sensitivity of cloned inward rectifier K^+ channels to intracellular spermine. FEBS Lett 1994;356:199–203.
41. Shao Z, Mellor IR, Brierley MJ, et al. Potentiation and inhibition of nicotinic acetylcholine receptors by spermine in the TE671 human muscle cell line. J Pharmacol Exp Ther 1998;186:1269–76.
42. Koh DS, Burnashev N, Jonas P. Block of native Ca(2+)-permeable AMPA receptors in rat brain by intracellular polyamines generates double rectification. J Physiol 1995;486:305–12.
43. Koenig H, Goldstone AD, Lu CY, et al. Brain polyamines are controlled by N-methyl-D-aspartate receptors during ischemia and recirculation. Stroke 1990;21:III98–102.
44. Lynch JW. Rectification of the olfactory cyclic nucleotide-gated channel by intracellular polyamines. J Membr Biol 1999;170:213–27.
45. Huang CJ, Moczydlowski E. Cytoplasmic polyamines as permeant blockers and modulators of the voltage-gated sodium channel. Biophys J 2001;80: 1262–79.
46. Antonov SM, Gmiro VE, Johnson JW. Binding sites for permeant ions in the channel of NMDA receptors and their effects on channel block. Nat Neurosci 1998;1(6):451–61.
47. Davies MS, Baganoff MP, Grishin EV, et al. Polyamine spider toxins are potent uncompetitive antagonists of rat cortex excitatory amino acid receptors. Eur J Pharmacol 1992;227(1):51–6.
48. Donevan SD, Rogawski MA. Intracellular polyamines mediate inward rectification of Ca(2+)-permeable alpha-amino-3-hydroxy-5-methyl-4-isoxazolepropionic acid receptors. Proc Natl Acad Sci U S A 1995;92:9298–302.
49. Vataev SI, Oganesian GA, Lukomskaia NI, et al. The action of ionotropic glutamate receptor channel blockers on effects of sleep deprivation in rats. Ross Fiziol Zh Im I M Sechenova 2013;99(5):575–85 [in Russian].
50. Abushik PA, Sibarov DA, Eaton MJ, et al. Kainate-induced calcium overload of cortical neurons in vitro: dependence on expression of AMPAR GluA2-subunit and down-regulation by subnanomolar ouabain. Cell Calcium 2013;54(2):95–104.
51. Benveniste M, Mayer ML. Multiple effects of spermine on N-methyl-D-aspartic acid receptor responses of rat cultured hippocampal neurones. J Physiol 1993;464:131–63.
52. Bahring R, Bowie D, Benveniste M, et al. Permeation and block of rat GluR6 glutamate receptor channels by internal and external polyamines. J Physiol 1997;502:575–89.

53. Araneda RC, Lan JY, Zheng X, et al. Spermine and arcaine block and permeate N-methyl-D-aspartate receptor channels. Biophys J 1999;76:2899–911.
54. Quinn SJ, Ye CP, Diaz R, et al. The Ca2+-sensing receptor: a target for polyamines. Am J Physiol 1997;273:C1315–23.
55. Jiang X, Newell EW, Schlichter LC. Regulation of a TRPM7-like current in rat brain microglia. J Biol Chem 2003;278:42867–76.
56. Rozov A, Burnashev N. Polyamine-dependent facilitation of postsynaptic AMPA receptors counteracts paired-pulse depression. Nature 1999;401:594–8.
57. Isa T, Iion M, Itazawa S, et al. Spermine mediates inward rectification of Ca(2+)-permeable AMPA receptor channels. Neuroreport 1996;6:2045–8.
58. Mott DD, Washburn MS, Zhang S, et al. Subunit-dependent modulation of kainate receptors by extracellular protons and polyamines. J Neurosci 2003;23:1179–88.
59. Lindquist TD, Sturman JA, Gould RM, et al. Axonal transport of polyamines in intact and regenerating axons of the rat sciatic nerve. J Neurochem 1985;44:1913–9.
60. Gilad GM, Balakrishnan K, Gilad VH. The course of putrescine immunocytochemical appearance in neurons, astroglia and microglia in rat brain cultures. Neurosci Lett 1999;268:33–6.
61. Araque A, Parpura V, Sanzgiri RP, et al. Tripartite synapses: glia, the unacknowledged partner. Trends Neurosci 1999;22:208–15.
62. Perea G, Araque A. Astrocytes potentiate transmitter release at single hippocampal synapses. Science 2007;317:1083–6.
63. Bacaj T, Tevlin M, Lu Y, et al. Glia are essential for sensory organ function in C. elegans. Science 2008;322:744–7.
64. Keyser DO, Pellmar TC. Synaptic transmission in the hippocampus: critical role of glia. Glia 1994;10:237–43.
65. Fonnum F, Johnsen A, Hassel B. Use of fluorocitrate and fluoroacetate in the study of brain metabolism. Glia 1997;21:106–13.
66. Zonta M, Angulo MC, Gobbo S, et al. Neuron-to-astrocyte signaling is central to the dynamic control of brain microcirculation. Nat Neurosci 2003;6:43–50.
67. Attwell D, Buchan AM, Charpak S, et al. Glial and neuronal control of brain blood flow. Nature 2010;468(7321):232–43.
68. Norenberg MD, Neary JT, Bender AS, et al. Hepatic encephalopathy: a disorder in glial-neuronal communication. Prog Brain Res 1992;94:261–9.
69. Dubois-Dauphin M, Poitry-Yamate C, de Bilbao F, et al. Early postnatal Müller cell death leads to retinal but not optic nerve degeneration in NSE-Hu-Bcl-2 transgenic mice. Neuroscience 2000;95:9–21.
70. Orkand RK, Nicholls JG, Kuffler SW. Effect of nerve impulses on the membrane potential of glial cells in the central nervous system of amphibia. J Neurophysiol 1966;29:788–806.
71. Newman EA, Frambach DA, Odette LL. Control of extracellular potassium levels by retinal glial cell K+ siphoning. Science 1984;225(4667):1174–5.
72. Kofuji P, Ceelen P, Zahs KR, et al. Genetic inactivation of an inwardly rectifying potassium channel (Kir4.1 subunit) in mice: phenotypic impact in retina. J Neurosci 2000;20:5733–40.
73. Kucheryavykh YV, Kucheryavykh LY, Nichols CG, et al. Downregulation of Kir4.1 inward rectifying potassium channel subunits by RNAi impairs potassium transfer and glutamate uptake by cultured cortical astrocytes. Glia 2007;55:274–81.
74. Djukic B, Casper JB, Philpot BD, et al. Conditional knock-out of Kir4.1 leads to glial membrane depolarization, inhibition of potassium and glutamate uptake, and enhanced short-term synaptic potentiation. J Neurosci 2007;27:11354–65.

75. Stevens ER, Esguerra M, Kim PM, et al. D-serine and serine racemase are present in the vertebrate retina and contribute to the physiological activation of NMDA receptors. Proc Natl Acad Sci U S A 2003;100(11):6789–94.

76. Newman EA. Glial cell inhibition of neurons by release of ATP. J Neurosci 2003;23:1659–66.

77. Newman EA. Glial control of synaptic transmission in the retina. Glia 2004;47:268–74.

78. Parpura V, Basarsky TA, Liu F, et al. Glutamate-mediated astrocyte-neuron signaling. Nature 1994;369:744–7.

79. Araque A, Carmignoto G, Haydon PG. Dynamic signaling between astrocytes and neurons. Annu Rev Physiol 2001;63:795–813.

80. Ye ZC, Wyeth MS, Baltan-Tekkok S, et al. Functional hemichannels in astrocytes: a novel mechanism of glutamate release. J Neurosci 2003;23:3588–96.

81. Filosa JA, Bonev AD, Straub SV, et al. Local potassium signaling couples neuronal activity to vasodilation in the brain. Nat Neurosci 2006;9:1397–403.

82. Metea MR, Kofuji P, Newman EA. Neurovascular coupling is not mediated by potassium siphoning from glial cells. J Neurosci 2007;27:2468–71.

83. Miller RF. D-Serine as a glial modulator of nerve cells. Glia 2005;47(3):275–83.

84. Sullivan SJ, Miller RF. AMPA receptor-dependent, light-evoked D-serine release acts on retinal ganglion cell NMDA receptors. J Neurophysiol 2012;108(4):1044–51.

85. Viviani B, Corsini E, Galli CL, et al. Glia increase degeneration of hippocampal neurons through release of tumor necrosis factor-alpha. Toxicol Appl Pharmacol 1998;150(2):271–6.

86. Halassa MM, Fellin T, Haydon PG. Tripartite synapses: roles for astrocytic purines in the control of synaptic physiology and behavior. Neuropharmacology 2009;57(4):343–6.

87. Burnashev N. Dynamic modulation of AMPA receptor mediated synaptic transmission by polyamines in principal neurons. Focus on polyamines modulate AMPA receptor-dependent synaptic response in immature layer V pyramidal neurons. J Neurophysiol 2005;93:2371–86.

88. Washburn MS, Numberger M, Zhang S, et al. Differential dependence on GluR2 expression of three characteristic features of AMPA receptors. J Neurosci 1997;17:9393–406.

89. Noh KM, Yokota H, Mashiko T, et al. Blockade of calcium-permeable AMPA receptors protects hippocampal neurons against global ischemia-induced death. Proc Natl Acad Sci U S A 2005;102:12230–5.

90. Mulle C, Sailer A, Swanson GT, et al. Subunit composition of kainate receptors in hippocampal interneurons. Neuron 2000;28:475–84.

91. Liu B, Liao M, Mielke JG, et al. Ischemic insults direct glutamate receptor subunit 2-lacking AMPA receptors to synaptic sites. J Neurosci 2006;26:5309–19.

92. Bell JD, Ai J, Chen Y, et al. Mild in vitro trauma induces rapid GluR-2 endocytosis, robustly augments calcium permeability and enhances susceptibility to secondary excitotoxic insult in cultured Purkinje cells. Brain 2007;130:2528–42.

93. Dingledine R, Borges K, Bowie D, et al. The glutamate receptor ion channels. Pharmacol Rev 1999;51(1):7–61.

94. Bowie D. Redefining the classification of AMPA-selective ionotropic glutamate receptors. J Physiol 2012;590(Pt 1):49–61.

95. Sibarov DA, Bolshakov AE, Abushik PA, et al. Na+,K+-ATPase functionally interacts with the plasma membrane Na+,Ca2+ exchanger to prevent Ca2+

overload and neuronal apoptosis in excitotoxic stress. J Pharmacol Exp Ther 2012;343(3):596–607.

96. Eisenberg T, Knauer H, Schauer A, et al. Induction of autophagy by spermidine promotes longevity. Nat Cell Biol 2009;11(11):1305–14.

97. Soda K, Dobashi Y, Kano Y, et al. Polyamine-rich food decreases age-associated pathology and mortality in aged mice. Exp Gerontol 2009;44(11): 727–32.

98. Soda K. Polyamine intake, dietary pattern, and cardiovascular disease. Med Hypotheses 2010;75(3):299–301.

99. Soda K, Kano Y, Chiba F, et al. Increased polyamine intake inhibits age-associated alteration in global DNA methylation and 1,2-dimethylhydrazine-induced tumorigenesis. PLoS One 2013;8(5):e64357.

100. Gupta VK, Scheunemann L, Eisenberg T, et al. Restoring polyamines protects from age-induced memory impairment in an autophagy-dependent manner. Nat Neurosci 2013;16:1453–60.

101. Liu P, Fleete MS, Jing Y, et al. Altered arginine metabolism in Alzheimer's disease brains. Neurobiol Aging 2014;35(9):1992–2003.

102. Cervós-Navarro J, Diemer NH. Selective vulnerability in brain hypoxia. Crit Rev Neurobiol 1991;6:149–82.

103. Velloso NA, Dalmolin GD, Fonini G, et al. Spermine attenuates behavioral and biochemical alterations induced by quinolinic acid in the striatum of rats. Brain Res 2008;1198:107–14.

104. Benedikt J, Inyushin M, Kucheryavykh YV, et al. Intracellular polyamines enhance astrocytic coupling. Neuroreport 2012;23(17):1021–5.

105. Shalaby IA, Chenard BL, Prochniak MA, et al. Neuroprotective effects of the N-methyl-D-aspartate receptor antagonists ifenprodil and SL-82, 0715 on hippocampal cells in culture. J Pharmacol Exp Ther 1992;260:925–32.

106. Sparapani M, Dall'Olio R, Gandolfi O, et al. Neurotoxicity of polyamines and pharmacological neuroprotection in cultures of rat cerebellar granule cells. Exp Neurol 1997;148:157–66.

107. Adachi K, Izumi M, Osano Y, et al. Polyamine concentrations in the brain of vitamin B12-deficient rats. Exp Biol Med 2003;228:1069–71.

108. Ferchmin PA, Pérez D, Biello M. Spermine is neuroprotective against anoxia and N-methyl-D-aspartate in hippocampal slices. Brain Res 2000;859:273–9.

109. Gilad GM, Gilad VH. Polyamines can protect against ischemia-induced nerve cell death in gerbil forebrain. Exp Neurol 1991;111:349–55.

110. Watanabe S, Kusama-Eguchi K, Kobayashi H, et al. Estimation of polyamine binding to macromolecules and ATP in bovine lymphocytes and rat liver. J Biol Chem 1991;266:20803–9.

111. Seiler N. Formation, catabolism and properties of the natural polyamines. In: Carter C, editor. The neuropharmacology of polyamines. New York; London: Academic; Harcourt Brace; 1994. p. 1–36.

112. Seiler N, Delcros JG, Moulinoux JP. Polyamine transport in mammalian cells. An update. Int J Biochem Cell Biol 1996;28:843–61.

113. Masuko T, Kusama-Eguchi K, Sakata K, et al. Polyamine transport, accumulation and release in brain. J Neurochem 2003;84:610–7.

114. Ingoglia NA, Sturman JA, Eisner RA. Axonal transport of putrescine, spermidine and spermine in normal and regenerating goldfish optic nerve. Brain Res 1977; 130:433–45.

115. Ingoglia NA, Sharma SC, Pilchman J, et al. Axonal transport and transcellular transfer of nucleosides and polyamines in intact and regenerating optic nerves

of goldfish: speculation on the axonal regulation of periaxonal cell metabolism. J Neurosci 1982;2:1412–23.

116. Ingoglia NA, Sturman JA, Jaggard P, et al. Association of spermine and 4S RNA during axonal transport in regenerating optic nerves of goldfish. Brain Res 1982; 238:341–51.

117. Cohen SS. Introduction to the polyamines. Englewood Cliffs (NJ): Prentice-Hall; 1971.

118. Wallace HM. The polyamines: past, present and future. Essays Biochem 2009; 46:1–9.

119. Krauss M, Langnaese K, Richter K, et al. Spermidine synthase is prominently expressed in the striatal patch compartment and in putative interneurons of matrix compartments. J Neurochem 2006;1:174–89.

120. Krauss M, Weiss T, Langnaese K, et al. Cellular and subcellular rat brain spermidine synthase expression patterns suggest region-specific roles for polyamines, including cerebellar pre-synaptic function. J Neurochem 2007;103: 679–93.

121. Gilad GM, Gilad VH. Polyamine uptake, binding and release in rat brain. Eur J Pharmacol 1991;193(1):41–6.

122. Laschet J, Grisar T, Bureau M, et al. Characteristics of putrescine uptake and subsequent GABA formation in primary cultured astrocytes from normal C57BL/6J and epileptic DBA/2J mouse brain cortices. Neuroscience 1992;48: 151–7.

123. Laschet J, Trottier S, Leviel V, et al. Heterogeneous distribution of polyamines in temporal lobe epilepsy. Epilepsy Res 1999;35:161–72.

124. Dot J, Lluch M, Blanco I, et al. Polyamine uptake in cultured astrocytes: characterization and modulation by protein kinases. J Neurochem 2000;75: 1917–26.

125. Dot J, Danchev N, Blanco I, et al. Polyamine uptake is necessary for a normal biochemical maturation of astrocytes in culture. Neuroreport 2002;13:1083–7.

126. De La Hera DP, Corradi GR, Adamo HP, et al. Parkinson's disease-associated human P5B-ATPase ATP13A2 increases spermidine uptake. Biochem J 2013; 450(1):47–53.

127. Valentino TL, Lukasiewicz PD, Romano C. Immunocytochemical localization of polyamines in tiger salamander retina. Brain Res 1996;713:278–85.

128. Cintra A, Fuxe K, Agnati LF, et al. Evidence for the existence of ornithine decarboxylase-immunoreactive neurons in the rat brain. Neurosci Lett 1987;76: 269–74.

129. Dorn A, Müller M, Bernstein HG, et al. Immunohistochemical localization of L-ornithine decarboxylase in developing rat brain. Int J Dev Neurosci 1987;5:145–50.

130. Fujiwara K, Bai G, Kitagawa T. Polyamine-like immunoreactivity in rat neurons. Brain Res 1997;767:166–71.

131. Soulet D, Gagnon B, Rivest S, et al. A fluorescent probe of polyamine transport accumulates into intracellular acidic vesicles via a two-step mechanism. J Biol Chem 2004;279(47):49355–66.

132. Poulin R, Casero RA, Soulet D. Recent advances in the molecular biology of metazoan polyamine transport. Amino Acids 2012;42(2–3):711–23.

133. De Keyser J, Mostert JP, Koch MW. Dysfunctional astrocytes as key players in the pathogenesis of central nervous system disorders. J Neurol Sci 2008; 267(1–2):3–16.

134. Ricci G, Volpi L, Pasquali L, et al. Astrocyte-neuron interactions in neurological disorders. J Biol Phys 2009;35(4):317–36.

135. Suzuki M, Van Paesschen W, Stalmans I, et al. Defective membrane expression of the Na(+)-HCO(3)(-) cotransporter NBCe1 is associated with familial migraine. Proc Natl Acad Sci U S A 2010;107(36):15963–8.

136. Kettenmann H, Ransom BR, editors. Neuroglia. 3rd edition. New York: Oxford University Press; 2012.

137. Cooper MS. Intercellular signaling in neuronal-glial networks. Biosystems 1995; 34(1–3):65–85.

138. Cooper ZD, Jones JD, Comer SD. Glial modulators: a novel pharmacological approach to altering the behavioral effects of abused substances. Expert Opin Investig Drugs 2012;21(2):169–78.

139. Verkhratsky A, Orkand RK, Kettenmann H. Glial calcium: homeostasis and signaling function. Physiol Rev 1998;78(1):99–141.

140. Verkhratsky A, Noda M, Parpura V, et al. Sodium fluxes and astroglial function. Adv Exp Med Biol 2013;961:295–305.

141. Verkhratsky A, Rodríguez JJ, Parpura V. Astroglia in neurological diseases. Future Neurol 2013;8(2):149–58.

142. Verkhratsky A, Rodríguez JJ, Steardo L. Astrogliopathology: a central element of neuropsychiatric diseases? Neuroscientist 2013. [Epub ahead of print].

143. Seidl R, Beninati S, Cairns N, et al. Polyamines in frontal cortex of patients with Down syndrome and Alzheimer disease. Neurosci Lett 1996;206(2–3):193–5.

144. Seitz R, Ohlmann A, Tamm ER. The role of Müller glia and microglia in glaucoma. Cell Tissue Res 2013;353(2):339–45.

145. Turner JR, Ecke LE, Briand LA, et al. Cocaine-related behaviors in mice with deficient gliotransmission. Psychopharmacology (Berl) 2013;226(1):167–76.

146. Dalkara T, Kiliç K. How does fasting trigger migraine? A hypothesis. Curr Pain Headache Rep 2013;17(10):368.

147. Zeidán-Chuliá F, Salmina AB, Malinovskaya NA, et al. The glial perspective of autism spectrum disorders. Neurosci Biobehav Rev 2014;38:160–72.

148. Scofield MD, Kalivas PW. Astrocytic dysfunction and addiction: consequences of impaired glutamate homeostasis. Neuroscientist 2014. [Epub ahead of print].

149. Clasadonte J, McIver SR, Schmitt LI, et al. Chronic sleep restriction disrupts sleep homeostasis and behavioral sensitivity to alcohol by reducing the extracellular accumulation of adenosine. J Neurosci 2014;34(5):1879–91.

150. Jo WK, Law AC, Chung SK. The neglected co-star in the dementia drama: the putative roles of astrocytes in the pathogeneses of major neurocognitive disorders. Mol Psychiatry 2014;19(2):159–67.

151. Classic pages in obstetrics and gynecology. Observationes...de natis è seminegenitali animalculis. Antoni Van Leeuwenhoek. Philosophical Transactions of the Royal Society (London), vol. 12, pp. 1040-1043, 1678-1679. Am J Obstet Gynecol 1978;131(4):469–70.

152. Dudley HW, Rosenheim O, Starling WW. The chemical constitution of spermine. III. Structure and synthesis. Biochem J 1926;20:1082–94.

153. Bachrach U. The early history of polyamine research. Plant Physiol Biochem 2010;48(7):490–5.

154. Redgate ES, Boggs S, Grudziak A, et al. Polyamines in brain tumor therapy. J Neurooncol 1995;25:167–79.

155. Minois N. Molecular basis of the 'anti-aging' effect of spermidine and other natural polyamines–a mini-review. Gerontology 2014;60(4):319–26.

156. LaRocca TJ, Gioscia-Ryan RA, Hearon CM Jr, et al. The autophagy enhancer spermidine reverses arterial aging. Mech Ageing Dev 2013;134(7–8):314–20.

157. Heby O. Role of polyamines in the control of cell proliferation and differentiation. Differentiation 1981;19:1–20.
158. Johnson TD. Modulation of channel function by polyamines. Trends Pharmacol Sci 1996;17:22–7.
159. Nichols CG, Lopatin AN. Inward rectifier potassium channels. Annu Rev Physiol 1997;59:171–91.
160. Skatchkov SN, Buldakova S, Kucheryavykh YV, et al. Neuronal network regulation in ca1 hippocampus: role of glial polyamines and hemichannels. J Neurochem 2006;96(Suppl 1, Symposium 08):138.
161. Rubin MA, Boemo RL, Jurach A, et al. Intrahippocampal spermidine administration improves inhibitory avoidance performance in rats. Behav Pharmacol 2000; 11:57–62.
162. Rubin MA, Stiegemeier JA, Volkweis MA, et al. Intra-amygdala spermidine administration improves inhibitory avoidance performance in rats. Eur J Pharmacol 2001;423:35–9.
163. Rubin MA, Berlese DB, Stiegemeier JA, et al. Intra-amygdala administration of polyamines modulates fear conditioning in rats. J Neurosci 2004;24: 2328–34.
164. Velloso NA, Dalmolin GD, Gomes GM, et al. Spermine improves recognition memory deficit in a rodent model of Huntington's disease. Neurobiol Learn Mem 2009;92(4):574–80.
165. Genedani S, Piccinini G, Bertolini A. Putrescine has analgesic activity, in rats. Life Sci 1984;34:2407–12.
166. Kolhekar R, Meller ST, Gephart GF. N-methyl-D-aspartate receptor-mediated changes in thermal nociception: allosteric modulation at glycine and polyamine recognition sites. Neuroscience 1994;63:925–36.
167. Adibhatla RM, Hatcher JF, Sailor K, et al. Polyamines and central nervous system injury: spermine and spermidine decrease following transient focal cerebral ischemia in spontaneously hypertensive rats. Brain Res 2002;938: 81–6.
168. Clarkson AN, Liu H, Pearson L, et al. Neuroprotective effects of spermine following hypoxic-ischemic-induced brain damage: a mechanistic study. FASEB J 2004;2004(18):1114–6.
169. Yin HZ, Tang DT, Weiss JH. Intrathecal infusion of a Ca(2+)-permeable AMPA channel blocker slows loss of both motor neurons and of the astrocyte glutamate transporter, GLT-1 in a mutant SOD1 rat model of ALS. Exp Neurol 2007; 207:177–85.
170. Ongur D, Drevets WC, Price JL. Glial reduction in the subgenual prefrontal cortex in mood disorders. Proc Natl Acad Sci U S A 1998;95(22):13290–5.
171. Zomkowski AD, Santos AR, Rodrigues AL. Putrescine produces antidepressant-like effects in the forced swimming test and in the tail suspension test in mice. Prog Neuropsychopharmacol Biol Psychiatry 2005;30:1419–25.
172. Bellé NA, Dalmolin GD, Fonini G, et al. Polyamines reduces lipid peroxidation induced by different pro-oxidant agents. Brain Res 2004;1008:245–51.
173. Shaw GG, Pateman AJ. The regional distribution of the polyamines spermidine and spermine in brain. J Neurochem 1973;20:1225–30.
174. Halaris A, Piletz JE. Relevance of imidazoline receptors and agmatine to psychiatry: a decade of progress. Ann N Y Acad Sci 2003;1009:1–20.
175. Peters D, Berger J, Langnaese K, et al. Arginase and arginine decarboxylase—where do the putative gate keepers of polyamine synthesis reside in rat brain? PLoS One 2013;8(6):e66735.

176. Bernstein HG, Müller M. The cellular localization of L-ornithine decarboxylase-polyamine system in the normal and diseased central nervous system. Prog Neurobiol 1999;57:485–505.

177. Bernstein HG, Steiner J, Bogerts B. Glial cells in schizophrenia: pathophysiological significance and possible consequences for therapy. Expert Rev Neurother 2009;9(7):1059–71.

178. Bernstein HG, Derst C, Stich C, et al. The agmatine-degrading enzyme agmatinase: a key to agmatine signaling in rat and human brain? Amino Acids 2011; 40:453–65.

179. Bernstein HG, Stich C, Jäger K, et al. Agmatinase, an inactivator of the putative endogenous antidepressant agmatine, is strongly upregulated in hippocampal interneurons of subjects with mood disorders. Neuropharmacology 2012; 62(1):237–46.

180. Abdulhussein AA, Wallace HM. Polyamines and membrane transporters. Amino Acids 2014;46(3):655–60.

181. Pegg AE. Mammalian polyamine metabolism and function. IUBMB Life 2009;61: 880–94.

182. Pegg AE. The function of spermine. IUBMB Life 2014;66(1):8–18.

183. Virgili M, Crochemore C, Pena-Altamira E, et al. Regional and temporal alterations of ODC/polyamine system during ALS-like neurodegenerative motor syndrome in G93A transgenic mice. Neurochem Int 2006;48:201–7.

184. Tracey KJ. The inflammatory reflex. Nature 2002;429:853–9.

185. Sequeira A, Gwadry FG, Ffrench-Mullen JM, et al. Implication of SSAT by gene expression and genetic variation in suicide and major depression. Arch Gen Psychiatry 2006;63:35–48.

186. Withrow C, Ashraf S, O'Leary T, et al. Effect of polyamine depletion on cone photoreceptors of the developing rabbit retina. Invest Ophthalmol Vis Sci 2002;43: 3081–90.

187. Jänne J, Alhonen L, Keinänen TA, et al. Animal disease models generated by genetic engineering of polyamine metabolism. J Cell Mol Med 2005;9: 865–82.

188. Jänne J, Alhonen L, Pietilä M, et al. Genetic manipulation of polyamine catabolism in rodents. J Biochem 2006;139:155–60.

189. Madai VI, Poller WC, Peters D, et al. Synaptic localisation of agmatinase in rat cerebral cortex revealed by virtual pre-embedding. Amino Acids 2012;43(3): 1399–403.

190. Gilad GM, Gilad VH, Finberg JP, et al. Neurochemical evidence for agmatine modulation of 1-methyl-4-phenyl-1,2,3,6-tetrahydropyridine (MPTP) neurotoxicity. Neurochem Res 2005;30(6–7):713–9.

191. Inazu M, Takeda H, Maehara K, et al. Functional expression of the organic cation/carnitine transporter 2 in rat astrocytes. J Neurochem 2006;97:424–34.

192. Sala-Rabanal M, Li DC, Inyushin M, et al. Polyamine transport by the polyspecific organic cation transporters OCT1, OCT2 and OCT3. Mol Pharm 2013; 10(4):1450–8.

193. Medeiros R, Laferla FM. Astrocytes: conductors of the Alzheimer disease neuroinflammatory symphony. Exp Neurol 2012;239:133–8.

194. Iliff JJ, Wang M, Liao Y, et al. A paravascular pathway facilitates CSF flow through the brain parenchyma and the clearance of interstitial solutes, including amyloid β. Sci Transl Med 2012;4(147):147ra111.

195. Sigrist SJ, Carmona-Gutierrez D, Gupta VK, et al. Spermidine-triggered autophagy ameliorates memory during aging. Autophagy 2014;10(1):178–9.

196. Nilsen LH, Witter MP, Sonnewald U. Neuronal and astrocytic metabolism in a transgenic rat model of Alzheimer's disease. J Cereb Blood Flow Metab 2014. http://dx.doi.org/10.1038/jcbfm.2014.37.

197. Johansson A, Engler H, Blomquist G, et al. Evidence for astrocytosis in ALS demonstrated by [11C](L)-deprenyl-D2 PET. J Neurol Sci 2007;255(1–2):17–22.

198. Martorana F, Brambilla L, Valori CF, et al. The BH4 domain of Bcl-X(L) rescues astrocyte degeneration in amyotrophic lateral sclerosis by modulating intracellular calcium signals. Hum Mol Genet 2012;21(4):826–40.

199. Sunyach C, Michaud M, Arnoux T, et al. Olesoxime delays muscle denervation, astrogliosis, microglial activation and motoneuron death in an ALS mouse model. Neuropharmacology 2012;62(7):2346–52.

200. Messing A, Brenner M, Feany MB, et al. Alexander disease. J Neurosci 2012; 32(15):5017–23.

201. Vila M, Jackson-Lewis V, Guégan C, et al. The role of glial cells in Parkinson's disease. Curr Opin Neurol 2001;14(4):483–9.

202. Rempe DA, Nedergaard M. Targeting glia for treatment of neurological disease. Neurotherapeutics 2010;7(4):335–7.

203. Cisbani G, Freeman TB, Soulet D, et al. Striatal allografts in patients with Huntington's disease: impact of diminished astrocytes and vascularization on graft viability. Brain 2013;136(Pt 2):433–43.

204. Chakraborty J, Singh R, Dutta D, et al. Quercetin improves behavioral deficiencies, restores astrocytes and microglia, and reduces serotonin metabolism in 3-nitropropionic acid-induced rat model of Huntington's disease. CNS Neurosci Ther 2014;20(1):10–9.

205. Srivastava R, Aslam M, Kalluri SR, et al. Potassium channel KIR4.1 as an immune target in multiple sclerosis. N Engl J Med 2012;367:115–23.

206. Palumbo S, Bosetti F. Alterations of brain eicosanoid synthetic pathway in multiple sclerosis and in animal models of demyelination: role of cyclooxygenase-2. Prostaglandins Leukot Essent Fatty Acids 2013;89(5):273–8.

207. Hinterkeuser S, Schroder W, Hager JG, et al. Astrocytes in the hippocampus of patients with temporal lobe epilepsy display changes in potassium conductances. Eur J Neurosci 2000;12:2087–96.

208. Bockenhauer D, Feather S, Stanescu HC, et al. Epilepsy, ataxia, sensorineural deafness, tubulopathy, and KCNJ10 mutations. N Engl J Med 2009;360:1960–70.

209. Inyushin M, Kucheryavykh LY, Kucheryavykh YV, et al. Potassium channel activity and glutamate uptake are impaired in astrocytes of seizure susceptible DBA/2 mice. Epilepsia 2010;51(9):1707–13.

210. Sala-Rabanal M, Kucheryavykh LY, Skatchkov SN, et al. Molecular mechanisms of EAST/SeSAME syndrome mutations in Kir4.1 (KCNJ10). J Biol Chem 2010; 285:36040–8.

211. Wallraff A, Köhling R, Heinemann U, et al. The impact of astrocytic gap junctional coupling on potassium buffering in the hippocampus. J Neurosci 2006; 26:5438–47.

212. Steinhäuser C, Seifert G, Bedner P. Astrocyte dysfunction in temporal lobe epilepsy: K+ channels and gap junction coupling. Glia 2012;60:1192–202.

213. Steinhäuser C, Boison D. Epilepsy: crucial role for astrocytes. Glia 2012;60(8):1191.

214. Boison D. Adenosine dysfunction in epilepsy. Glia 2012;60(8):1234–43.

215. Hines DJ, Schmitt LI, Hines RM, et al. Antidepressant effects of sleep deprivation require astrocyte-dependent adenosine mediated signaling. Transl Psychiatry 2013;3:e212.

216. Takano K, Ogura M, Nakamura Y, et al. Neuronal and glial responses to poly-amines in the ischemic brain. Curr Neurovasc Res 2005;2(3):213–23.
217. D'Ambrosio R, Maris DO, Grady MS, et al. Impaired K(+) homeostasis and altered electrophysiological properties of post-traumatic hippocampal glia. J Neurosci 1999;19(18):8152–62.
218. Zhang RL, Zhang ZG, Wang Y, et al. Stroke induces ependymal cell transforma-tion into radial glia in the subventricular zone of the adult rodent brain. J Cereb Blood Flow Metab 2007;27(6):1201–12.
219. Kucheryavykh LY, Kucheryavykh YV, Inyushin M, et al. Ischemia increases TREK-2 channel expression in astrocytes: relevance to glutamate clearance. Open Neurosci J 2009;3:40–7.
220. Quirié A, Demougeot C, Bertrand N, et al. Effect of stroke on arginase expres-sion and localization in the rat brain. Eur J Neurosci 2013;37(7):1193–202.
221. Sword J, Masuda T, Croom D, et al. Evolution of neuronal and astroglial disrup-tion in the peri-contusional cortex of mice revealed by in vivo two-photon imag-ing. Brain 2013;136(Pt 5):1446–61.
222. Zhang M, Caragine T, Wang H, et al. Spermine inhibits proinflammatory cytokine synthesis in human mononuclear cells: a counterregulatory mechanism that re-strains the immune response. J Exp Med 1997;185(10):1759–68.
223. Zhang M, Borovikova LV, Wang H, et al. Spermine inhibition of monocyte activa-tion and inflammation. Mol Med 1999;55:595–605.
224. Olsen ML, Sontheimer H. Mislocalization of Kir channels in malignant glia. Glia 2004;46(1):63–73.
225. Olsen ML, Sontheimer H. Functional implications for Kir4.1 channels in glial biology: from K+ buffering to cell differentiation. J Neurochem 2008;107: 589–601.
226. Kucheryavykh L, Rolón-Reyes K, Kucheryavykh Y, et al. Glioblastoma develop-ment in mouse brain: general reduction of OCTs and mislocalization of OCT3 transporter and subsequent uptake of ASP+ substrate to the nuclei. J Neurosci Neuroeng 2014;3(1):3–9.
227. Goodenberger ML, Jenkins RB. Genetics of adult glioma. Cancer Genet 2012; 205(12):613–21.
228. Nelson PG, McCune SK, Ades AM, et al. Glial-neurotrophic mechanisms in Down syndrome. J Neural Transm 2001;(61):85–94.
229. Cason AL, Ikeguchi Y, Skinner C, et al. X-linked spermine synthase gene (SMS) defect: the first polyamine deficiency syndrome. Eur J Hum Genet 2003;11:937–44.
230. Ikeguchi Y, Bewley MC, Pegg AE. Aminopropyltransferases: function, structure and genetics. J Biochem 2006;139:1–9.
231. Scholl UI, Choi M, Liu T, et al. Seizures, sensorineural deafness, ataxia, mental retardation, and electrolyte imbalance (SeSAME syndrome) caused by muta-tions in KCNJ10. Proc Natl Acad Sci U S A 2009;106(14):5842–7.
232. Iliff JJ, Nedergaard M. A link between glial Ca2+ signaling and hypoxia in ag-ing? J Cereb Blood Flow Metab 2013;33(2):170.
233. Kilpeläinen P, Rybnikova E, Hietala O, et al. Expression of ODC and its regula-tory protein antizyme in the adult rat brain. J Neurosci Res 2000;62:675–85.
234. Junttila T, Hietanen-Peltola M, Rechardt L, et al. Ornithine decarboxylase-like immunoreactivity in rat spinal motoneurons and motoric nerves. Brain Res 1993;609:149–53.
235. Stout CE, Costantin JL, Naus CC, et al. Intercellular calcium signaling in astro-cytes via ATP release through connexin hemichannels. J Biol Chem 2002;277: 10482–8.

236. Contreras JE, Sáez JC, Bukauskas FF, et al. Functioning of Cx43 hemichannels demonstrated by single channel properties. Cell Commun Adhes 2003;10: 245–9.
237. Pannicke T, Faude F, Reichenbach A, et al. A function of delayed rectifier potassium channels in glial cells: maintenance of an auxiliary membrane potential under pathological conditions. Brain Res 2000;862:187–93.
238. Zhou M, Kimelberg HK. Freshly isolated hippocampal CA1 astrocytes comprise two populations differing in glutamate transporter and AMPA receptor expression. J Neurosci 2001;21:7901–8.
239. Bao L, Locovei S, Dahl G. Pannexin membrane channels are mechanosensitive conduits for ATP. FEBS Lett 2004;572:65–8.
240. Huang Y, Grinspan JB, Abrams CK, et al. Pannexin1 is expressed by neurons and glia but does not form functional gap junctions. Glia 2007;55:46–56.
241. Makarov V, Kucheryavykh L, Kucheryavykh Y, et al. Transport reversal during heteroexchange: a kinetic study. J Biophys 2013;2013:683256.
242. Rossi DJ, Oshima T, Attwell D. Glutamate release in severe brain ischaemia is mainly by reversed uptake. Nature 2000;403:316–21.
243. Sulzer D, Chen TK, Lau YY, et al. Amphetamine redistributes dopamine from synaptic vesicles to the cytosol and promotes reverse transport. J Neurosci 1995;15:4102–8.
244. Sulzer D. How addictive drugs disrupt presynaptic dopamine neurotransmission. Neuron 2011;69(4):628–49.
245. Kucheryavykh YV, Pearson WL, Kurata H, et al. Unique features of Kir4.1 channel rectification. Channels (Austin) 2007;1:172–8.
246. Lalo U, Palygin O, Rasooli-Nejad S, et al. Exocytosis of ATP from astrocytes modulates phasic and tonic inhibition in the neocortex. PLoS Biol 2014;12(1): e1001747.
247. Iglesias R, Dahl G, Qiu F, et al. Pannexin 1: the molecular substrate of astrocyte "hemichannels". J Neurosci 2009;29:7092–7.
248. Wang F, Smith NA, Xu Q, et al. Photolysis of caged Ca2+ but not receptor-mediated Ca2+ signaling triggers astrocytic glutamate release. J Neurosci 2013;33(44):17404–12.
249. Bennett MV, Contreras JE, Bukauskas FF, et al. New roles for astrocytes: gap junction hemichannels have something to communicate. Trends Neurosci 2003;26:610–7.
250. Bennett MV, Garré JM, Orellana JA, et al. Connexin and pannexin hemichannels in inflammatory responses of glia and neurons. Brain Res 2012;1487:3–15.
251. Enkvetchakul D, Ebihara L, Nichols CG. Polyamine flux in Xenopus oocytes through hemi-gap junctional channels. J Physiol 2003;553(Pt 1):95–100.
252. Musa H, Veenstra RD. Voltage-dependent blockade of connexin40 gap junctions by spermine. Biophys J 2003;84:205–19.
253. Musa H, Fenn E, Crye M, et al. Amino terminal glutamate residues confer spermine sensitivity and affect voltage gating and channel conductance of rat connexin40 gap junctions. J Physiol 2004;557:863–78.
254. Pelegrin P, Surprenant A. Pannexin-1 mediates large pore formation and interleukin-1b release by the ATP-gated P2X7 receptor. EMBO J 2006;25:5071–82.
255. Skatchkov SN, Inyushin M, Kucheryavykh YV, et al. Multiple pathways of polyamine accumulation in glia. Proceedings of the Annual Meetings of Society for Neuroscience. SFN Abstr. 138.7. Chicago (IL); 2009.
256. Alvarez-Maubecin V, Garcia-Hernandez F, Williams JT, et al. Functional coupling between neurons and glia. J Neurosci 2000;20:4091–8.

257. Rivera Y, YV Kucheryavykh, J Benedikt, et al. Polyamine fluxes through Cx43-hemichannels in freshly isolated astrocytes and Müller glia. Proceedings of the Annual Meetings of Society for Neuroscience. SFN Abstr. 536.16. New Orleans (LA); 2012.

258. Rivera Y, Inyushin M, Kucheryavykh YV, et al. Pathways for physiological accumulation of polyamines in astrocytes. Proceedings of the Annual Meetings of Society for Neuroscience. SFN Abstr. 521.06. San Diego (CA): 2013.

259. Busch AE, Wuester S, Ulzheimer JC, et al. Electrogenic properties and substrate specificity of the polyspecific rat cation transporter rOCT1. J Biol Chem 1996;271:32599–604.

260. Gründemann D, Koster S, Kiefer N, et al. Transport of monoamine transmitters by the organic cation transporter type 2, OCT2. J Biol Chem 1998;273:30915–20.

261. Gründemann D, Schömig E. Gene structures of the human non-neuronal monoamine transporters EMT and OCT2. Hum Genet 2000;106:627–35.

262. Schömig E, Spitzenberger F, Engelhardt M, et al. Molecular cloning and characterization of two novel transport proteins from rat kidney. FEBS Lett 1998;425:79–86.

263. Koepsell H, Lips K, Volk C. Polyspecific organic cation transporters: structure, function, physiological roles, and biopharmaceutical implications. Pharm Res 2007;24:1227–51.

264. Takeda H, Inazu M, Matsumiya T. Astroglial dopamine transport is mediated by norepinephrine transporter. Naunyn Schmiedebergs Arch Pharmacol 2002;366:620–3.

265. Inazu M, Takeda H, Matsumiya T. The role of glial monoamine transporters in the central nervous system. Nihon Shinkei Seishin Yakurigaku Zasshi 2003;23:171–8.

266. Inyushin M, Kucheryaykh Y, Kucheryavykh L, et al. Membrane potential and pH-dependent accumulation of decynium-22 (1,1'-diethyl-2,2'-cyanine iodide) fluorescence through OCT transporters in astrocytes. Bol Asoc Med P R 2010;102(3):5–12.

267. Autere AM, Lamsa K, Kaila K, et al. Synaptic activation of GABAA receptors induces neuronal uptake of Ca2+ in adult rat hippocampal slices. J Neurophysiol 1999;81:811–6.

268. Fedirko N, Avshalumov M, Rice ME, et al. Regulation of postsynaptic Ca^{2+} influx in hippocampal CA1 pyramidal neurons via extracellular carbonic anhydrase. J Neurosci 2007;27:1167–75.

269. Ballanyi K, Grafe P, Ten Bruggencate G. Ion activities and potassium uptake mechanisms of glial cells in guinea-pig olfactory cortex slices. J Physiol 1987;382:159–74.

270. Siemkowicz E, Hansen AJ. Brain extracellular ion composition and EEG activity following 10 minutes ischemia in normo- and hyperglycemic rats. Stroke 1981;12(2):236–40.

271. Nilsson P, Laursen H, Hillered L, et al. Calcium movements in traumatic brain injury: the role of glutamate receptor-operated ion channels. J Cereb Blood Flow Metab 1996;16(2):262–70.

272. Hansen AJ, Nedergaard M. Brain ion homeostasis in cerebral ischemia. Neurochem Pathol 1988;9:195–209.

273. Hansen AJ, Zeuthen T. Extracellular ion concentrations during spreading depression and ischemia in the rat brain cortex. Acta Physiol Scand 1981;113(4):437–45.

274. Parpura V, Scemes E, Spray DC. Mechanisms of glutamate release from astrocytes: gap junction "hemichannels", purinergic receptors and exocytotic release. Neurochem Int 2004;45:259–64.

275. Spray DC, Ye ZC, Ransom BR. Functional connexin "hemichannels": a critical appraisal. Glia 2006;54(7):758–73.

276. Roth M, Obaidat A, Hagenbuch B. OATPs, OATs and OCTs: the organic anion and cation transporters of the SLCO and SLC22A gene superfamilies. Br J Pharmacol 2012;165(5):1260–87.

277. Ivanova S, Botchkina GI, Al-Abed Y, et al. Identification of enzymatically formed 3-aminopropanal as an endogenous mediator of neuronal and glial cell death. J Exp Med 1998;188:327–40.

278. Bell MR, Belarde JA, Johnson HF, et al. A neuroprotective role for polyamines in a *Xenopus* tadpole model of epilepsy. Nat Neurosci 2011;14:505–12.

279. Antony T, Hoyer W, Cherny D, et al. Cellular polyamines promote the aggregation of alpha-synuclein. J Biol Chem 2003;278:3235–40.

280. Goers J, Uversky VN, Fink AL. Polycation-induced oligomerization and accelerated fibrillation of human alpha-synuclein in vitro. Protein Sci 2003;12:702–7.

281. Mandal S, Mandal A, Johansson HE, et al. Depletion of cellular polyamines, spermidine and spermine, causes a total arrest in translation and growth in mammalian cells. Proc Natl Acad Sci U S A 2013;110(6):2169–74.

282. Nishimura K, Shiina R, Kashiwagi K, et al. Decrease in polyamines with aging and their ingestion from food and drink. J Biochem 2006;139:81–90.

283. Arshavsky YI. Alzheimer disease and cellular mechanisms of memory storage. J Neuropathol Exp Neurol 2014;73(3):192–205.

284. Matthews HR. Polyamines, chromatin structure and transcription. Bioessays 1993;15(8):561–6.

285. Kondapalli KC, Hack A, Schushan M, et al. Functional evaluation of autism-associated mutations in NHE9. Nat Commun 2013;4:2510.

286. Zhu HJ, Appel DI, Gründemann D, et al. Evaluation of organic cation transporter 3 (SLC22A3) inhibition as a potential mechanism of antidepressant action. Pharm Res 2012;65(4):491–6.

287. Torres-Platas SG, Hercher C, Davoli MA, et al. Astrocytic hypertrophy in anterior cingulate white matter of depressed suicides. Neuropsychopharmacology 2011;36(13):2650–8.

288. Gomes GM, Mello CF, da Rosa MM, et al. Polyaminergic agents modulate contextual fear extinction in rats. Neurobiol Learn Mem 2010;93(4):589–95.

289. Morrison LD, Kish SJ. Brain polyamine levels are altered in Alzheimer's disease. Neurosci Lett 1995;197(1):5–8.

290. Inoue K, Tsutsui H, Akatsu H, et al. Metabolic profiling of Alzheimer's disease brains. Sci Rep 2013;3:2364.

291. Grabenauer M, Bernstein SL, Lee JC, et al. Spermine binding to Parkinson's protein alpha-synuclein and its disease-related A30P and A53T mutants. J Phys Chem B 2008;112(35):11147–54.

292. Lewandowski NM, Ju S, Verbitsky M, et al. Polyamine pathway contributes to the pathogenesis of Parkinson disease. Proc Natl Acad Sci U S A 2010;107(39):16970–5.

293. Paik MJ, Ahn YH, Lee PH, et al. Polyamine patterns in the cerebrospinal fluid of patients with Parkinson's disease and multiple system atrophy. Clin Chim Acta 2010;411(19–20):1532–5.

294. Lesort M, Chun W, Tucholski J, et al. Does tissue transglutaminase play a role in Huntington's disease? Neurochem Int 2002;40(1):37–52.

295. Colton CA, Xu Q, Burke JR, et al. Disrupted spermine homeostasis: a novel mechanism in polyglutamine-mediated aggregation and cell death. J Neurosci 2004;24:7118–27.

296. Acevedo-Torres K, Berríos L, Rosario N, et al. Mitochondrial DNA damage is a hallmark of chemically induced and the R6/2 transgenic model of Huntington's disease. DNA Repair (Amst) 2009;8:126–36.

297. Tong X, Ao Y, Faas GC, et al. Astrocyte Kir4.1 ion channel deficits contribute to neuronal dysfunction in Huntington's disease model mice. Nat Neurosci 2014. http://dx.doi.org/10.1038/nn.3691.

298. Gomes-Trolin C, Nygren I, Aquilonius SM, et al. Increased red blood cell polyamines in ALS and Parkinson's disease. Exp Neurol 2002;177(2):515–20.

299. Ferchmin PA, Eterović VA, Rivera EM, et al. Spermine increases paired-pulse facilitation in area CA1 of hippocampus in a calcium-dependent manner. Brain Res 1995;689(2):189–96.

300. Casero RA, Pegg AE. Polyamine catabolism and disease. Biochem J 2009;421: 323–38.

301. Fiori LM, Wanner B, Jomphe V, et al. Association of polyaminergic loci with anxiety, mood disorders, and attempted suicide. PLoS One 2010;5(11):e15146.

302. Le Roy C, Laboureyras E, Laulin JP, et al. A polyamine-deficient diet opposes hyperalgesia, tolerance and the increased anxiety-like behaviour associated with heroin withdrawal in rats. Pharmacol Biochem Behav 2013;103(3):510–9.

303. Gilad GM, Gilad VH. Overview of the brain polyamine-stress-response: regulation, development, and modulation by lithium and role in cell survival. Cell Mol Neurobiol 2003;23(4–5):637–49.

304. Kossel A. Über das Agmatin. Zeitschrift für Physiologische Chemie 1910;66: 257–61 [in German].

305. Bardócz S, Duguid TJ, Brown DS, et al. The importance of dietary polyamines in cell regeneration and growth. Br J Nutr 1995;73(6):819–28.

306. Kalač P. Health effects and occurrence of dietary polyamines: a review for the period 2005-mid 2013. Food Chem 2014;161:27–39.

307. Gorboulev V, Ulzheimer JC, Akhoundova A, et al. Cloning and characterization of two human polyspecific organic cation transporters. DNA Cell Biol 1997; 16(7):871–81.

308. Kimura N, Masuda S, Katsura T, et al. Transport of guanidine compounds by human organic cation transporters, hOCT1 and hOCT2. Biochem Pharmacol 2009; 77(8):1429–36.

309. Becker ML, Visser LE, van Schaik RH, et al. OCT1 polymorphism is associated with response and survival time in anti-Parkinsonian drug users. Neurogenetics 2011;12(1):79–82.

310. Cui M, Aras R, Christian WV, et al. The organic cation transporter-3 is a pivotal modulator of neurodegeneration in the nigrostriatal dopaminergic pathway. Proc Natl Acad Sci U S A 2009;106(19):8043–8.

The Importance of Glia in Dealing with Stress

Michel A. Woodbury-Fariña, MD, DFAPA, FAIS

KEYWORDS

- Glia • Intelligence • Environmental enrichment • Drug abuse • Astroglia • Microglia
- NG2 glia • Oligodendrocytes • S100B
- Immune theory of mental illness-Glymphatics

KEY POINTS

- Glia are the equal of neurons.
- Glia are a buffer against stress because of effects on intelligence.
- Glia's effect on stress can be maximized with environmental enrichment and exercise.
- Glia establish cerebral dominance and can increase or decrease stress depending on the dominance.
- NG2 glia establish cerebral dominance.
- Oligodendrocytes are important in stress reactions.
- Glia are implicated in depression and schizophrenia.
- Glia and the immune theory of mental illness.
- S100B as a marker for suicidal behavior.
- Microglia are not just immune cells and can modulate many functions, including being implicated in addictive behavior.
- There are numerous microglial modulators, especially cAMP agonists, such as PDE-4 inhibitors, as well as minocycline.
- There possibly is a glymphatic (glial-lymphatic) system in human brains that helps to take out the day's debris every night while we sleep.

INTRODUCTION

More than 100 years ago, glia were relegated to a backseat role in the brain. Their contribution to the stress response was believed to be minimal, because it was believed that they could only feed and clean up while the real work of the neurons was being done. Initially, glia were believed to be only the cement of the brain; glia is the name given to them in 1858 by Virchow[1–3] and means glue. Glial research

---

Disclosure: Speaker for Pfizer.

Department of Psychiatry, University of Puerto Rico School of Medicine, 307 Calle Eleonor Roosevelt, San Juan, PR 00918-2720, USA

E-mail address: michel.woodbury@upr.edu

Psychiatr Clin N Am 37 (2014) 679–705

http://dx.doi.org/10.1016/j.psc.2014.08.003

psych.theclinics.com

Abbreviations	
ATP	Adenosine triphosphate
BBB	Blood-brain barrier
BD	Bipolar disorder
BDNF	Brain-derived neurotropic factor
cAMP	Cyclic adenosine monophosphate
CSF	Cerebrospinal fluid
DG	Dentate gyrus
dlPFC	Dorsolateral prefrontal cortex
EE	Environmental enrichment
EEG	Electroencephalographic
GABA	Gamma-aminobutyric acid
GAFP	Glial fibrillary acidic protein
GDNF	Glial cell-derived neurotrophic factor
IL	Interleukin
KYNA	Kynurenic acid
LTP	Long-term potentiation
MD	Mood disorder
Met	Methionine
mPFC	Medial prefrontal cortex
NDRG2	N-myc downstream regulated gene 2
NMDA	N-Methyl-D-aspartate
NOase	Nitric oxide synthesase
PDE	Phosphodiesterase
PFC	Prefrontal cortex
QUIN	Quinolinic acid
SSRI	Selective serotonin reuptake inhibitor
TGFb	Transforming growth factor beta
TNF-α	Tumor necrosis factor α
Val	Valine

has evolved from showing that they only give support and sustenance to the neuron to the present knowledge that they have been shown to be the equal of neurons, controlling synaptic connections and transmission as well as providing the nutrients to support the activity of the neurons.[4,5] This observation does not mean that everyone has integrated this view. Most of the research is still concentrated on neurons, because the neuron doctrine[6] of the late 1800s and early 1900s is still dominant. I wanted to publish this article for psychiatrists so that we as a specialty can understand the importance of glia in health and illness. To show that glia are a factor in modulating stress, their role in intelligence is pointed out, because of intelligence being such an important buffer against stress. Ways to improve intelligence by environmental enrichment (EE) and exercise are in a sense ways to increase glia's ability to help us deal with stress. Glia form the basis of cerebral dominance as well as having an important role in stress and disease and can even be used to predict suicidality via S100B serum levels. The immune theory of stress includes the role of microglia and has directed the treatment of mental illness towards controlling the microglia. The role of the glia in sleep is reviewed.

GLIA AND INTELLIGENCE

The view that glia can be involved in intelligence is a recent development. For instance, in 1960, when glia were thought to be 90% of the brain and neurons 10%, the conclusion was that we use only 10% of our brains, because all the important functions involved only neurons. There is evidence that this breakdown is not based on any specific study. I was unable to find an original study establishing this theory. The most recent consensus using new technology[7] has glia/neuron ratio in the whole brain closer to 1:1, with large discrepancies found within the brain, (eg, 3.76:1 in the cerebral cortex and 1:4.3 in the cerebellum).[8]

Even with all the information about glia, there was a tendency to relegate them to being a support structure, with little to do with intelligence. R. Douglas Fields, PhD has published on the evolutionary adaptations that the human brain has undergone to increase processing capabilities,[9] and he believes that glia are important players. There is an experiment that even Dr Fields[10] believes establishes this link. Before discussing this experiment, I want to point out that Dr Fields has made an important contribution to popularizing the importance of glia as the head of the Nervous System Development and Plasticity Section of the National Institute of Child Health and Human Development since 2001, giving lectures to doctors free of charge, including to the psychiatrists of Puerto Rico (myself included) and the author of a layman-oriented book on glia called *The Other Brain: The Scientific and Medical Breakthroughs That Will Heal Our Brains and Revolutionize Our Health*.[11] He has been actively promoting the wonders of glia such as the fact that although astrocytes are electrically inert, thanks to calcium imaging technology, they have been shown to participate in synaptic signaling via increases in calcium concentrations.[12] The glia use these increases in calcium to send messages to other glia (you can see these waves in actions by going to rdouglasfields.wordpress.com), without necessarily being connected to the other glia.[13,14] In his writings,[11] Fields directs us to the study of the brain of a genius, whose glia turned out to be unusually prominent. In 1985, Marion C. Darmon, PhD found that Einstein had the same number of neurons as her controls. However, not only did Einstein's brain have many more glia than neurons but also he had more glia than each of the 11 normal male individuals whom she had as controls. However, the study reached statistical significance only in the left inferior parietal area,[15,16] which is responsible for mathematical thought[17] and has been found to be larger in mathematicians.[18] Could the increase here and in mathematicians be seen as a sign that there are more glia in those areas that are most stimulated? Jorge Colombo later reported[19] that the type of glia that was increased in Albert Einstein's brain were astrocytes. Einstein not only had more astrocytes, but in the cerebral cortex, he had the typically large type that Colombo had earlier established are seen only in primates and humans, called intralaminar astrocytes.[20] Increased numbers, increased size, and possibly increased intelligence? Up to now these have been interesting associations that were not seen as definitive proof that could ascribe glia a role in intelligence. However, for the past 15 years, researchers such as Alfonso Araque[21,22] have shown that there exist all the elements needed to associate glia with synaptic transmission and plasticity, which means that they must be involved in learning. Glia are part of the tripartite synapse (glia, presynaptic, and postsynaptic neuron [or quadripartite, if the blood vessels are included]) and have been shown to modulate the transmission of the signals that the neurons send. Plasticity has to do with the changes in the postsynaptic neuronal membrane that ensure that that neuron fires quicker when stimulated again. This result is called long-term potentiation (LTP) and is the basis for learning.[23] Most of the glia and neuron studies have been performed using rodents. However, there are many differences between murine and human glia. For instance, human protoplasmic astrocytes are larger and complex, being 2.5 times larger and having 10 times more processes than the astrocytes of rodents.[24] The result is that 1 human astrocyte can contact up to 2 million synapses versus 20 to 120,000 in the rodent.[25,26] What could help support the fact that glia are crucial for learning in humans? What if murine glia could be replaced by human glia in these animals? What if these hybrid mice were to be smarter than those without the human glia? These experiments have been carried out, and the mice that had their glia replaced by human glia turned out to be smarter.[27] In a creative experiment, human glial progenitor cells (GPCs) were successfully grafted into the brains of neonatal mice. Because these mice were made to be immunodeficient, the cells took, grew into, and took over large areas of their brain. The GPCs developed into humanlike astrocytes that are found only in adult humans and apes.[26] Although these humanoid astrocytes worked faster than their unengrafted counterparts, never changing their humanoid structures, they were completely integrated in the murine brain.[28] As expected, the engrafted mice performed better on multiple hippocampal memory tests. To prove that the humanoid glia were responsible, a human glial blocker was given, which made the engrafted mice perform at the level of their unengrafted controls. As mentioned by Dr Fields, these results go far to show that all that involves learning and intelligence involves both neurons and glia, with astrocytes being an important part of our intelligence. There is now ample evidence that the evolution of their complexity and size has contributed to the increased capacity of the hominid brain.[24] Genomic studies have borne out that the biggest difference between humans and mice is that humans have more glial transcripts.[29] These results indicate that, as astrocytes increase in size and number, as is the case as one ascends the animal kingdom, so does cognition increases, with humans having the highest potential because we have more in number and more complex astroglia.[24] This finding might explain the different glia/neuron ratios in the brain that were mentioned earlier, with a high neuron/glia ratio in the phylogenically older cerebellum and a high glia/neuron ratio in the newer cerebral cortex.

GLIA AND ENVIRONMENTAL ENRICHMENT

Because it has been shown that glia participate in intelligence, it would be interesting to know if this intelligence can be manipulated to increase the ability to serve as a buffer against stress. The answer might be in EE studies. The initial study in rodents was by Donald Hebb, the same researcher who described a neuronal learning paradigm that bears his name[30] and that needs to have as few glia as possible to prove neuronal learning. Thus the research had to be performed on simple-celled invertebrate animals.[31] As for EE, Hebb noticed that his pet mice performed better on intelligence tests than the mice raised in his laboratory.[32] However, it was not until the 1960s that research was directed to assess the impact of the environment on brain development in animals. In one of the earliest studies, rats that were exposed to being handled and were allowed to be active in a well-equipped cage had heavier cerebral cortexes than the controls that were raised in isolation[33]; this study was replicated two years later.[34] In 1964, more information was published that showed that the increased weight was caused by having a thicker cerebral cortex and a greater number of synapses and glia.[35,36] At that time, news started to spread that an enriched environment must also be crucial for maximal human development, spawning numerous efforts to entertain children with as many activities as possible and as early as possible. Even in the late 1980s, I myself had a plastic barrel for our kids filled with toys that enriched every room. In human beings, being taught to read is part of an enriched environment that can promote so much brain development that the American Academy of Pediatrics has issued a policy statement that pediatricians in the office visit should promote reading at an early age, that is, from infancy to five years of age.[37] Research has gone on to show that there are many benefits for animals exposed to EE, because they show less aggression,[38] anxiety, fear, and emotional reactivity,[39–42] reduced signs of stress,[43–45] and better learning abilities, as seen by an increase in hippocampal neurons.[46] In rats and humans, attachment theory stresses the importance of maternal contact in the development of emotional health[47–49] (for a more detailed explanation of the amygdala response to the absence of caregiving see Ref.[50]). Variations in maternal care levels of offspring can induce epigenetic effects that produce long-lasting changes in the way they handle stress in adulthood, for instance, by altering hippocampal structure and function (for a review see Refs.[51,52]). In one seminal study with mice, offspring of mothers showing higher levels of licking and grooming behavior during a certain critical period grew up to show increased exploratory behavior, reduced anxietylike behavior, and increased glucocorticoid receptors in the hippocampus, leading to an increase in the feedback control on hypothalamic-pituitary-adrenal axis as well as increased synaptic plasticity in the hippocampus when compared with those that were exposed to less licking.[53–55] In mice, enriched environments after weaning are effective in protecting from or reversing the negative effect of a stressor in highly emotional or anxious animals.[56,57]

In neural development, positive experiences increase the number and size of synapses per neuron,[36,58] increase synaptic activity,[59] increase dendritic complexity,[60–62] and can restore neurogenesis.[63,64] Glia have been shown to participate in these changes. EE increases capillary vascularization, which provides the glia and neurons with more nutrients and energy. The ensuing increase in size and number of glia promotes the glia to activate more synapses and increase their activity.[59] Enrike Aragandoña and his group have contributed extensively to this field.[65] These investigators believe that EE includes all stimulation that is sensory, cognitive, and motor and that has been shown to promote activation, signaling, and neuronal plasticity in all brain areas. EE improves learning and memory,[66,67] as well as decreasing cognitive impairment caused by aging.[64] These changes include not only neurons but also astrocytes, which have been shown to increase in size and density with EE. These investigators have also found that the neuron, glia, and even the blood vessels are so interrelated that they should be known as the neurogliovascular unit (or neuropil).[68] Thus, as mentioned earlier, an update on the tripartite synapse is that it is now the quadripartite synapse, when one adds the vascular component. The maturation/stimulation of the sensory system involves not only neurons, glia, blood vessels and their connections[69] but also the substances they share, which are called angioglioneurins.[70] All the angioglioneurins are cytokines, small nonantibody proteins, which were first believed to be produced by the immune system but were found to come from other cells, which are important in signaling and have been shown to have proliferative and protective effects on all components of the neurovascular unit. For instance, the proangiogenic vascular endothelial growth factor has been found to be particularly important in this system, not only because of obvious angiogenic effects but also because of neurotropic, neuroprotective, and astrocyte proliferative effects. Others include brain-derived neurotropic factor (BDNF), insulinlike growth factor 1, and the glycoprotein erythropoietin.[71] Because of studies showing that physical exercise is the major neurogenic and neurotropic stimulus that is most likely mediated by the angioglioneurins,[70] to maximize the effect of EE, exercise most likely has to be included.[72,73] EE is known to help reverse the effects of sensory deprivation on glia in rats.[74] When exercise was added to EE, the astrocyte density increased,[74] meaning that exercise and EE were the best ways to overcome the provoked sensory deficits. Other studies have supported these findings.[75,76] These interactions are being studied in humans to examine the effects on glia. In humans, the effect of EE in the form of continuous learning, novel experiences, and being aerobically fit increases cognitive performance and decreases the chance that there will be cognitive decline,[77–79] a concept that has been called cognitive resilience. As mentioned earlier, EE stabilized mice that had developed dysfunctional emotional behaviors in their early development as a result of being exposed to stressful events. EE not only mitigated the effect of stress but also helped the mice be calmer, more animated, and smarter than controls that were not exposed to stress in their youth.[80] Although the contribution of what exercise alone can do remains to be clarified,[81] there are experiments that show that being fit and exercising diminishes the negative cognitive and neurobiological consequences of stress,[82] by keeping another glial type called microglia inactivated. Before elaborating on this glial type, how glia are believed to be involved in major stress paradigms based on dominance is discussed.

GLIAL HEMISPHERIC DOMINANCE AND STRESS

Boldizsár Czéh and his group in Göttingen, Germany have an interesting view. In humans and primates, the area associated with regulating the stress response, and showing changes with stress, is the dorsolateral prefrontal cortex (dlPFC),[83,84] which in rodents corresponds to the medial prefrontal cortex (mPFC).[85] These investigators found that normally, the rat hippocampus was associated mainly with neurogenesis, whereas the mPFC was associated with gliogenesis and a little endothelial genesis. However, after chronic stress, there was suppression of both gliogenesis in the mPFC and neurogenesis in the hippocampus. Nowhere else were there signs of suppression. These effects were reversed with the antidepressant fluoxetine.[86] Studies on cerebral dominance have shed more light. Frontal hemispheric dominance is well known, with the left frontal hemisphere usually being dominant in humans and in rodents.[87–89] There is evidence that the dominance pattern can be affected by psychiatric conditions.[90,91] In normal healthy conditions, the right hemisphere is considered the one that starts to analyze a problem, and the left resolves it. In animal behavior, the right is the part that coordinates approach behaviors and the left with withdrawal behaviors. The right is considered negative and depressive and the left positive and euphoric.[89] Studies on brain lesions support this theory, with depression being associated with left hemispheric lesions and the lesioned right with mania.[92–94] In humans, it is believed that in depression, there is less left hemispheric control, and this gives rise to suicidal ideation. What needs to be clarified is that the left frontal hemisphere is still trying to solve a problem but because it is not working as efficiently as it should because of a decrease in working memory, it offers suicide as an option. Thus, more information on cerebral dominance would be crucial. Boldizsár Czéh and his group went on to establish that there is asymmetry in the number of frontal glia in rats.[86] Having more glia in the left mPFC establishes the left mPFC as a dominant hemisphere. With stress, there was a suppression of the gliogenesis on the left hemisphere, with an increase in the right, effectively reversing the dominance. Nondominant activation has been associated with anxiety.[89,94] Fluoxetine corrected this problem in the frontal cortexes as well as in the hippocampus. There are some human studies that could give credence to these findings. For instance, electroencephalographic (EEG) studies in depressed humans tend to show decreased left hemispheric activation, with anxious humans showing overactivation of the right hemisphere.[89,94] Hypometabolism and decreased volumes of the left prefrontal cortex (PFC) have been found in depression.[95,96] Animals have been shown to have the same tendencies to show lateralization of the mPFC in stress paradigms.[89] Animals that were fearful and had increased cortisol levels showed increased right frontal activity on the EEG,[97] giving further support to the association of the right hemisphere with anxious behavior. Other studies in rodents have supported the results of the studies of Boldizsár Czéh and his group.[89,94] Again, the glia are shown to be intimately involved in the stress response, possibly orchestrating the intellectual responses to stress through lateralization.[98]

NG2 GLIA

The cerebral dominance that was described earlier might be explained by NG2 cells, because this was the type of cell that changed in number. The glia found to be increased in the left mPFC of unstressed rats were the NG2 glia, with stress increasing the NG2 glia in the right mPFC, in the latter case, resulting in the right mPFC having more NG2 glia than the left mPFC. Here, too, fluoxetine can neutralize the effect of stress.[86,99] Changes with the use of antidepressants as well as corticosterone and electroconvulsive therapy are seen in the NG2 glia. This is a common type of glia found throughout the central nervous system,[100,101] which has been a bit of a mystery. Not much was known about these glia except that they could turn into oligodendrocytes.[100,101] Because of this fact, this cell line was not believed to be a distinct one. However, not only are these cells too complex to be oligodendrocyte precursors, but they also, have a structure similar to astrocytes, can form links to neurons, astrocytes, myelin structures, and oligodendrocytes,[100,101] can monitor glial-neuronal signals, and can act like neurons,[101] complete with synaptic junctions with the axons in the gray and white matter.[102,103] The NG2 cell synapses are electrophysiologically similar to synapses.[104] The consensus has been that they are the fifth element, that is, the fifth participant in synaptic activity, along with astrocytes, oligodendrocytes, microglia, and neurons.[100,101]

OLIGODENDROCYTES AND STRESS

I have not mentioned all of the glia and glial transmitters that are involved in stress because every day it seems that new links with stress and glia are being found. The laboratory of Diane Kaufer is studying the molecular and cellular changes seen in acute and chronic stress.[105] This research includes the effect of one glia that I have not mentioned much in stress, which is the oligodendrocyte. In these investigators' latest study on mice, the stress of immobilization increased the number of oligodendrocytes and decreased the number of neurons in the dentate gyrus (DG) of the hippocampus.[106] The stem cells of the DG that are constantly being produced were believed to turn only into astrocytes or neurons. The significance of having the oligodendrocyte, a cell that is involved in synapse and myelin formation, show up under stress is that whatever connections are made by the oligodendrocytes at that moment of stress are strengthened (eg, to the amygdala), and others ignored if not present (eg, to the PFC). Fear activates the amygdala (for an excellent review, see Ref.[107]). It is up to the PFC to relay inhibitory signals to the amygdala to prevent us from always being afraid. When there is an exposure to an initially fearful, stressful event, the PFC is bypassed, with the amygdala and the hippocampus dominating, which means that the fight-flight sympathetic response is set off and we feel afraid. If the danger turns out to be unthreatening, the PFC, which is where we receive help to attenuate the response to the stressful stimuli, modulates the amygdala, so that the amygdala stops setting off the fight-flight response, thus ensuring that we are no longer afraid. However, when the oligodendrocytes increase the fear circuits of the amygdala, the PFC has less inhibitory control of the amygdala, meaning that even if the stressful event is found to be unthreatening, the amygdala can continue to keep up the fear response. Repeated exposure results in the oligodendrocytes making this connection pattern even stronger and more permanent. This enhanced link from the hippocampus to the amygdala could explain flashbacks, thus explaining acute and chronic stress models such as posttraumatic stress disorder. This result implies that even the intelligent who have been exposed to adequate amounts of EE-can still be prone to excessive anxiety if they are exposed to extremely stressful situations. This scenario should be considered as another risk factor in the stress/resilience models that include the discovery that a short allele polymorphism in the serotonin receptor transporter promoter region can increase the likelihood that a stressful life event causes depression[108] as well as the work showing that a substituted methionine (Met) for valine (Val) in the BDNF gene, Val66Met, prevents the PFC from being efficient in extinguishing repeated nonthreatening fear stimuli in both mice and humans.[109] It should be pointed out that thanks to the work of those like Diane Kaufer, progress is being undertaken to develop therapies for anxiety disorders that target the amygdala and not the PFC.

GLIA AND DEPRESSION

Although neither definitive glial pathology nor neurodegeneration is found in human depression, it is logical to assume that if glia are such an active part of the brain, they must be involved. At first, only neurons were believed to be involved in the shrinkage that was found in the brain after stress and depression. When it was found that there was less BDNF, a neurotrophin that controls the growth, differentiation, and survival of neurons, in the postmortem examinations of the brains of depressed humans, this growth factor was believed to explain this shrinkage. Thus, a decrease of BDNF was surmised to be one of the important causes of depression. Because BDNF and other neurotrophins are involved, this theory is known as the neurotrophin theory of depression,[110] which can be corrected by antidepressants.[111–114] This was big news when the selective serotonin reuptake inhibitors (SSRIs) first appeared, that is, that the SSRIs were increasing BDNF, resulting in neurogenesis or at least an increase in neuronal arboralization that results in improved neuronal function.[115] In depression, it is the astrocyte that stops producing several neurogliotrophins including BDNF.[116] Antidepressants, such as the SSRI fluoxetine, not only restore the ability of the astrocyte to produce BDNF[115] but also help them increase their use of glucose and, as a consequence, increase the release of lactate.[117] These initial glial deficits may be the result of altered gliogenesis, because various factors that impair glial cell proliferation are likely to be altered in the cortex in depression. Among the known factors that regulate proliferation of glia with the potential to affect the neurophysiology of depression are growth and differentiation proteins in the developing and adult brain, stress-related hormones, glucocorticoids, gonadal steroids, and neurosteroids,[118] neurotransmitters like glutamate[24] or noradrenaline, ethanol,[119] and blood vessel–derived factors. This situation is especially complicated, because astrocytes can be both excitatory or inhibitory.[120] Also unresolved is that when these changes do occur, are they causal or seen only in illness? Because stressful life events can lead to depressive disorders,[121,122] many studies of the effects of stress and depression have shown glial involvement, usually in the form of a decrease in number in the frontal cortical regions, including the orbitofrontal cortex,[98,123] PFC,[124] and anterior cingulate cortex.[125] As has usually been the case, the bulk of the research has been performed on animals (for good reviews, see Refs.[110,126]). The goal is always to see which part of the glial structure should be studied to obtain a good idea of the effects of stress. One positive study chose glial fibrillary acidic protein (GAFP) and N-myc downstream regulated gene 2 (NDRG2).[126] GFAP is a cytoskeleton protein that is involved in astrocyte-neuron communication,[127] and NDRG2 is found in the astrocyte.[127] In a social defeat model of chronic stress,[126] stress decreased GAFP and increased NDRG2 in the rat hippocampus. Citalopram was not able to influence these changes. The implications are that chronic stress in rats caused signs of significant changes in the hippocampal astroglia that are not affected by one of the antidepressants that most increases serotonin.[128] Because the stressed rats did do better with citalopram, the positive effect was possibly mediated by other mechanisms such as direct neuronal effects or preventing the neuronal protein syntaxin 1A from being increased by stress.[126] That the astrocytes did not change has been believed to mean that the initial improvements in mood are not permanent; it is not enough to normalize the function of neurons, because astrocytes would have to change to prevent a relapse. This situation might help explain why patients relapse after discontinuing their antidepressant medications too early.

GLIA AND SCHIZOPHRENIA

As for the glial changes in schizophrenia, most studies show lower numbers of glia,[129,130] with antipsychotics increasing them. Not much was attempted at first to follow up on these results, because glia were not seen as important in this condition. Now that glia are known to be a major factor in synaptic transmission, more studies are being performed.[131] For instance, after 40 days of consecutive daily administration of chlorpromazine to rats, there was an increased number of astrocytes and a reduced number of synapses in the arcuate nucleus of the hypothalamus.[131] This decrease in synapses was caused by the astrocytes surrounding the neurons and neutralizing their synapses. This effect was reversed when the chlorpromazine was discontinued, that is, without chlorpromazine the astrocytes unwrapped themselves, leaving the neurons as bare as they were before, thus giving a possible explanation as to why symptoms return after stopping medication. Atypical and typical antipsychotics affected the astrocytes in other parts of the brain. The greatest astrocyte response of all the antipsychotics was in the central part of the nucleus accumbens, with a moderate response in the cingulate cortex of the atypical group, some increases in the hypothalamus and stratum, and little changes in the hippocampus and amygdala of both groups.[131] It is interesting to speculate on the main effect on the nucleus accumbens, because this is the pleasure center. This factor might explain some of the antimanic, antipleasure-seeking effects of these mood stabilizers. The results of studies like these again stress the importance of studying how to modulate astrocytes pharmacologically, hoping to find a way to make the glial responses more permanent.

MICROGLIA AND STRESS

Microglia are another glial type that have been shown to be important in stress and cognition. They make up between 5% and 20% of the glia and are found throughout the central nervous system.[132] There has been a significant change in our understanding of the role of these glia in the brain.[133] Microglia were initially believed to be concerned only with coordinating the immune response, because in embryonic development, monocytes enter the brain, develop processes, and become microglia.[92] They retain their ability to be phagocytotic and go around the brain picking up foreign debris as well as sick or dead cells. Their association with synaptic signaling was only surmised because they had neurotransmitter receptors.[134] Only recently have studies shown that they contribute to synaptic signaling.[133,134] Microglia even have most of the excitatory and inhibitory receptors as well as ion channels as seen in synapses (for more see Kettlenmann and Pocock).[135,136] There is evidence that chronic stress negatively activates microglia in rat mPFC.[137] Madeleine Hinwood and her group[138] coordinated some of the initial experiments on the role of microglia that proved that microglia are key players in the neuronal and behavioral responses to chronic psychological stress. To choose what to study, these investigators point out that working memory in the rat is very sensitive to stress[139–142] and is routinely attenuated in emotional diseases such as depression.[143,144] As mentioned before, in humans and primates, the area associated with regulating the stress response, and showing changes with stress, is the dlPFC,[83,84] which in rodents corresponds to the mPFC,[85] a fact verified by these investigators. The results showed that in a chronic stress paradigm, changes in neuronal activation in the mPFC were associated with microglia activation, which in turn decreased working memory. This activation was blocked by minocycline, a tetracycline class antibiotic that passes the blood-brain barrier (BBB) easily and has been shown to be a microglia modulator.[145,146] The result was that minocycline increased working memory and, logically, the ability to deal with stress effectively. This finding has led the way to study the role of microglia in psychiatric disease states.

Changes that result in mood disturbances are felt to occur when the natural balance between the microglia, astrocytes, neurons and oligodendrocytes is upset. (For an excellent review on this subject see Maletic V and colleagues[147] and Salter MW and colleagues.[148] In a non-stressed model, the oligodendrocytes are stabilizing the neuronal signals while the neurons are stimulated, releasing glutamate at the synapses.[147] This glutamate would destabilize the system except for the astrocytes that pick it up. The astrocytes also contribute specifically to the stability of the microglia with ATP, GABA, and TGFb and generally to the stabilization of the microglia, neurons and oligodendrocytes with BDNF and GDNF. The microglia are busy promoting memory, by not pruning those synaptic spines that are produced by important events that are novel and important, possibly by fractalkine, a chemokine which originates from neurons and goes on to stimulate microglia, the only cells that have the fractalkine receptor CX_3CR1 in the healthy brain.[149] In fact this system might explain the changes seen in environmental enrichment as knockout mice ($CX_3CR1^{KO/KO}$) that did not have the fractalkine receptor CX_3CR1 did not benefit from this enrichment, performing poorly in the test given, with no increase in LTP nor hippocampal neurogenesis seen.[150] At the same time, microglia will be pruning or stripping unwanted synapses according to the presence of C1Q and C3 that tag "weak" synapses.[151,152]

MICROGLIA, MOOD DISORDERS AND INFLAMMATION

In a stressed model, there is evidence that we are programmed to become depressed because of the cytokine-induced sickness behavior system[153] that we have developed to deal with infections. This system makes sure that we have to stay in bed to rest due to the onslaught of immune cell attack that results in the production of proinflammatory cytokines interleukin 1 (IL-1), IL-6, and tumor necrosis factor α (TNF-α),[153] which results in slowness, fatigue, poor concentration, hypersomnia, reduction in appetite, little desire to socialize, and poor personal grooming habits seen when we are sick. It is now believed that stress also induces the immune response to the point at which these same behavioral symptoms are present, complete with all the cytokines and activated microglia are present[154,155] without there being an infection. Thus, in this immune based stress paradigm, the microglia agitate the astroglia with ATP, cytokines, chemokines, reactive nitrogen species and reactive oxygen species, starting a vicious cycle whereby the astrocytes become over activated which also makes them secrete cytokines and chemokines that further stimulate the microglia. Astrocytes when activated become inefficient and become unable to control their communications with the blood vessels as well as become unable to control glutamate levels. Glutamate then starts to increase in the synapse, leak out and to stimulate extrasynaptic N-methyl-D-aspartate (NMDA) receptors. At the same time activated astrocytes produce less GABA which actually changes the shape of the microglia; they become more mobile and thus spread their toxic products elsewhere. The activated astrocytes start to produce less BDNF and GDNF which further destabilizes the whole unit. Microglia become even more activated, attacking the oligodendrocytes, demyelinating the neurons and promoting neuronal apoptosis. This thinking forms the basis for the inflammatory theory of depression. Bipolar disorders (BDs) and mood disorders (MDs) are conditions that have been particularly associated with inflammation. In one excellent review,[156] the investigators made the point that all of the systemic[153,157] (including cardiovascular[158]), autoimmune, and neuroendocrine[159,160] inflammatory disorders are associated with an increase in the incidence of MDs. People with BD who are not taking lithium have an increase in premature natural deaths.[157] BD is associated with an increase in multiple markers of inflammation,[161] including proinflammatory cytokines and C-reactive protein, as well as with positive antidepressant responses to various antiinflammatories, such as the omega-3 fatty acids[162] and cyclooxygenase 2 inhibitors.[163] Chronic treatment with interferon-γ treatment of hepatitis C caused in an increase in cytokines, which has resulted in hypomanic and manic behavior in previously unaffected individuals.[161] As has been noted, by orchestrating the production of cytokines, the microglia are deemed to be the cause of the MDs in the inflammatory conditions that have just been mentioned. This inflammation is believed to drive the microglia to cause degeneration of the PFC and anterior cingulate cortex[164,165] because there are decreased numbers and sizes of microglia in these areas in postmortem studies of MD.[164,165] The investigators point out that the literature suggests that the decrease in microglia is a specific marker for the presence of an MD, with the degeneration possibly preceding the exacerbation of the illness. Many studies[161,166–168] show that the state of microglia and cytokines can predict when a relapse of depression or mania will occur, as well as serve as a measure of response to therapeutic interventions. When the microglia are primed, they change and are called activated microglia. As previously mentioned, these activated microglia have cytokines that in this case stimulate cascades that increase the metabolism of tryptophan, which in turn starts a chain of reactions that end up decreasing serotonin levels[169,170] and serotonin transporters.[40,164,165,171] The resultant alterations in tryptophan production increase the levels of excitotoxins and cytokines, which in turn increase glutamate to the point that even the NMDA receptors are affected. Microglia have the NMDA receptor agonist quinolinic acid (QUIN), whereas the astrocytes have kynurenic acid (KYNA), an NMDA receptor antagonist.[172] Cytokine-provoked depression as well as major depressive disorder are associated with increased blood and cerebrospinal fluid (CSF) levels of QUIN,[173,174] implying microglia activation in both. On the other hand, schizophrenia is associated with increased KYNA production, implying astroglial involvement. Antidepressants such as the SSRIs have both proinflammatory and antiinflammatory effects on microglia, with physiological relevant doses showing proinflammatory effects.[175] The implication is that the SSRIs can modulate serotonin through the control of microglia. Although reaching the right balance between antiinflammatory and proinflammatory effects might be a therapeutic goal, this has never even been contemplated, because only the serotonin inhibition properties of these medications have been targeted for study.[175]

GLIA AND S100B

There has been a lot of interest in S100B, because it has been found to be an excellent biomarker for suicidal behavior. S100B is a protein that is part of the S100 family of proteins, which bind to calcium in the cytoplasm of numerous cells but are actively secreted by astrocytes and adipocytes (for a review, see Ref.[176]). In some behavioral disorders, cells can have more S100B. In a study of paranoid schizophrenics, there were more astrocytes with S100B as well as more oligodendrocytes with S100B in the white matter when compared with control individuals.[177] This finding might explain why schizophrenics have higher levels of S100B in the blood and CSF.[178–180] Although S100B increases when there is cell damage, here the increase is believed to be caused by the astrocytes producing more S100B than usual for reasons not understood. Some think that this increased S100B is caused by having been activated by prenatal maternal infections and is part of the inflammatory disease cascade associated with the development of schizophrenia. Increased S100B can reduce LTP, and LTP is reduced in schizophrenia. The effects of S100B on memory are complex because, on the other hand, it has been shown that S100B increases neurogenesis in the hippocampus, with an ability to improve cognition after induced traumatic brain injury.[181,182] For a review of the role of S100B in memory, see Refs.[183–185] There are various ways to increase S100B: by giving 5HT1A agonists,[186] natural antioxidants,[187] and risperidone,[188] by increasing glutamate,[189] TNF-α,[190] during metabolic stress,[191] and after intense physical exercise,[192] to name a few of those relevant to our field. Increased serum levels are seen with melanomas,[193] after heart ischemia[194] and non-brain trauma.[195] Neurologists use serum levels of S100B, because serum levels increase during the initial stages of brain trauma and decrease as the brain recovers; this way they are able to follow the course of the injury.[182] Recently, it has been shown that in brain trauma, brain S100B levels do not necessarily increase and are not necessarily bad, as mentioned earlier. Instead, the increased serum levels reflect the outflow of S100B due to the increased permeability of the BBB,[182,196] which is manned by astrocytes and microglia.[197] In suicidal patients, it is believed that this increase in permeability is caused by an inflammatory process that involves the microglia, because inflammatory conditions can increase permeability.[197] There is evidence that suicidality has been associated with microglial activation[198] and neuroinflammation.[155] A recent study showed that a normal serum level of S100B in a suicidal patient rules out any concerns that suicide is pending.[199] As the levels increase so does the suicide risk, no matter whether the patients are schizophrenic or depressed.[199] The average levels that were associated with a low risk were 0.152 +/− 0.02 ng/mL, and a high risk was seen at 0.354 +/− 0.044 ng/mL.[199]

MICROGLIA AND MEDICATIONS

Minocycline is a second-generation tetracycline, which has the ability to enter the brain and reaches brain levels that are 11% to 56% of the plasma concentration,[200] because it is fat soluble.[201] A further analysis of the effect of minocycline on glia includes preventing microglia from releasing proinflammatory cytokines such as IL-6B, TNF-α, and p38,[202] the first two by inhibiting the matrix enzymes that produce them[200] and stimulating the release of antiinflammatory IL-10 cytokine.[202] Minocycline neutralizes reactive oxygen species as well as nitric oxide synthesase (NOase).[203] NOase increases presynaptic glutamate release (into the synapse) but inhibits glial glutamate transporters (which take out glutamate), which can result in an excess of glutamate in the synapse, thereby increasing the chance of excitotoxicity and cell death.[204] Thus, inhibiting NOase can be protective against cell death. The antiinflammatory effect of minocycline in helping to remediate psychiatric illnesses has been another addition to the view that psychiatric illness is an inflammatory disease. Continued research seems to be bearing out that minocycline can help in schizophrenia.[205] To prove how popular the notion of minocycline as a psychiatric medication is, there have been various proof of concept studies of whether minocycline can ameliorate psychiatric illnesses, one with low-dose aspirin to study the effect in bipolar depression[206] after reports that in a double-blind study, minocycline helped the negative symptoms and cognition in early schizophrenia.[207] The National Institute of Mental Health is also conducting trials, one with minocycline and clozaril (http://clinicaltrials.gov/ct2/show/NCT01433055) and another using minocycline for the treatment of negative and cognitive symptoms in early phase schizophrenia (http://clinicaltrials.gov/ct2/show/NCT00733057).

There are many ways to suppress microglia. Glucocorticoids[208] are obvious, because of their known antiinflammatory actions. Also, any substance that increases cyclic adenosine monophosphate (cAMP) can modulate the microglia, such as adrenergic agonists (isoproterenol[209]), prostaglandins,[210] and adenosine.[211] Phosphodiesterase (PDE) type inhibitors, the most well known being caffeine and aminophylline, also increase cAMP. There are nonspecific (such as coffee and aminophylline) and specific PDEs. Not all inhibit the microglia and astrocytes. (For an extensive review, especially on the isoforms, see Ref.[212]) Of the different PDEs, PDE4 inhibitors are the most effective in increasing cAMP in microglia and astrocytes.[213] PDE4s in general have been implicated in psychosis mainly because of positive effects seen with rolipram (a selective PDE4 inhibitor[214])[215–218] and propentofylline (a mixed PDE inhibitor/adenosine agonist[219]).[220,221] Mesembrine, an alkaloid that has been found in the herb *Sceletium tortuosum*,[222] is yet another specific PDE4 inhibitor that is being studied in psychiatry. I was on the team that showed no undue physical (with one exception) or mental problems in a safety study of a subtherapeutic dose of *Sceletium tortuosum* in middle-aged normal volunteers,[223] which also was shown to be safe in another study.[224] Because *Sceletium tortuosum* has a strong serotonin effect, any addition of another medication/supplement that increases serotonin should be avoided, because this can theoretically induce a serotonergic syndrome. We had one mild case with a patient on risedronate sodium, which has been associated with this syndrome. We did find a statistically significant increase in cognitive flexibility and executive functions.

MICROGLIA AND DRUG ABUSE

Microglia seem to be intimately involved in the development of drug abuse. Ibudilast, yet another specific PDE4 inhibitor that can inhibit microglia, was used in a study of how maternal rearing practices in neonatal mice were protective for adult drug abuse.[225] While the risks of addiction are multifactorial, with genetic, experience, and biological factors being important, here the environment was studied. Stressful, events in early life have been shown to be so important; in rats, such stress can increase drug abuse.[226–228] Having the mother mouse lick her pups is a stress-reducing event, already discussed earlier, that decreases drug abuse in adulthood.[227,228] As mentioned earlier, stressful life events can permanently alter the immune functions of the brain.[225] Morphine can act like stress, altering glial activation and affecting reward behavior.[229] In the nucleus accumbens, morphine needs to activate the microglia to produce what is known as the reinstatement response months after the initial use.[225] This process means that morphine primes and changes even the morphology of the microglia in such a way that when the rodent is reexposed to morphine (reinstatement) later, there is an increased intent of the rodent to abuse morphine (response), because of the new changes in the microglia. This situation occurs because morphine causes an inflammatory response by increasing the release of proinflammatory cytokines and chemokines from the microglia.[229,230] Because these actions cause permanent changes in the microglia, the microglia remain more sensitive to the use of morphine later. To understand how this situation can be prevented, the immune response has to be understood. Initially, when activated, the immune system responds with proinflammatory substances, followed by the need to decrease this proinflammatory response by using antiinflammatories such as cytokines. One of the antiinflammatory cytokines in the brain is called cytokine IL-10. If IL-10 in the microglia is increased before being exposed to morphine, morphine is prevented from activating the proinflammatory response.[225] The specific epigenetic phenomenon that occurs is that the IL-10 area of the DNA is methylated (activated) by these interventions. Because the change is at the DNA level, the increased IL-10 effect is long lasting, if not permanent. Thus, the morphine reinstatement is attenuated, because the negative permanent changes, which would have occurred had the proinflammatory changes been allowed to take place in the microglia, were prevented from occurring. In the study on the effects of neonatal handling and drug abuse,[225] factors that were found to increase IL-10 and thus be protective against morphine reinstatement were: not being exposed to morphine in the neonatal period, neonatal handling, PDE4 inhibitors, minocycline, propentofylline, and ibudilast. Early exposure to morphine without neonatal handling or medication was a risk factor for morphine reinstatement when reaching adulthood. Even the adult mice that were never exposed to morphine in their neonatal period were less at risk for morphine abuse than those that had been exposed. As for the importance of increased neonatal handling, IL-10 levels in this group were 4 times more than their controls. The implications for the development of addictive behavior in general is that children need loving homes and should not be exposed to morphine early in life. How these findings apply to the use of anesthesia in youth is conjecture. It remains to be seen if these findings apply to humans, and if so, what interventions might help. There is one recent study in humans that could be understood by these findings. Early pseudomature adolescents who were the cool kids in early adolescence abused drugs early and had major problems as adults with drug abuse.[231] Being pseudomature was the strongest risk factor for adult drug abuse, more than early drug abuse among the nonpseudomature. Because pseudomaturity is associated with ineffectual parenting,[232] it can be hypothesized that those early adolescents who were exposed to effectual parenting had their glia primed to resist later drug abuse, with the pseudomature being at risk for drug abuse because of poor parenting. It is unfortunate that parenting effectiveness was not studied in the pseudomature study to see if these conjectures are valid.

Another example of how the proinflammatory cytokines of the brain can prime the microglia for life is the way that infections in young mice can permanently make the microglia produce an excess amount of IL-1β, a cytokine that is associated with learning in the hippocampus.[233] Too much[234,235] or too little IL-1β[236,237] decreases memory, so with the increase seen with early life infections, these memory deficits last throughout life, long after the infection is over. Thus, these studies in rats point to the need to study whether memory impairments in adult humans can be prevented if infections that make microglia produce an excess of IL-1β are avoided in early development.

GLIA, SLEEP, AND STRESS

Sleep is important in reducing stress. One of the latest findings in murine research is that in sleep there is a clearance phenomenon that uses convection to move liquids from the interstitial fluid of the brain to the cerebral spinal fluid and on to the bloodstream, thus cleaning out the brain. In the brains of mice when asleep or anesthetized, this fluid system was found to increase 60%, possibly because of the shrinkage of the astrocytes.[238,239] This increase allows the brain to effectively drain unwanted debris, including amyloid, into the bloodstream. If applicable to humans, this cleansing could explain why we are more efficient on awakening. Because glia seem to be involved, it has been called the glymphatic system and has the potential to help understand the development of degenerative diseases.

Sleep deprivation is known to cause memory deficits in many ways, but often, the deficits are related to a decrease of cAMP. One study[240] found that in mice, memory problems were in part caused by the buildup of forebrain adenosine, produced by astrocytes, which in turn stimulates the adenosine1 receptor that inhibits cAMP. In sleep deprivation, a PDE4 enzyme starts to inhibit cAMP in the hippocampus.[241] The research group increased the memory in these sleep-deprived mice with a PDE4 inhibitor. Even although they believed that a PDE4A5 inhibitor, which has not been developed, would have been better, rolipram was used successfully. At least rolipram works in rats.

SUMMARY

I hope that you have a clearer view of the role of glia in stress and illness. I encourage you to keep up with all the latest advances so as to understand the underpinning of our patients' behaviors. I hope that you realize that the rules that glia follow are different from those of neurons. Because osmotic pressure is the way glia control the synapses, they are exquisitely sensitive to hydration, with dietary potassium and taurine being important solutes that improve glial function, areas that my clinic is studying. Because astrocytes are wrapped around the blood vessels, they are sensitive to changes in nutrients, hydration and oxygen supplies. We now have a new reason to enrich our environment, get exercise, eat well and get enough sleep. Finally, there are still many psychiatric illnesses that are not controlled by conventional pharmacology. The answer might be in the better understanding of the role of glia in stress and psychiatric illness.

REFERENCES

1. Virchow R. Über das granulierte anschen der Wandungen der Gehirnventrikel. Allg Z Psychiat 1846;3:242–50 [in German].
2. Virchow R, editor. Gesammelte Abhandlungen zur wissenschaftlichen Medizin. Frankfurt am Main (Germany): Meidinger; 1856 [in German].
3. Virchow R. Die Cellularpathologie in ihrer Begründung auf physiologische und pathologische Gewebelehre. Berlin: Verlag von August Hirschwald; 1859 [in German].
4. Perea G, Araque A. Communication between astrocytes and neurons: a complex language. J Physiol Paris 2002;96(3–4):199–207.
5. Volterra A, Meldolesi J. Astrocytes, from brain glue to communication elements: the revolution continues. Nat Rev Neurosci 2005;6(8):626–40.
6. Golgi C. The neuron doctrine—theory and facts, Nobel lecture. December 11, 1906.
7. Herculano-Houzel S, Lent R. Isotropic fractionator: a simple, rapid method for the quantification of total cell and neuron numbers in the brain. J Neurosci 2005;25(10):2518–21.
8. Azevedo FA, Carvalho LR, Grinberg LT, et al. Equal numbers of neuronal and nonneuronal cells make the human brain an isometrically scaled-up primate brain. J Comp Neurol 2009;513(5):532–41.

9. Fields RD. The other half of the brain. Sci Am 2004;290(4):54–61.

10. Fields R. Unusual brain cell (astrocytes) boost learning. Posted: March 8, 2013. Available at: http://www.huffingtonpost.com/dr-douglas-fields/unusual-brain-cell-astroc_b_2810871.html.

11. Fields RD. The other brain. New York: Simon and Schuster; 2011.

12. Parpura V, Basarsky TA, Liu F, et al. Glutamate-mediated astrocyte–neuron signalling. Nature 1994;369:744–7.

13. Fields RD, Burnstock G. Purinergic signaling in neuron-glia interactions. Nat Rev Neurosci 2006;7:423–36.

14. Fields RD. Visualizing calcium signaling in astrocytes. Sci Signal 2010;3(147):tr5.

15. Diamon MC, Scheibel AB, Murphy GM Jr, et al. On the brain of a scientist: Albert Einstein. Exp Neurol 1985;88:198–204.

16. Diamond MC. Why Einstein's brain? Lecture at Doe Library, January 8, 1999.

17. Dehaene S, Spelke E, Pinel P, et al. Sources of mathematical thinking: behavioral and brain imaging evidence. Science 1999;284(5416):970–4.

18. Aydin K, Ucar A, Oguz KK, Okur OO, et al. Increased gray matter density in the parietal cortex of mathematicians: a voxel-based morphometry study. AJNR Am J Neuroradiol 2007;28(10):1859–64.

19. Colombo JA, Reisin HD, Miguel-Hidalgo JJ, et al. Cerebral cortex astroglia and the brain of a genius: a propos of A Einstein's. Brain Res Rev 2006;52(2):257–63.

20. Colombo JA, Reisin HD. Interlaminar astroglia of the cerebral cortex: a marker of the primate brain. Brain Res 2004;1006:126–31.

21. Pérez-Alvarez A, Araque A. Astrocyte-neuron interaction at tripartite synapses. Curr Drug Targets 2013;14(11):1220–4.

22. Araque A, Navarrete M. Glial cells in neuronal network function. Philos Trans R Soc Lond B Biol Sci 2010;365(1551):2375–81.

23. Lee YS, Silva AJ. The molecular and cellular biology of enhanced cognition. Nat Rev Neurosci 2009;10:126–40.

24. Oberheim NA, Wang X, Goldman S, et al. Astrocyte complexity distinguishes the human brain. Trends Neurosci 2006;29(10):547–53.

25. Bushong EA, Martone ME, Jones YZ, et al. Protoplasmic astrocytes in CA1 stratum radiatum occupy separate anatomical domains. J Neurosci 2002;22(1):183–92.

26. Oberheim NA, Takano T, Han X, et al. Uniquely hominid features of adult brain astrocyte. J Neurosci 2009;29(10):3276–87.

27. Han X, Chen M, Wang F. Forebrain engraftment by human glial progenitor cells enhances synaptic plasticity and learning in adult mice. Cell Stem Cell 2013;12:342–53.

28. Windrem MS, Moyle C, Chandler-Militello D, et al. Neonatally-implanted human glial progenitor cells out-compete endogenous glial progenitor cells to generate fully humanized glial-chimeric mouse brains. Society for Neuroscience Online. Poster presentation, Program No. 12621/A48. Neuroscience Meeting Planner. Chicago (IL), 2009.

29. Miller JA, Horvath S, Geschwind DH. Divergence of human and mouse brain transcriptome highlights Alzheimer disease pathways. Proc Natl Acad Sci U S A 2010;107:12698–703.

30. Hebb DO. The organization of behavior. New York: Wiley; 1949.

31. Antonov I, Antonova I, Kandel ER, et al. Activity-dependent presynaptic facilitation and Hebbian LTP are both required and interact during classical conditioning in aplysia. Neuron 2003;37(1):135–47.

32. Hebb D. The effects of early experience on problem solving at maturity. Am Psychol 1947;2:306–7.
33. Krech D, Rosenzweig MR, Bennett EL. Effects of environmental complexity and training on brain chemistry. J Comp Physiol Psychol 1960;53:509–19.
34. Rosenzweig MR, Krech D, Bennett EL, et al. Effects of environmental complexity and training on brain chemistry and anatomy: a replication and extension. J Comp Physiol Psychol 1962;55(4):429–37.
35. Altman J, Das GD. Autoradiographic examination of the effects of enriched environment on the rate of glial multiplication in the adult rat brain. Nat Rev Neurosci 1964;204(4964):1161–3.
36. Diamond MC, Krech D, Rosenzweig MR. The effects of an enriched environment on the histology of the rat cerebral cortex. J Comp Neurol 1964;123:111–20.
37. High PC, Klass P. Literacy promotion: an essential component of primary care pediatric practice. Pediatrics 2014;134(2):1384.
38. Armstrong KR, Clark TR, Peterson MR. Use of corn-husk nesting material to reduce aggression in caged mice. Contemp Top Lab Anim Sci 1998;37(4):64–6.
39. Chapillon P, Manneché C, Belzung C, et al. Rearing environmental enrichment in 2 inbred strains of mice: 1. Effects on emotional reactivity. Behav Genet 1999; 29(1):41–6.
40. Engellenner WJ, Goodlett CR, Burright RG, et al. Environmental enrichment and restriction: effects on reactivity, exploration and maze learning in mice with septal lesions. Physiol Behav 1982;29(5):885–93.
41. Hansen LT, Berthelsen H. The effect of environmental enrichment on the behaviour of caged rabbits (*Oryctolagus cuniculus*). Appl Anim Behav Sci 2000;68(2): 163–78.
42. Sharp J, Zammit T, Azar T, et al. Stress-like responses to common procedures in individually and group-housed female rats. Contemp Top Lab Anim Sci 2003; 42(1):9–18.
43. Chamove AS. Cage design reduces emotionality in mice. Lab Anim 1989;23(3): 215–9.
44. Van Loo PL, Van der Meer E, Kruitwagen CL, et al. Long-term effects of husbandry procedures on stress-related parameters in male mice of two strains. Lab Anim 2004;38(2):169–77.
45. Huang-Brown KM, Guhad FA. Chocolate, an effective means of oral drug delivery in rats. Lab Anim 2002;31(10):34–6.
46. Kempermann G, Kuhn HG, Gage FH. More hippocampal neurons in adult mice living in an enriched environment. Nature 1997;386(6624):493–5.
47. Bowlby J. Pathological mourning and childhood mourning. J Am Psychoanal Assoc 1963;11(3):500–41.
48. Hofer MA. Hidden regulators in attachment, separation, and loss. Monogr Soc Res Child Dev 1994;59(2–3):192–207.
49. Hofer MA. Early relationships as regulators of infant physiology and behavior. Acta Paediatr Suppl 1994;83(397):9–18.
50. Tottenham N. Human amygdala development in the absence of species-expected caregiving. Dev Psychobiol 2012;54(6):598–611.
51. Zhang TY, Labonte B, Wen XL, et al. Epigenetic mechanisms for the early environmental regulation of hippocampal glucocorticoid receptor gene expression in rodents and humans. Neuropsychopharmacology 2013;38:111–23.
52. Meaney MJ, Szyf M. Environmental programming of stress responses through DNA methylation: life at the interface between a dynamic environment and a fixed genome. Dialogues Clin Neurosci 2005;7(2):103–23.

53. Liu D, Diorio J, Tannenbaum B, et al. Maternal care, hippocampal glucocorticoid receptors, and hypothalamic-pituitary-adrenal responses to stress. Science 1997;277:1659–62.
54. Liu D, Diorio J, Day JC, et al. Maternal care, hippocampal synaptogenesis and cognitive development in rats. Nat Neurosci 2000;3:799–806.
55. Meaney MJ, Mitchell JB, Aitken DH, et al. The effects of neonatal handling on the development of the adrenocortical response to stress: implications for neuropathology and cognitive deficits in later life. Psychoneuroendocrinology 1991;16:85–103.
56. Levine S. Maternal and environmental influences on the adrenocortical response to stress in weanling rats. Science 1967;156:258–60.
57. Laviola G, Rea M, Morley-Fletcher S, et al. Beneficial effects of enriched environment on adolescent rats from stressed pregnancies. Eur J Neurosci 2004;20:1655–64.
58. Diamond MC, Law F, Rhodes H, et al. Increases in cortical depth and glia numbers in rats subjected to enriched environment. J Comp Neurol 1966;128(1):117–26.
59. Sirevaag AM, Greenough WT. Differential rearing effects on rat visual cortex synapses III. Neuronal and glial nuclei, boutons, dendrites, and capillaries. Brain Res 1987;424(2):320–32.
60. Greenough WT, Volkmar FR. Pattern of dendritic branching in occipital cortex of rats reared in complex environments. Exp Neurol 1973;40(2):491–504.
61. Volkmar FR, Greenough WT. Rearing complexity affects branching of dendrites in the visual cortex of the rat. Science 1972;176(4042):1445–7.
62. Wallace CS, Kilman VL, Withers GS, et al. Increases in dendritic length in occipital cortex after 4 days of differential housing in weanling rats. Behav Neural Biol 1992;58(1):64–8.
63. Fan Y, Liu Z, Weinstein PR, et al. Environmental enrichment enhances neurogenesis and improves functional outcome after cranial irradiation. Eur J Neurosci 2007;25(1):38–46.
64. Speisman RB, Kumar A, Rani A, et al. Environmental enrichment restores neurogenesis and rapid acquisition in aged rats. Neurobiol Aging 2013;34(1):263–74.
65. Argandoña EG, Bengoetxea H, Ortuzar N, et al. Vascular endothelial growth factor: adaptive changes in the neuroglial vascular unit. Curr Neurovasc Res 2012;9(1):72–81.
66. van Praag H, Kempermann G, Gage FH. Neural consequences of environmental enrichment. Nat Rev Neurosci 2000;1(3):191–8.
67. Escorihuela RM, Tobeña A, Fernandez-Teruel A. Environmental enrichment reverses the detrimental action of early inconsistent stimulation and increases the beneficial effects of postnatal handling on shuttlebox learning in adult rats. Behav Brain Res 1994;61(2):169–73.
68. Figley CR, Stroman PW. The role(s) of astrocytes and astrocyte activity in neurometabolism, neurovascular coupling, and the production of functional neuroimaging signals. Eur J Neurosci 2011;33:577–88.
69. Hensch TK, Fagiolini M. Excitatory-inhibitory balance and critical period plasticity in developing visual cortex. Prog Brain Res 2005;147:115–24.
70. Lafuente JV, Ortuzar N, Bengoetxea H, et al. Vascular endothelial growth factor and other angioglioneurins: key molecules in brain development and restoration. Int Rev Neurobiol 2012;102:317–46.
71. Zacchigna S, Lambrechts D, Carmeliet P. Neurovascular signalling defects in neurodegeneration. Nat Rev Neurosci 2008;9:169–81.

72. Will B, Galani R, Kelche C, et al. Recovery from brain injury in animals: relative efficacy of environmental enrichment, physical exercise or formal training. Prog Neurobiol 2004;72:167–82.
73. Xie H, Wu Y, Jia J, et al. Enrichment-induced exercise to quantify the effect of different housing conditions: a tool to standardize enriched environment protocols. Behav Brain Res 2013;249:81–9.
74. Bengoetxea H, Ortuzar N, Bulnes S, et al. Enriched and deprived sensory experience induces structural changes and rewires connectivity during the postnatal development of the brain. Neural Plast 2012;2012:305693.
75. Fabel K, Wolf SA, Ehninger D, et al. Additive effects of physical exercise and environmental enrichment on adult hippocampal neurogenesis in mice. Front Neurosci 2009;3:50.
76. Mustroph ML, Chen S, Desai SC, et al. Aerobic exercise is the critical variable in an enriched environment that increases hippocampal neurogenesis and water maze learning in male C57BL/6J mice. Neuroscience 2012;219:62–71.
77. Colcombe SJ, Kramer AF, Erickson KI, et al. Cardiovascular fitness, cortical plasticity, and aging. Proc Natl Acad Sci U S A 2004;101:3316–21.
78. Griesbach GS, Hovda DA, Molteni R, et al. Voluntary exercise following traumatic brain injury: brain-derived neurotrophic factor upregulation and recovery of function. Neuroscience 2004;125:129–39.
79. Cruise KE, Bucks RS, Loftus AM, et al. Exercise and Parkinson's: benefits for cognition and quality of life. Acta Neurol Scand 2011;123:13–9.
80. Ilin Y, Richter-Levin G. Enriched environment experience overcomes learning deficits and depressive-like behavior induced by juvenile stress. PLoS One 2009;4(1):e4329.
81. Kobilo T, Liu QR, Gandhi K, et al. Running is the neurogenic and neurotrophic stimulus in environmental enrichment. Learn Mem 2011;18:605–9.
82. Fleshner M, Greenwood BN, Yirmiya R. Current topics in behavioral neurosciences. In: Geyer M, Ellenbroek B, Marsden C, editors. Neuronal-glial mechanisms of exercise-evoked stress robustness. Berlin; Heidelberg (Germany): Springer; 2014. [Epub ahead of print].
83. Uylings HB, Groenewegen HJ, Kolb B. Do rats have a prefrontal cortex? Behav Brain Res 2003;146:3–17.
84. Sawaguchi T, Goldman-Rakic PS. The role of D1-dopamine receptor in working memory: local injections of dopamine antagonists into the prefrontal cortex of rhesus monkeys performing an oculomotor delayed-response task. J Neurophysiol 1994;71:515–28.
85. Moghaddam B. Stress activation of glutamate neurotransmission in the prefrontal cortex: implications for dopamine-associated psychiatric disorders. Biol Psychiatry 2002;51:775–87.
86. Czeh B, Müller-Keuker JI, Rygula R, et al. Chronic social stress inhibits cell proliferation in the adult medial prefrontal cortex: hemispheric asymmetry and reversal by fluoxetine treatment. Neuropsychopharmacology 2007;32:1490–503.
87. Sullivan RM. Hemispheric asymmetry in stress processing in rat prefrontal cortex and the role of mesocortical dopamine. Stress 2004;7:131–43.
88. Sullivan RM, Gratton A. Lateralized effects of medial prefrontal cortex lesions on neuroendocrine and autonomic stress responses in rats. J Neurosci 1999;19:2834–40.
89. Sullivan RM, Gratton A. Prefrontal cortical regulation of hypothalamic-pituitary-adrenal function in the rat and implications for psychopathology: side matters. Psychoneuroendocrinology 2002;27:99–114.

90. Bench CJ, Friston KJ, Brown RG, et al. The anatomy of melancholia-focal abnormalities of cerebral blood flow in major depression. Psychol Med 1992;22:607–15.

91. Davidson RJ. Anterior cerebral asymmetry and the nature of emotion. Brain Cogn 1992;20:125–51.

92. Rotenberg VS. The peculiarity of the right-hemisphere function in depression: solving the paradoxes. Prog Neuropsychopharmacol Biol Psychiatry 2004;28: 1–13.

93. Starkstein SE, Robinson RG. Lateralized emotional response following stroke. In: Kinsbourne M, editor. Cerebral hemisphere function in depression. Washington, DC: American Psychiatric Press; 1988. p. 33–43.

94. Shenal BV, Harrison DW, Demaree HA. The neuropsychology of depression: a literature review and preliminary model. Neuropsychol Rev 2003;13: 33–42.

95. Drevets WC. Functional anatomical abnormalities in limbic and prefrontal cortical structures in major depression. Prog Brain Res 2000;126:413–31.

96. Drevets WC, Price JL, Simpson JR Jr, et al. Subgenual prefrontal cortex abnormalities in mood disorders. Nature 1997;386:824–7.

97. Kalin NH, Larson C, Shelton SE, et al. Asymmetric frontal brain activity, cortisol, and behavior associated with fearful temperament in rhesus monkeys. Behav Neurosci 1998;112:286–92.

98. Öngür D, Drevets WC, Price JL. Glial reduction in the subgenual prefrontal cortex in mood disorders. Proc Natl Acad Sci U S A 1998;95:13290–5.

99. Banasr M, Valentine GW, Li XY, et al. Chronic unpredictable stress decreases cell proliferation in the cerebral cortex of the adult rat. Biol Psychiatry 2007; 62:496–504.

100. Butt AM, Hamilton N, Hubbard P, et al. Synantocytes: the fifth element. J Anat 2005;207:695–706.

101. Butt AM, Kiff J, Hubbard P, et al. Synantocytes: new functions for novel NG2 expressing glia. J Neurocytol 2002;31:551–65.

102. Ge WP, Zhou W, Luo Q, et al. Dividing glial cells maintain differentiated properties including complex morphology and functional synapses. Proc Natl Acad Sci U S A 2009;106:328–33.

103. Lin SC, Huck JH, Roberts JD, et al. Climbing fiber innervation of NG2-expressing glia in the mammalian cerebellum. Neuron 2005;46:773–85.

104. Bergles DE, Jabs R, Steinhauser C. Neuron-glia synapses in the brain. Brain Res Rev 2010;63:130–7.

105. Sanders R. New evidence that chronic stress predisposes brain to mental illness. Media Relations. Neuroscience News. February 12, 2014.

106. Chetty S, Friedman AR, Taravosh-Lahn K, et al. Stress and glucocorticoids promote oligodendrogenesis in the adult hippocampus. Mol Psychiatry 2014. [Epub ahead of print].

107. Shin LM, Liberzon I. The neurocircuitry of fear, stress, and anxiety disorders. Neuropsychopharmacology 2010;35(1):169–91.

108. Caspi A, Sugden K, Moffitt TE, et al. Influence of life stress on depression: moderation by a polymorphism in the 5-HTT gene. Science 2003;301:386–9.

109. Frielingsdorf H, Bath KG, Soliman F, et al. Variant brain-derived neurotrophic factor Val66Met endophenotypes: implications for posttraumatic stress disorder. Ann N Y Acad Sci 2010;1208:150–7.

110. Czéh B, Fuchs E, Flügge G. Altered glial plasticity in animal models for mood disorders. Curr Drug Targets 2013;14:1–13.

111. Castren E. Is mood chemistry? Nat Rev Neurosci 2005;6:241–6.

112. Duman RS, Monteggia LM. A neurotrophic model for stress-related mood disorders. Biol Psychiatry 2006;59:1116–27.
113. Hashimoto K, Shimizu E, Iyo M. Critical role of brain-derived neurotrophic factor in mood disorders. Brain Res Brain Res Rev 2004;45:104–14.
114. Martinowich K, Manji H, Lu B. New insights into BDNF function in depression and anxiety. Nat Neurosci 2007;10:1089–93.
115. Castrén E, Rantamäki T. Neurotrophins in depression and antidepressant effects. Novartis Found Symp 2008;289:43–52.
116. Czeh B, Di Benedetto B. Antidepressants act directly on astrocytes: evidences and functional consequences. Eur Neuropsychopharmacol 2013; 23(3):171–85.
117. Allaman I, Fiumelli H, Magistretti PJ, et al. Fluoxetine regulates the expression of neurotrophic/growth factors and glucose metabolism in astrocytes. Psychopharmacology 2011;216:75–84.
118. Garcia-Segura LM, Chowen JA, Naftolin F. Endocrine glia: roles of glial cells in the brain actions of steroid and thyroid hormones and in the regulation of hormone secretion. Front Neuroendocrinol 1996;17(2):180–211.
119. Udomuksorn W, Mukem S, Kumarnsit E, et al. Effects of alcohol administration during adulthood on parvalbumin and glial fibrillary acidic protein immunoreactivity in the rat cerebral cortex. Acta Histochem 2011;113(3):283–9.
120. Butt AM, Colquhoun K, Berry M. Confocal imaging of glial cells in the intact rat optic nerve. Glia 1994;10:315–22.
121. Kendler KS, Kuhn J, Prescott CA. The interrelationship of neuroticism, sex, and stressful life events in the prediction of episodes of major depression. Am J Psychiatry 2004;161:631–6.
122. McEwen BS, Magarinos AM, Reagan LP. Studies of hormone action in the hippocampal formation: possible relevance to depression and diabetes. J Psychosom Res 2002;53:883–90.
123. Miguel-Hidalgo JJ, Waltzer R, Whittom AA, et al. Glial and glutamatergic markers in depression, alcoholism, and their comorbidity. J Affect Disord 2010;127:230–40.
124. Rajkowska G, Miguel-Hidalgo JJ. Gliogenesis and glial pathology in depression. CNS Neurol Disord Drug Targets 2007;6:219–33.
125. Cotter D, Mackay D, Landau S, et al. Reduced glial cell density and neuronal size in the anterior cingulate cortex in major depressive disorder. Arch Gen Psychiatry 2001;58:545–53.
126. Araya-Callís C, Hiemke C, Abumaria N, et al. Chronic psychosocial stress and citalopram modulate the expression of the glial proteins GFAP and NDRG2 in the hippocampus. Psychopharmacology 2012;224(1):209–22.
127. Nedergaard M, Ransom B, Goldman SA. New roles for astrocytes: redefining the functional architecture of the brain. Trends Neurosci 2003;26:523–30.
128. Hiemke C, Hartter S. Pharmacokinetics of selective serotonin reuptake inhibitors. Pharmacol Ther 2000;85:11–28.
129. Selemon LD, Lidow MS, Goldman-Rakic PS. Increased volume and glial density in primate prefrontal cortex associated with chronic antipsychotic drug exposure. Biol Psychiatry 1999;46:161–72.
130. Jellinger K. Neuropathologic findings after neuroleptic long-term therapy. In: Roizin L, Shirakl H, Grcevic N, editors. Neurotoxicology. New York: Raven Press; 1977. p. 25–42.
131. Blázquez Arroyo JL, Fraile Malmierca E, Casadiego Cubides A, et al. Glial reactivity after antipsychotic treatment. An experimental study in rats and its implications for psychiatry. Actas Esp Psiquiatr 2010;38(5):278–84.

132. Brodal P, editor. The central nervous system. 4th edition. New York: Oxford University Press; 2010. p. 19–26.
133. Graeber MB. Changing face of microglia. Science 2010;330:783–8.
134. Wake H, Moorhouse AJ, Jinno S, et al. Resting microglia directly monitor the functional state of synapses in vivo and determine the fate of ischemic terminals. J Neurosci 2009;29:3974–80.
135. Kettenmann H, Hanisch UK, Noda M, et al. Physiology of microglia. Physiological Reviews 2011;91(2):461–553.
136. Pocock JM, Kettenmann H. Neurotransmitter receptors on microglia. Trends in Neurosciences 2007;30(10):527–35.
137. Tynan RJ, Naicker S, Hinwood M, et al. Chronic stress alters the density and morphology of microglia in a subset of stress-responsive brain regions. Brain Behav Immun 2010;24:1058–68.
138. Hinwood M, Morandini J, Day TA, et al. Evidence that microglia mediate the neurobiological effects of chronic psychological stress on the medial prefrontal cortex. Cereb Cortex 2012;22(6):1442–54.
139. Bessa JM, Ferreira D, Melo I, et al. The mood-improving actions of antidepressants do not depend on neurogenesis but are associated with neuronal remodeling. Mol Psychiatry 2009;14:764–73.
140. Arnsten AF, Goldman-Rakic PS. Noise stress impairs prefrontal cortical cognitive function in monkeys: evidence for a hyperdopaminergic mechanism. Arch Gen Psychiatry 1998;55:362–8.
141. Cerqueira JJ, Mailliet F, Almeida OF, et al. The prefrontal cortex as a key target of the maladaptive response to stress. J Neurosci 2007;27:2781–7.
142. Qin S, Hermans EJ, van Marle HJ, et al. Acute psychological stress reduces working memory-related activity in the dorsolateral prefrontal cortex. Biol Psychiatry 2009;66:25–32.
143. Elliott R, Sahakian BJ, McKay AP, et al. Neuropsychological impairments in unipolar depression: the influence of perceived failure on subsequent performance. Psychol Med 1996;26:975–89.
144. Weiland-Fiedler P, Erickson K, Waldeck T, et al. Evidence for continuing neuropsychological impairments in depression. J Affect Disord 2004;82:253–8.
145. Tikka T, Fiebich BL, Goldsteins G, et al. Minocycline, a tetracycline derivative, is neuroprotective against excitotoxicity by inhibiting activation and proliferation of microglia. J Neurosci 2001;21:2580–8.
146. Colovic M, Caccia SJ, Chromatogr B. Liquid chromatographic determination of minocycline in brain-to-plasma distribution studies in the rat. J Chromatogr B Analyt Technol Biomed Life Sci 2003;791:337–43.
147. Maletic V, Raison C. Integrated neurobiology of bipolar disorder. Front Psychiatry 2014;5:98. eCollection 2014.
148. Salter MW, Beggs S. Sublime microglia: expanding roles for the guardians of the CNS. Cell 2014;158(1):15–24.
149. Nishiyori A, Minami M, Ohtani Y, et al. Localization of fractalkine and CX3CR1 mRNAs in rat brain: does fractalkine play a role in signaling from neuron to microglia? FEBS Lett 1998;429(2):167–72.
150. Maggi L, Scianni M, Branchi I, et al. CX(3)CR1 deficiency alters hippocampal-dependent plasticity phenomena blunting the effects of enriched environment. Front Cell Neurosci 2011;5:22. eCollection 2011.
151. Schafer DP, Lehrman EK, Kautzman A, et al. Microglia sculpt postnatal neural circuits in an activity and complement-dependent manner. Neuron 2012;74(4): 691–705.

152. Tremblay ME, Lowery RL, Majewska AK. Microglial interactions with synapses are modulated by visual experience. PLoS Biology 2010;8(11):e1000527.
153. Dantzer R, O'Connor JC, Freund GG, et al. From inflammation to sickness and depression: when the immune system subjugates the brain. Nat Rev Neurosci 2008;9:46–56.
154. Lindqvist D, Janelidze S, Hagell P, et al. Interleukin-6 is elevated in the cerebrospinal fluid of suicide attempters and related to symptom severity. Biol Psychiatry 2009;66:287–92.
155. Steiner J, Bielau H, Brisch R, et al. Immunological aspects in the neurobiology of suicide: elevated microglial density in schizophrenia and depression is associated with suicide. J Psychiatr Res 2008;42:151–7.
156. Watkins CC, Sawa A, Pomper MG. Glia and immune cell signaling in bipolar disorder: insights from neuropharmacology and molecular imaging to clinical application. Transl Psychiatry 2014;4:e350.
157. Tsai SY, Lee CH, Kuo CJ, et al. A retrospective analysis of risk and protective factors for natural death in bipolar disorder. J Clin Psychiatry 2005;66:1586–91.
158. Otte C, McCaffery J, Ali S, et al. Association of a serotonin transporter polymorphism (5-HTTLPR) with depression, perceived stress, and norepinephrine in patients with coronary disease: the Heart and Soul Study. Am J Psychiatry 2007; 164:1379–84.
159. McIntyre RS, Rasgon NL, Kemp DE, et al. Metabolic syndrome and major depressive disorder: co-occurrence and pathophysiologic overlap. Curr Diab Rep 2009;9:51–9.
160. Ridker PM. Inflammatory biomarkers and risks of myocardial infarction, stroke, diabetes, and total mortality: implications for longevity. Nutr Rev 2007;65(Pt 2): S253–9.
161. Miller AH, Maletic V, Raison CL. Inflammation and its discontents: the role of cytokines in the pathophysiology of major depression. Biol Psychiatry 2009;65: 732–41.
162. Montgomery P, Richardson AJ. Omega-3 fatty acids for bipolar disorder. Cochrane Database Syst Rev 2008;(16):CD005169.
163. Nery FG, Monkul ES, Hatch JP, et al. Celecoxib as an adjunct in the treatment of depressive or mixed episodes of bipolar disorder: a double-blind, randomized, placebo-controlled study. Hum Psychopharmacol 2008;23(2):87–94.
164. Cotter DR, Pariante CM, Everall IP. Glial cell abnormalities in major psychiatric disorders: the evidence and implications. Brain Res Bull 2001;55:585–95.
165. Rajkowska G. Postmortem studies in mood disorders indicate altered numbers of neurons and glial cells. Biol Psychiatry 2000;48:766–77.
166. Munkholm K, Vinberg M, Vedel Kessing L. Cytokines in bipolar disorder: a systematic review and meta-analysis. J Affect Disord 2013;144:16–27.
167. Goldstein BI, Kemp DE, Soczynska JK, et al. Inflammation and the phenomenology, pathophysiology, comorbidity, and treatment of bipolar disorder: a systematic review of the literature. J Clin Psychiatry 2009;70:1078–90.
168. Watkins CC, Endres CJ, Rosenberg PB, et al. In vivo PET imaging of glial activation in normal aging. Presented at Annual Meeting of the Society for Neuroscience. New Orleans (LA), 2012.
169. Wierzba-Bobrowicz T, Lewandowska E, Kosno-Kruszewska E, et al. Degeneration of microglial cells in frontal and temporal lobes of chronic schizophrenics. Folia Neuropathol 2004;42:157–65.
170. Wierzba-Bobrowicz T, Lewandowska E, Lechowicz W, et al. Quantitative analysis of activated microglia, ramified and damage of processes in the frontal

and temporal lobes of chronic schizophrenics. Folia Neuropathol 2005;43: 81–9.

171. Rajkowska G, Halaris A, Selemon LD. Reductions in neuronal and glial density characterize the dorsolateral prefrontal cortex in bipolar disorder. Biol Psychiatry 2001;49:741–52.

172. Steiner J, Mawrin C, Ziegeler A, et al. Distribution of HLA-DR-positive microglia in schizophrenia reflects impaired cerebral lateralization. Acta Neuropathol 2006;112:305–16.

173. Sisask M, Varnik A, Kolves K, et al. Subjective psychological well-being (WHO-5) in assessment of the severity of suicide attempt. Nord J Psychiatry 2008;62: 431–5.

174. Bayard-Burfield L, Alling C, Blennow K, et al. Impairment of the blood-CSF barrier in suicide attempters. Eur Neuropsychopharmacol 1996;6:195–9.

175. Tynan RJ, Weidenhofer J, Hinwood M, et al. A comparative examination of the anti-inflammatory effects of SSRI and SNRI antidepressants on LPS stimulated microglia. Brain Behav Immun 2012;26:469–79.

176. Donato R, Sorci G, Riuzzi F, et al. S100B's double life: intracellular regulator and extracellular signal. Biochim Biophys Acta 2009;1793(6):1008–22.

177. Steiner J, Bernstein HG, Bielau H, et al. S100B-immunopositive glia is elevated in paranoid as compared to residual schizophrenia: a morphometric study. J Psychiatr Res 2008;42(10):868–76.

178. Rothermundt M, Ponath G, Arolt G. S100B in schizophrenic psychosis. Int Rev Neurobiol 2004;59:445–70.

179. van Beveren NJ, van der Spelt JJ, de Haan L, et al. Schizophrenia-associated neural growth factors in peripheral blood. A review. Eur Neuropsychopharmacol 2006;16:469–80.

180. Liu J, Shi Y, Tang J, et al. SNPs and haplotypes in the S100B gene reveal association with schizophrenia. Biochem Biophys Res Commun 2005;328: 335–41.

181. Kleindienst A, McGinn MJ, Harvey HB, et al. Enhanced hippocampal neurogenesis by intraventricular S100B infusion is associated with improved cognitive recovery after traumatic brain injury. J Neurotrauma 2005;22:645–55.

182. Kleindienst A, Ross Bullock M. A critical analysis of the role of the neurotrophic protein S100B in acute brain injury. J Neurotrauma 2006;23:1185–200.

183. Donato R. S100: a multigenic family of calcium-modulated proteins of the EF-hand type with intracellular and extracellular functional roles. Int J Biochem Cell Biol 2001;33:637–68.

184. Shapiro LA, Whitaker-Azmitia PM. Expression levels of cytoskeletal proteins indicate pathological aging of S100B transgenic mice: an immunohistochemical study of MAP-2, drebrin and GAP-43. Brain Res 2004;1019:39–46.

185. Kielbinski M, Soltys Z. S100B protein, astrocytes and memory. Adv Cell Biol 2009;1(1):1–11.

186. Whitaker-Azmitia PM, Murphy R, Azmitia EC. S100 protein is released from astroglial cells by stimulation of 5-HT1A receptors. Brain Res 1990;528: 155–8.

187. de Almeida LM, Piñeiro CC, Leite MC, et al. Resveratrol increases glutamate uptake, glutathione content, and S100B secretion in cortical astrocyte cultures. Cell Mol Neurobiol 2007;27:661–8.

188. Quincozes-Santos A, Abib RT, Leite MC, et al. Effect of the atypical neuroleptic risperidone on morphology and S100B secretion in C6 astroglial lineage cells. Mol Cell Biochem 2008;314:59–63.

189. Ciccarelli R, Di Iorio P, Bruno V, et al. Activation of A1 adenosine or mGlu3 metabotropic glutamate receptors enhances the release of nerve growth factor and S100β protein from cultured astrocytes. Glia 1999;27:275–81.
190. Edwards MM, Robinson SR. TNF-α affects the expression of GFAP and S100B: implications for Alzheimer's disease. J Neural Transm 2006;113:1709–15.
191. Gerlach R, Demel G, König HG, et al. Active secretion of S100B from astrocytes during metabolic stress. Neuroscience 2006;141:1697–701.
192. Dietrich MO, Tort AB, Schaf DV, et al. Increase in serum S100B protein level after a swimming race. Can J Appl Physiol 2003;28:710–6.
193. Cochran AJ, Lu HF, Li PX, et al. S-100 protein remains a practical marker for melanocytic and other tumours. Melanoma Res 1993;3:325–30.
194. Mazzini GS, Schaf DV, Oliveira AR, et al. The ischemic rat heart releases S100B. Life Sci 2005;77:882–9.
195. Anderson RE, Hansson LO, Nilsson O, et al. High serum S100B levels for trauma patients without head injuries. Neurosurgery 2001;48:1255–8.
196. Marchi N, Cavaglia M, Fazio V, et al. Peripheral markers of blood-brain barrier damage. Clin Chim Acta 2004;342:1–12.
197. Prat A, Biernacki K, Wosik K, et al. Glial cell influence on the human blood-brain barrier. Glia 2001;36(2):145–55.
198. Bayer TA, Buslei R, Havas L, et al. Evidence for activation of microglia in patients with psychiatric illnesses. Neurosci Lett 1999;271:126–8.
199. Falcone F, Fazio V, Lee C, et al. Serum S100B: a potential biomarker for suicidality in adolescents? PLoS One 2010;5(6):e11089.
200. Elewa HF, Hilali H, Hess DC, et al. Minocycline for short-term neuroprotection. Pharmacotherapy 2006;26:515–21.
201. Zemke D, Majid A. The potential of minocycline for neuroprotection in human neurologic disease. Clin Neuropharmacol 2004;27:293–8.
202. Hailer NP. Immunosuppression after traumatic or ischemic CNS damage: it is neuroprotective and illuminates the role of microglial cells. Prog Neurobiol 2008;84:211–33.
203. Pae CU, Marks DM, Han C, et al. Does minocycline have antidepressant effect? Biomed Pharmacother 2008;62:308–11.
204. Wang Y, Qin ZH. Molecular and cellular mechanisms of excitotoxic neuronal death. Apoptosis 2010;15:1382–402.
205. Chaudhry IB, Hallak J, Husain N, et al. Minocycline benefits negative symptoms in early schizophrenia: a randomised double-blind placebo-controlled clinical trial in patients on standard treatment. J Psychopharmacol 2012; 26(9):1185–93.
206. Savitz J, Preskorn S, Teague TK, et al. Minocycline and aspirin in the treatment of bipolar depression: a protocol for a proof-of-concept, randomised, double-blind, placebo-controlled, 2×2 clinical trial. BMJ Open 2012;2(1): e000643.
207. Levkovitz Y, Mendlovich S, Riwkes S, et al. A double-blind, randomized study of minocycline for the treatment of negative and cognitive symptoms in early-phase schizophrenia. J Clin Psychiatry 2010;71:138–49.
208. Rock RB, Gekker G, Hu S, et al. Role of microglia in central nervous system infections. Clin Microbiol Rev 2004;17(4):942–64.
209. Colton A, Chernyshev ON. Inhibition of microglial superoxide anion production by isoproterenol and dexamethasone. Neurochem Int 1996;29:43–53.
210. Aloisi F, De Simone R, Columba-Cabezas S, et al. Opposite effects of interferon-γ and prostaglandin E2 on tumor necrosis factor and interleukin-10 production

in microglia: a regulatory loop controlling microglia pro- and anti-inflammatory activities. J Neurosci Res 1999;56:571–80.

211. Kust BM, Biber K, Van Calker D, et al. Regulation of K+ channel mRNA expression by stimulation of adenosine A2a-receptors in cultured rat microglia. Glia 1999;25:120–30.

212. Halpin DM. ABCD of the phosphodiesterase family: interaction and differential activity in COPD. Int J Chron Obstruct Pulmon Dis 2008;3(4):543–61.

213. Zhang B, Yang L, Konishi Y, et al. Suppressive effects of phosphodiesterase type IV inhibitors on rat cultured microglial cells: comparison with other types of cAMP-elevating agents. Neuropharmacology 2002;42(2):262–9.

214. Semmler J, Wachtel H, Endres S. The specific type IV phosphodiesterase inhibitor rolipram suppresses tumor necrosis factor-α production by human mononuclear cells. Int J Immunopharmacol 1993;15:409–13.

215. Davis JA, Gould TJ. Rolipram attenuates MK-801-induced deficits in latent inhibition. Behav Neurosci 2005;119:595–602.

216. Kanes SJ, Tokarczyk J, Siegel SJ, et al. Rolipram: a specific phosphodiesterase 4 inhibitor with potential antipsychotic activity. Neuroscience 2007; 144:239–46.

217. Millar JK, Mackie S, Clapcote SJ, et al. Disrupted in schizophrenia 1 and phosphodiesterase 4B: towards an understanding of psychiatric illness. J Physiol 2007;584(Pt 2):401–5.

218. Millar JK, Pickard BS, Mackie S, et al. DISC1 and PDE4B are interacting genetic factors in schizophrenia that regulate cAMP signaling. Science 2005;310:1187–91.

219. Noble S, Wagstaff AJ. Propentofylline. CNS Drugs 1997;8:257–64.

220. Salimi S, Fotouhi A, Ghoreishi A, et al. A placebo controlled study of the propentofylline added to risperidone in chronic schizophrenia. Prog Neuropsychopharmacol Biol Psychiatry 2008;32(3):726–32.

221. Frampton M, Harvey RJ, Kirchner V. Propentofylline for dementia. Cochrane Database Syst Rev 2003;(2):CD002853.

222. Harvey AL, Young LC, Viljoen AM, et al. Pharmacological actions of the South African medicinal and functional food plant Sceletium tortuosum and its principal alkaloids. J Ethnopharmacol 2011;137:1124–9.

223. Chiu S, Gericke N, Badmaev V, et al. Proof of concept RCT of Sceletium tortuosum extract targeting PDE4 (phosphodiesterase subtype-4) in regulating cognition and mood in normal subjects: implications for Alzheimer dementia and mood disorders. Presented at World Psychiatric Association Congress. Prague, 2012.

224. Nell H, Siebert M, Chellan P, et al. A randomized, double-blind, parallel-group, placebo-controlled trial of extract Sceletium tortuosum (Zembrin) in healthy adults. J Altern Complement Med 2013;19(11):898–904.

225. Schwarz JM, Hutchinson MR, Bilbo SD. Early-life experience decreases drug-induced reinstatement of morphine CPP in adulthood via microglial-specific epigenetic programming of anti-inflammatory IL-10 expression. J Neurosci 2011;31(49):17835–47.

226. Kosten TA, Miserendino MJ, Kehoe P. Enhanced acquisition of cocaine self-administration in adult rats with neonatal isolation stress experience. Brain Res 2000;875:44–50.

227. Moffett MC, Vicentic A, Kozel M, et al. Maternal separation alters drug intake patterns in adulthood in rats. Biochem Pharmacol 2007;73:321–30.

228. Jaworski JN, Francis DD, Brommer CL, et al. Effects of early maternal separation on ethanol intake, GABA receptors and metabolizing enzymes in adult rats. Psychopharmacology 2005;181:8–15.

229. Hutchinson MR, Northcutt AL, Chao LW, et al. Minocycline suppresses morphine-induced respiratory depression, suppresses morphine-induced reward, and enhances systemic morphine-induced analgesia. Brain Behav Immun 2008;22: 1248–56.

230. Bland ST, Hutchinson MR, Maier SF, et al. The glial activation inhibitor AV411 reduces morphine-induced nucleus accumbens dopamine release. Brain Behav Immun 2009;23:492–7.

231. Allen JP, Schad MM, Oudekerk B, et al. What ever happened to the "cool" kids? Long-term sequelae of early adolescent pseudomature behavior. Child Dev 2014. [Epub ahead of print].

232. Nolte L. Becoming visible: the impact of parental mental health difficulties on children. In: Loshak R, editor. Out of the mainstream: helping the children of parents with a mental illness. New York: Routledge; 2013. p. 31–44.

233. Schneider H, Pitossi F, Balschun D, et al. A neuromodulatory role of interleukin-1beta in the hippocampus. Proc Natl Acad Sci U S A 1998;95:7778–83.

234. Barrientos RM, Higgins EA, Sprunger DB, et al. Memory for context is impaired by a post context exposure injection of interleukin-1 beta into dorsal hippocampus. Behav Brain Res 2002;134:291–8.

235. Barrientos RM, Frank MG, Hein AM, et al. Time course of hippocampal IL-1 beta and memory consolidation impairments in aging rats following peripheral infection. Brain Behav Immun 2009;23:46–54.

236. Goshen I, Kreisel T, Ounallah-Saad H, et al. A dual role for interleukin-1 in hippocampal-dependent memory processes. Psychoneuroendocrinology 2007; 32:1106–15.

237. Spulber S, Mateos L, Oprica M, et al. Impaired long term memory consolidation in transgenic mice overexpressing the human soluble form of IL-1ra in the brain. J Neuroimmunol 2009;208(1–2):46–53.

238. Xie L. Sleep drives metabolite clearance from the adult brain. Science 2013; 342(6156):373–7.

239. Mendelsohn AR, Larrick JW. Sleep facilitates clearance of metabolites from the brain: glymphatic function in aging and neurodegenerative diseases. Rejuvenation Res 2013;16(6):518–23.

240. Havekes R, Vecsey CG, Abel T. The impact of sleep deprivation on neuronal and glial signalling pathways important for memory and synaptic plasticity. Cell Signal 2012;24(6):1251–60.

241. Vecsey CG, Baillie GS, Jaganath D, et al. Sleep deprivation impairs cAMP signalling in the hippocampus. Nature 2009;461:1122–5.

Index

Note: Page numbers of article titles are in **boldface** type.

Psychiatr Clin N Am 37 (2014) 707–714
http://dx.doi.org/10.1016/S0193-953X(14)00092-6
0193-953X/14/$ – see front matter © 2014 Elsevier Inc. All rights reserved.

United States Postal Service

Statement of Ownership, Management, and Circulation
(All Periodicals Publications Except Requestor Publications)

1. Publication Title
Psychiatric Clinics of North America

2. Publication Number
0 0 0 - 7 0 3

3. Filing Date
9/14/14

4. Issue Frequency
Mar, Jun, Sep, Dec

5. Number of Issues Published Annually
4

6. Annual Subscription Price
$300.00

7. Complete Mailing Address of Known Office of Publication (Not printer) (Street, city, county, state, and ZIP+4®)

Elsevier Inc.
360 Park Avenue South
New York, NY 10010-1710

Contact Person
Stephen R. Bushing
Telephone (Include area code)
215-239-3688

8. Complete Mailing Address of Headquarters or General Business Office of Publisher (Not printer)

Elsevier Inc., 360 Park Avenue South, New York, NY 10010-1710

9. Full Names and Complete Mailing Addresses of Publisher, Editor, and Managing Editor (Do not leave blank)

Publisher (Name and complete mailing address)

Linda Belfus, Elsevier, Inc., 1600 John F. Kennedy Blvd. Suite 1800, Philadelphia, PA 19103-2899

Editor (Name and complete mailing address)

Joanne Husovski, Elsevier, Inc., 1600 John F. Kennedy Blvd. Suite 1800, Philadelphia, PA 19103-2899

Managing Editor (Name and complete mailing address)

Adrianne Brigido, Elsevier, Inc., 1600 John F. Kennedy Blvd. Suite 1800, Philadelphia, PA 19103-2899

10. Owner (Do not leave blank. If the publication is owned by a corporation, give the name and address of the corporation immediately followed by the names and addresses of all stockholders owning or holding 1 percent or more of the total amount of stock. If not owned by a corporation, give the names and addresses of the individual owners. If owned by a partnership or other unincorporated firm, give its name and address as well as those of each individual owner. If the publication is published by a nonprofit organization, give its name and address.)

Full Name	Complete Mailing Address
Wholly owned subsidiary of	1600 John F. Kennedy Blvd, Ste. 1800
Reed/Elsevier, US holdings	Philadelphia, PA 19103-2899

11. Known Bondholders, Mortgagees, and Other Security Holders Owning or Holding 1 Percent or More of Total Amount of Bonds, Mortgages, or Other Securities. If none, check box ▸ None

Full Name	Complete Mailing Address
N/A	

12. Tax Status (For completion by nonprofit organizations authorized to mail at nonprofit rates) (Check one)
The purpose, function, and nonprofit status of this organization and the exempt status for federal income tax purposes:
☐ Has Not Changed During Preceding 12 Months
☐ Has Changed During Preceding 12 Months (Publisher must submit explanation of change with this statement)

PS Form 3526, August 2012 (Page 1 of 3 (Instructions Page 3)) PSN 7530-01-000-9931 PRIVACY NOTICE: See our Privacy policy in www.usps.com

---

13. Publication Title
Psychiatric Clinics of North America

14. Issue Date for Circulation Data Below
September 2014

15. Extent and Nature of Circulation

			Average No. Copies Each Issue During Preceding 12 Months	No. Copies of Single Issue Published Nearest to Filing Date
a. Total Number of Copies (Net press run)			796	814
b. Paid Circulation (By Mail and Outside the Mail)	(1)	Mailed Outside-County Paid Subscriptions Stated on PS Form 3541. (Include paid distribution above nominal rate, advertiser's proof copies, and exchange copies)	447	470
	(2)	Mailed In-County Paid Subscriptions Stated on PS Form 3541 (Include paid distribution above nominal rate, advertiser's proof copies, and exchange copies)		
	(3)	Paid Distribution Outside the Mails Including Sales Through Dealers and Carriers, Street Vendors, Counter Sales, and Other Paid Distribution Outside USPS®	149	151
	(4)	Paid Distribution by Other Classes Mailed Through the USPS (e.g. First-Class Mail®)		
c. Total Paid Distribution (Sum of 15b (1), (2), (3), and (4))		▸	596	621
d. Free or Nominal Rate Distribution (By Mail and Outside the Mail)	(1)	Free or Nominal Rate Outside-County Copies Included on PS Form 3541	65	67
	(2)	Free or Nominal Rate In-County Copies Included on PS Form 3541		
	(3)	Free or Nominal Rate Copies Mailed at Other Classes Through the USPS (e.g. First-Class Mail)		
	(4)	Free or Nominal Rate Distribution Outside the Mail (Carriers or other means)		
e. Total Free or Nominal Rate Distribution (Sum of 15d (1), (2), (3) and (4))		▸	65	67
f. Total Distribution (Sum of 15c and 15e)		▸	661	688
g. Copies not Distributed (See instructions to publishers #4 (page #3))		▸	135	126
h. Total (Sum of 15f and g)		▸	796	814
i. Percent Paid (15c divided by 15f times 100)		▸	90.17%	90.26%

16. Total circulation includes electronic copies. Report circulation on PS Form 3526-X worksheet.

17. Publication of Statement of Ownership
If the publication is a general publication, publication of this statement is required. Will be printed in the December 2014 issue of this publication.

18. Signature and Title of Editor, Publisher, Business Manager, or Owner

Stephen R. Bushing

Stephen R. Bushing – Inventory Distribution Coordinator

Date
September 14, 2014

I certify that all information furnished on this form is true and complete. I understand that anyone who furnishes false or misleading information on this form or who omits material or information requested on the form may be subject to criminal sanctions (including fines and imprisonment) and/or civil sanctions (including civil penalties).

PS Form 3526, August 2012 (Page 2 of 3)

Moving?

Make sure your subscription moves with you!

To notify us of your new address, find your **Clinics Account Number** (located on your mailing label above your name), and contact customer service at:

Email: journalscustomerservice-usa@elsevier.com

800-654-2452 (subscribers in the U.S. & Canada)
314-447-8871 (subscribers outside of the U.S. & Canada)

Fax number: 314-447-8029

Elsevier Health Sciences Division
Subscription Customer Service
3251 Riverport Lane
Maryland Heights, MO 63043

*To ensure uninterrupted delivery of your subscription, please notify us at least 4 weeks in advance of move.